# People of Vision

*The Unique History of Ophthalmology*
*in*
*South Texas*

by

**Diana Kleiner, Ph.D.**
**W.A.J. van Heuven, M.D.**

Jean-Paul Wayenborgh
Calle Presidente Franco, 1
3040 Piribebuy, Cordillera
Paraguay
ISBN 10: 90-6299-211-0
ISBN 13: 978-90-6299-211-9

Distributor: Kugler Publications
P.O. Box 20538
1001 NM Amsterdam, The Netherlands
Telefax (+31.20) 68 47 788
website: www.kuglerpublications.com

## PREFACE

History, if honestly remembered, accurately annotated, and carefully studied, can help us to understand why things occur and who we ourselves are. It can provide insight into how we as individuals fit into the greater scheme of things and it can help to give our lives meaning in a larger context. Particularly in rapidly developing and expanding intellectual or geographic areas, history can guide us to a more rapid achievement of our goals. For individuals wishing to contribute something positive to this world, the knowledge of specific segments of history can point to activities that are most likely to succeed and help institutions, disciplines, and regional areas grow more efficiently and effectively.

By documenting the massive changes that occurred in the rapidly growing region known as South Texas in little more than one hundred years, this history of ophthalmology offers the reader an account and an analysis of a unique period in medical history. By looking at a single branch of medicine, ophthalmology, it explains why medicine in South Texas developed as it did and documents the unusual conditions present in the region that made such change possible, including the recent independence of Texas, the simultaneous German invention of the ophthalmoscope in 1850 and the German influx into the region after a cholera epidemic nearly eliminated the entire population of the San Antonio area, the strong military influence throughout the region's history, and the longstanding presence of a largely Hispanic population.

From the vantage point of the beginning of the twenty-first centry, the history demonstrated by the microcosm of ophthalmology further shows how our short South Texas history is leading us rapidly into an era in which South Texas, with San Antonio as its headquarters, will play an increasingly important role in this hemisphere and in the world. San Antonio, the city where the NAFTA agreement was signed in 1994, is being thrust into the limelight as a headquarters for future Pan-American relations. In ophthalmology this means that, based on our understanding of how we reached this point, we can better rise to this historic occasion by facilitating the work that will make San Antonio a Pan-American center for education and research. Thus, the frontier days of South Texas are not over. In fact, South Texas continues to be a frontier town, although the frontier is now of hemispheric proportions.

While an understanding of South Texas ophthalmic history sheds light on these interests, however, it is the focus of this book primarily for two reasons: the first, because it seeks to fill the void that exists in medical history in the area of regional ophthalmology and, second, because of this writer's personal interest in ophthalmology. Brought up in Europe, educated along the American East Coast, and brought to Texas only in 1981, I have had the opportunity to observe the unique South Texas history of ophthalmology both from a distance and at first hand. As an ophthalmologist, the chairman of an academic ophthalmology department, and the son of a European and later American ophthalmologist, I have seen both private institutional and academic ophthalmology from many sides. Historically, I was fortunate to have a father who was trained at the historic Donders Eye Hospital (at the University of Utrecht), whose professor was Snellen, and whose friends and mentors included Gonin, Schepens, Weve and Duke-Elder, all major influences in the field of ophthalmology in the last hundred years. Thus, I have been surrounded by ophthalmic history from childhood on and I have been lucky to have known some of these great ophthalmologists personally. It has been, therefore, natural for me to want to record some of this history. Fortunately, I was able to find a talented Texas historian, Diana Kleiner, to research and write this treatise on the history of ophthalmology in South Texas.

The timing of this history is important, because we were able to interview personally many of the ophthalmologists in San Antonio and surrounding areas who have had some of the greatest influence on our region's ophthalmic history. These interviews were largely conducted by Sue McDonald of the Institute of Texan Cultures. Much of the book's historical content was obtained from these personal histories and memories, with extensive research done from available records to corroborate their testimony. As a result, if errors or omissions have occurred, I can assure you it is not for lack of historical research, but rather because memory fails all of us from time to time.

In particular, this book was made possible through the generous contributions of many people to whom we owe a debt of gratitude. The authors especially wish to thank the archivists and librarians of the Briscoe Library of the University of Texas Health Science Center for their assistance, and the archivists and reference librarians of the following military, university, and medical libraries who generously gave of their time and expertise: U.S. Army Medical Department (AMEDD) Museum, Fort Sam Houston, San Antonio; Bexar County Medical Society, San Antonio; The Center for American History, University of Texas at Austin; Daughters of the Republic of Texas Library, San Antonio; Fort Sam Houston Museum Archives, Fort Sam Houston, San Antonio; Hangar 9, Brooks Air Force Base, San Antonio; Houston Metropolitan Research Center; Institute of Texan Cultures Library, University of Texas at San Antonio; Robert B. Green Memorial Hospital Archives, San Antonio; Texana Collection, San Antonio Public Library; Stimson Library, U.S. Medical Department, Fort Sam Houston, San Antonio; Strughold Library, Brooks Air Force Base, San Antonio; Texas Medical Association Archives, Austin; Texas Ophthalmological Association Archives, Austin; Wilford Hall Hospital Department of Ophthalmology Archives, San Antonio. Finally, we wish to thank the many people who kindly agreed to be interviewed and whose knowledge and memory supplied many of the key facts and descriptions that enrich this history.

W. A. J. van Heuven, M.D.
Professor and Chair (1981 – 2006)
University of Texas Health Science Center
at San Antonio

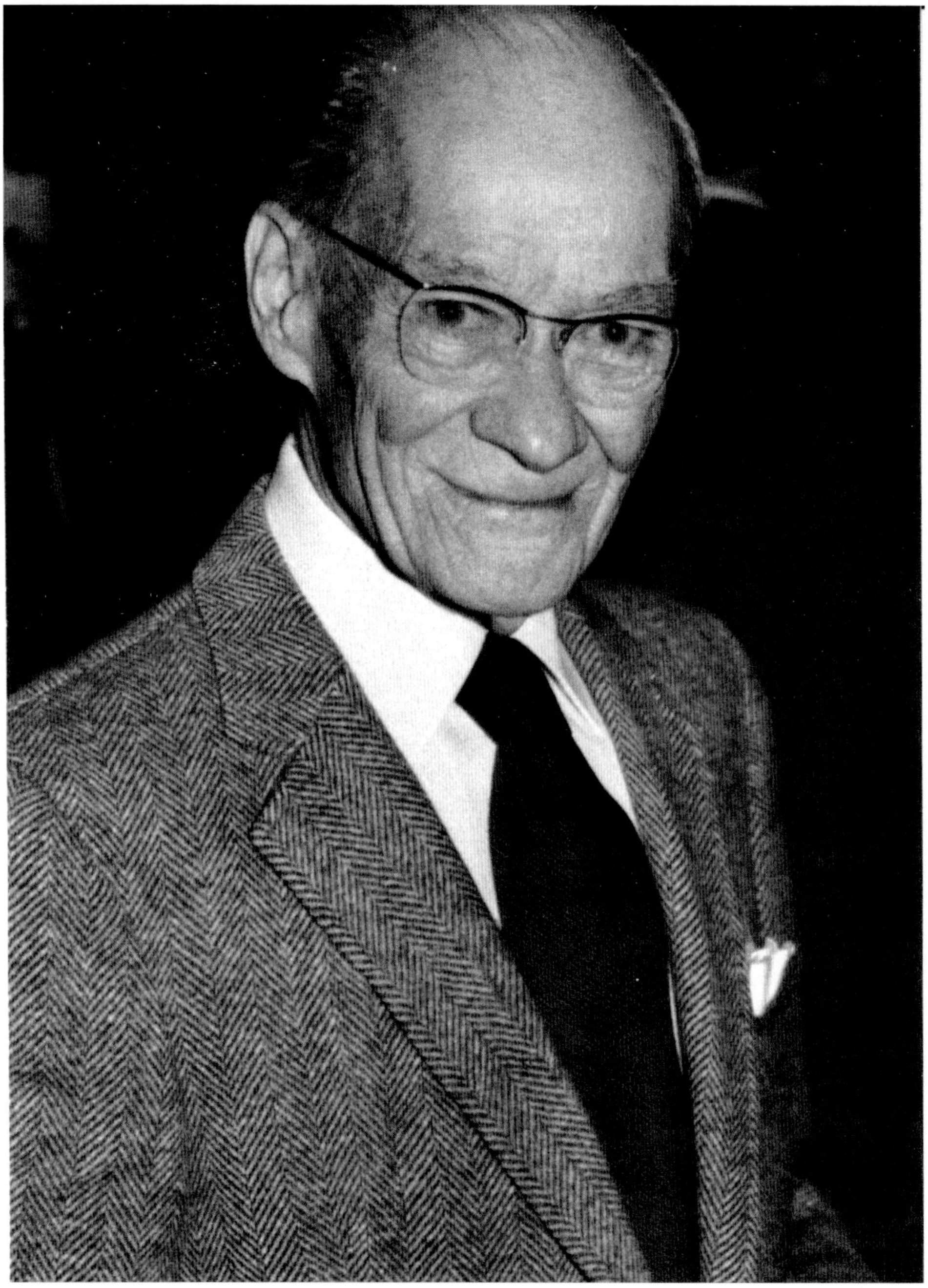

Dedicated
to

**John Larkin Matthews**
**1908 – 1995**

*A gentleman and an outstanding and ethical ophthalmologist who, with kindness and humility, brought, more than anyone else, modern ophthalmic practice, teaching and research to South Texas.*

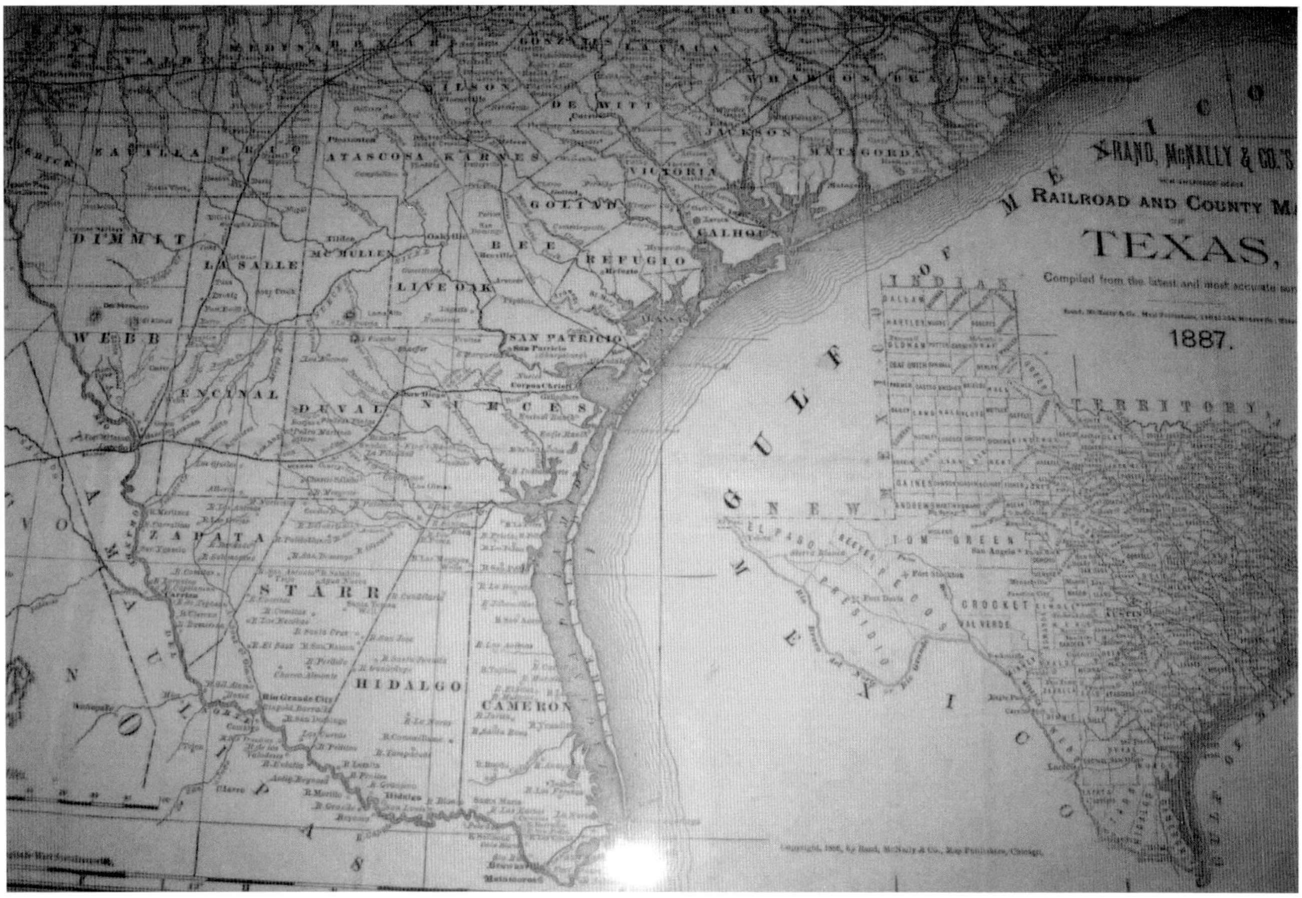
RAND, McNALLY & CO.'S
RAILROAD AND COUNTY MA
TEXAS,
1887.
GULF OF MEXICO
WILSON
DE WITT
ATASCOSA
KARNES
JACKSON
MATAGORDA
VICTORIA
GOLIAD
DIMMIT
LA SALLE
McMULLEN
BEE
REFUGIO
LIVE OAK
WEBB
SAN PATRICIO
ENCINAL
DUVAL
NUECES
ZAPATA
STARR
HIDALGO
CAMERON
TOM GREEN
CROCKET
NEW MEXICO

## Table of Contents

# CHAPTER 1

## NATIONAL AND SCIENTIFIC FRONTIERS: CREATING AN HISTORICAL PERSPECTIVE

*No real fulfillment of the role we play as ophthalmologists can be achieved unless we learn something of the origins of our thoughts about eye diseases and of the attitudes we assume toward the problems of what constitutes diagnosis, prognosis, and therapeutics—in short, of what constitutes ophthalmology and rational ophthalmological thought. The origins of these concepts . . . are clearly written on the pages of history.*

Arrington, History of Ophthalmology, 1

*The medical historian is charged with selecting representative material and individuals who best summarize his concept of the salient features of a given age.*

Arrington, History of Ophthalmology, 5

In the Fall of 1959, an Alamo Ironworks railroad car carrying a collection of old and valuable books wound its way northward toward San Antonio through the Rio Grande Valley of South Texas. The rare volumes had been gathered nearly a century before by physicians of the Burns family who had practiced in the early community that grew up at Cuero. Sent as a gift to a new regional medical complex then

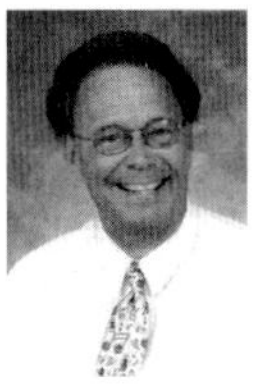

*Chester R. Burns arranged for the donation and transfer of the Burns Collection of medical books from Cuero to San Antonio, where it became the core collection of the Briscoe Library at the new San Antonio Medicine School.*

under construction in San Antonio, the books were destined to become the core collection of the Briscoe Library at the University of Texas Health Science Center. The collection's arrival drew little public attention, and it was quietly housed temporarily in the vaults of the municipal library. Yet because Cuero offered some of the earliest medical care on the South Texas frontier, the transfer of the Burns Collection marks the moment when stewardship over medicine in the region passed from one of its original centers to the Alamo City. Because Cuero was also the place where one of the region's first trained ophthalmologists began his career, the transfer of the Burns Collection serves as an emblem for the growth of professional ophthalmology in South Texas. (Alamo Ironworks, Inc. (1878-1923), a manufacturer of machinery at San Antonio, used its rail service to deliver raw materials inland from the valley. Alamo Ironworks vertical file, San Antonio Public Library).

Dr. John Smith Interview, April 5, 1996;
"Burns Memorial Library Dedication,"
University of Texas Health Science Center News Release, May 14, 1970,
Briscoe Library Archives.

The dusty volumes of the Burns Collection raise the central question this book seeks to answer. At their dedication, the volumes were described as "*an extraordinary collection for a community the size of Cuero*." Among them, several books bearing the title Ophthalmology, published by Schmidt and Rimpler in 1888, by Fuchs in 1893, and Duane in 1908, along with Norris's 1897 and Colburn's 1901 volumes entitled *Diseases of the Eye* in four volumes, May's 1907 *Disease of the Eye*, and others dealing with the ear, nose and throat, prove that early South Texas physicians practiced a relatively sophisticated level of medicine even when the region was still considered a no-man's land of isolated ranches, cattle thieves, and nomadic tribes of Native Americans. How, one asks, did the highly specialized science of ophthalmology develop so rapidly in a place that remained part of the frontier until almost 1900?

Inventory of the Burns Memorial Library, May 1, 1962, Briscoe Library Archives

The answer lies in the nature of the frontier experience. The rapid transfer of the most up-to-date ophthalmological practice to the American Southwest resulted from the convergence of powerful forces from outside the region. To understand how these events occurred, however, requires a look back at a world no longer clearly visible to the modern observer. This book, therefore, seeks to make the reader aware of influences that shaped the growth of medical specialization along the frontier, to explore the dimensions of a medical world different from our own, to understand the dynamics of that world, and to identify the particular circumstances in which ophthalmology developed distant from the nation's centers of medical science. Its goal, much like that of an earlier history of ophthalmology, is to achieve:

*"more than a simple recounting of momentous ophthalmological discoveries, to search for these eluding environmental influences and scientific trends . . . and, thereby, to weave the thread of ophthalmology through the intricate tapestry of medicine and human civilization."*

Burns Collection Catalog,
Briscoe Library,
University of Texas Health Science Center,
San Antonio;
Arrington, History of Ophthalmology, 4-5.

## THE SCIENCE OF OPHTHALMOLOGY

At a time when scientific knowledge about a subject is thought to constitute most of the important information about it, the history of ophthalmology frequently gets reduced to a litany of facts. From a purely scientific perspective, ophthalmology is most often defined as "*a surgical specialty concerned with the structure and function of the eye and the medical and surgical treatment of its defects*" or, more simply, "*a vast bulk of technical and medical information related to the eye, vision, and ocular diseases.*" Within the "*elaborate system of special-*

*ized knowledge, technical procedures, and rules of behavior*" that comprises all of modern medicine, specialized medicine in general and ophthalmology in particular are also described as the result of a necessary division of labor in medical science.

Arrington, 1;Chance, 1-5;
"Ophthalmology," Oxford Companion to Medicine;
"Ophthalmology," Encyclopedia of Medical History.

As a science, ophthalmology and ophthalmological history rest on a series of important discoveries, starting with sixteenth and seventeenth-century studies of physiological optics and the theory of vision. Johann Kepler discovered that vision occurs when light stimulates the eye and the lens forms an image on the retina—the basic knowledge needed to explain near and far-sightedness. The French philosopher Descartes, who was interested in vision as well as other ideas, found that changes in the lens caused by the action of the ciliary processes gave the eye its ability to accommodate various amounts of light. Descartes' contemporaries found that the image formed on the retina is inverted or upside down. They also identified a "*blind spot*" in the eye where no image is recorded. Further progress came when practitioners learned to apply cocaine and use the poison bella donna extracted from the nightshade plant to make atropine, a substance that relieved spasm and dilated the pupil of the eye. By the eighteenth century, doctors proficient in surgical skills also learned to perform iridotomy operations that made an artificial pupil within the iris when the pupillary opening had been closed by injury or disease.
Friedrich W.E. A.von Graefe introduced iridectomy for treating glaucoma, iritis, and iridochoroiditis, and devised an operation for strabismus.

"The Eye," 558-580.

History shows that doctors who chose to treat the human eye exclusively were the earliest to limit themselves in this way, making ophthalmology the first field of specialized medicine. Statistically, visual problems have always affected a substantial portion of the population. In 1975 one and a half million Americans were blind in one eye and three and a half million had only partial vision. The numbers of those afflicted in earlier centuries would have been even larger. Despite these facts, ophthalmology became a formal science separate from the rest of medicine only when the ophthalmoscope made it possible for a physician to observe the interior of the eyeball known as the ocular fundus. The German scientist, Hermann von Helmholtz, is credited with inventing the instrument in 1850 that made it possible to see this remarkable sight. Other specialized medical fields followed the ophthalmologists' lead until a full spectrum of professional specialties had been established. By 1930 there were 152,500 medical practitioners in the United States, of whom only 26% were specialists. Just twelve years later, specialists comprised 51% of the total, outdistancing general practitioners who numbered less than half (49%). Ophthalmology has continued to evolve, moreover, such that today's ophthalmologists divide themselves among seven sub-specialty areas ranging from pediatric ophthalmology to neuroophthalmology.

Starr, 2,3,54,60;
Atkinson, External Diseases, 3;
Rosen, iii, xi,1-3,6,8,30;
Edwards and Albert, 186-89;
"Ophthalmology,"
Encyclopedia of Medical History;
"Ophthalmology,"
Oxford Companion to Medicine.

Among other great discoveries that contributed to the modern science of ophthalmology was a study that showed the cornea, lens and vitreous are among a small number of tissues in the body lacking blood vessels, and that this "*avascularity*" makes vision possible. Because the eye tissues are transparent, light passes easily from the air through the eye fluids to produce an undistorted image on the retina. Discovery of the transparency resulting from the avascularity of eye tissues also led to the realization that many eye tissues are anatomically and physiologically "*isolated*" (the concept of immune privilege). Finally, early eye specialists learned that the eyes work together or are characterized by "paired functional interaction," and that one half of all the cranial nerves relate to eye function. Key discoveries about the eye representing many separate discoveries together make up the body of knowledge that defines ophthalmology, yet constitute only part of the larger story of how ophthalmology developed.

Cocaine was used to anesthetize the eye beginning with Koch's efforts in 1884, some years after the first use of general anesthesia.

Dammin, 1456

## THE IMPORTANCE OF CULTURE

From a cultural perspective, a strictly scientific approach reduces ophthalmological knowledge to pure information and overlooks the important role of culture in scientific advance. Medical historians believe explanations of ophthalmology that omit cultural contributions to its history are insufficient. Scientific fact still forms the backbone of knowledge about any scientific field, but the history of science sounds remarkably different when supported by an understanding of the culture in which a science developed. A cultural approach to scientific history, moreover, recognizes that some of history's most valuable lessons have been lost because of our preoccupation with results. According to historians and doctors who acknowledge the importance of culture, the story of how physicians arrived at medical results can be as important as the outcome of their efforts.

Dr. E.K. Manders Interview

Examples of this idea are numerous, since the eye has served as a powerful cultural symbol throughout history. Medical historian George Arrington acknowledged the link between science and culture and the powerful significance of vision in art and literature with the comment that, "*We recognize interrelationships of ophthalmology with the arts, cultural pursuits, and many intellectual human activities.*" Many cultures have employed scientific facts about the human eye for non-scientific purposes and associated vision as much with intention as perception. Vision has supplied the imagination with a rich catalog of metaphors linking sight with inner wisdom or insight for centuries. The blind writer, John Milton, penned perhaps the most memorable line about the moment the world began as one of "*no light, but rather darkness visible.*" Adages or proverbs such as "*beauty is in the eye of the beholder*" or phrases such as "*more than meets the eye*" are common in many cultures. The Bible expresses the oldest idea of justice as "*an eye for an eye,*" and other cultures have feared the "*evil eye.*" Tales of the blind seer Teresias, of Oedipus, and Lear use the experience of the loss of sight as a metaphorical gateway to self-knowledge. Poet Theodore Roethke expressed a similar idea with the phrase "*In a dark time, the eye begins to see.*" Finally, William Shakespeare, who claimed love added "*a precious seeing to the eye*," created an equally powerful image by linking the act of seeing with love.

Arrington, History of Ophthalmology, 8;
Atkinson, On External Diseases, 13;
Milton, John, Paradise Lost, l. 63;
Shakespeare, Love's Labors Lost, 4:3, 333;
Roethke, Theodore, In a Dark Time, 1964, st. 1.

To appreciate the cultural meaning of sight and appreciate ophthalmology from an historical standpoint, it also helps to recognize that people at different times have had different ideas about the reality of vision. Not only have visual standards changed to the point that the longevity of information about the human eye has shrunk from roughly ten years to approximately three, but ophthalmologists living in different periods have literally thought differently about what it means to see. The idea that people in particular cultures at different times have entertained different opinions about what they wished to see suggests another way to explore the science of ophthalmology. A better definition might be that ophthalmology—the science that deals with the human eye and its unique properties—is one of the most progressive fields in medicine because of the ophthalmologist's desire to solve problems relating to ever-new visual contexts. In this sense, the scientific practice of ophthalmology as we know it today is a relatively recent phenomenon. Today, ophthalmology moves forward through both improved clinical practice and research that literally expands man's ability to see in new dimensions. And this suggests that an understanding of history is essential if we are to appreciate the complex process by which ophthalmology has reached the sophisticated level of today's medical science.

In essence, this constitutes a phenomological approach to the field.
Dr. Jack Lee Interview;
Seifert, Josef, 1-50

Cultural studies of ophthalmological history show that people in early cultures believed the eye originates light, associated it with heat, or thought like the great Roman medical writer, Aulus Cornelius Celsus (AD3-CAD.64), that "*water enters it through the optic nerve and escapes as tears*." To the Greeks, the goddess Hygeia was the guardian of eyesight. The fact that other societies believed the eye clouds when a "*morbid humor of some sort*" flows down into a space that exists between the lens and iris, hence the name "*cataract*," helps us to understand an otherwise inexplicable terminology. Similarly, the familiar "*Rx*" sign used by today's pharmacists in prescriptions, signifying the phrase "*take thou*" or "*make up*," represents the distillation over time of a symbol that originated in ancient Egypt. The *Rx* began as a stylized design that recalled a myth about the god Horus who lost an eye in a battle with a demon. According to the story, the god of wisdom restored the injured eye, and henceforth any subsequent reference to the eye gave it mystical properties. When Greek physicians subsequently adopted the design and transformed it into the sign of Apollo to symbolize their profession, the original symbol came to stand for health and happiness. This sign was handed on down to the Romans when the emperor Nero bumped into the Greeks. Nero felt threatened by the symbol since it seemed to empower another authority than himself and ascribed it to the god Jupiter, knowing that by doing so Roman belief would support the subjugation of physicians to the state. How the eye of Horus became connected with medical prescriptions is unclear, but no doubt less a matter of science than of politics and culture. In this case, the stabilizing force of a specific cultural understanding for a particular society may have actually retarded the acceptance of scientific fact and medical discovery. Thus, purely scientific facts about ophthalmology fail to tell the entire story of how the field developed.

Chance, 8, 15-17;
Rosenberg, C., The Cholera Years;Numbers, R.L., 245-263;
Arrington, 37;
"The Eye of Horus," Australian Prescriber, 18:4 (1995), 84;
Rosen, 2

Another good example of a more complete picture of the history of ophthalmology depends on cultural understandings can be found at the place where culture and science overlap in techniques used to create works of art. Early painters, rather than scientists, were the first to learn the principles of perspective that allow artists to manipulate the visual sense to create the illusion of space. The artist's desire to control what the viewer sees when looking at a painting drove painter Michel Eugene Chevreul—whose notes are still used as a guide to painting—to discover the secrets of color theory. Chevreul not only found that colored light or optical mixtures of colors and contrasting colors achieved results equal to those obtained by mixing pigments, but explained why certain colors placed in proximity on a two dimensional canvas create a three-dimensional sense of space. By experimenting with colored yarns at the Gobelins tapestry works, Chevreul discovered universal principles of color harmony that led not only to pointillism and divisionism in painting, but to new understandings of related science. Ophthalmologists such as Dr. Donald Taylor Atkinson, one of the first South Texas doctors to limit his practice exclusively to ophthalmology, were among those who studied vision in this way.

Chevreul, M.E., 13-17; Dr. Joseph De Gasperi Interview.

While cultural information creates a different perspective on pure science, however, the order in which discoveries were made and cultural beliefs developed and expressed-- that is, the history of human thought and action relating to vision-- adds a further dimension to our understanding of science. An historical approach to ophthalmology recognizes that a Greek physician named Euelpides was once called "*the most famous oculist of our time*" and that King Cyrus of Persia once asked a fellow ruler, King Amasis, for a referral to a good oculist around 560 B.C.. What is meant by science, in other words, can be quite different at different moments in history. Eye care is believed to have become a separate branch of medicine in ancient times. The fact that specialization had already developed, according to following statement by Herodotus in the fifth century B.C., suggests that Helmholtz may not deserve all the credit.:

*"The art of medicine among them is distributed thus: each physician is a physician of one disease and no more;and the whole country is full of physicians, for some profess themselves to be physicians of the eyes, others of the head."*

Ferris and Hoppe, 214

Because skilled practitioners who treated eye problems remained itinerant and worked without formal training, licensing, or other marks of professional achievement for centuries, however, the field could not yet be fully considered a specialty.

This story is attributed to Herodotus. Rosen, 1;
Rothstein, 207-9;
Starr, 40-55;
Dunlop, 6.

At a fundamental level, an historical and cultural approach to ophthalmology enables the modern observer to uncover and appreciate the unique accomplishments of practitioners at different periods of history. According to instruments displayed at the British Museum, for example, we know that Egyptian doctors who removed cataracts knew very little, but succeeded nonetheless in treating patients. Physicians at Rome and Alexandria may have been the first true specialists since they restricted themselves solely to the "*couching*" of cataract, but the process involved simply pushing the offending material out of the patient's field of vision. Late nineteenth century doctors, living in what they considered the Golden Age of Ophthalmology, believed they already understood everything about the eye that could be known, but today seem primitive in their knowledge and practice. What most failed to realize was that, as people's visual needs changed, so too would the ophthalmologist's knowledge and objectives. The "*eye lane*," a twenty-foot room in a clinic for testing visual acuity according to visual standards, symbolizes only one concept of vision as do the giant national eyeglasses of the Hubbell telescope trained on the heavens. The importance of this dynamic—the fact that older ideas of vision have receded as newer ones rushed in to take their places—is key to understanding the science of ophthalmology. All of which suggests that, to fully understand the development of ophthalmology in South Texas, it is necessary to explore the cultural circumstances surrounding its development in this region.

## SOCIAL AND CULTURAL FACTORS CONTRIBUTING TO THE GROWTH OF SPECIALIZED MEDICINE

Recognizing that science develops in the context of culture, scholars have looked more closely at the ways in which medical advances have occurred in particular societies. According to medical historian George Rosenberg, "*specialization in any kind of cultural activity is a socially conditioned phenomenon.*" Rosenberg "*convincingly demonstrated the interdependence of medical and cultural history*" and developed a general model of how ophthalmology arose by looking at characteristics common to the appearance of medical specialization in different places. Key to understanding medical history, Rosen explained, is "*situating medical developments within their cul-*

*tural context*" and "exploring connections between ideas and institutions." Medicine did not develop uniformly everywhere and medical advances did not appear in all places simultaneously. It is important to examine social attitudes and the configuration of medical institutions existing at specific times in order to understand why particular developments occurred. By implication, it is logical to expect or to speculate that ophthalmology may have developed in certain unique ways in South Texas. The question for this history to answer, therefore, is "*Did the same conditions stimulate the growth of specialization in South Texas that caused ophthalmology to develop elsewhere?*" (Rosenberg was a student of historian Richard Hofstadter at Columbia University and the Institute of the History of Medicine affiliated with the Johns Hopkins Medical School).

Numbers, 250; Rothstein, 3.

Medical historians Paul Starr and George Rosen subsequently added a component to the conclusion reached by Rosenberg identifyed general patterns in the appearance of the medical specialties that reflect the "*growing solidarity and structural interdependence of society.*" This interdependence, they explained, is partly a result of "*social forces operating within the medical profession itself,*" but also of "*forces impinging on physicians from the larger environment of the society within which they operate(d).*" In general, they suggest, it is necessary to take into account the particular human context in which ophthalmology advanced in order to understand its history. What is important about this conclusion is that a matrix of people, places, ideas, and events representing a combination of scientific, social and cultural forces all apparently contribute to scientific development.

Starr, 2, 3, 54, 60;
Atkinson, External Diseases, 3;
Rosen, iii, vi, 1-3, 6, 8, 30;
Eye Report.

George Rosen has been inspired by W.H.R. Rivers, who explained specialization in part as a social phenomenon in the following passage that Rosen used in the Prologue of his book:

*Medicine is a social institution. It comprises a set of beliefs and practices which only become possible when held and carried out by members of an organized society, among whom a high degree of the division of labor and specialization of the social function has come into being. Any principles and methods found to be of value in the study of social institutions in general cannot be ignored by the historian of medicine.*

According to Starr's theory, "*medical instrumentation*" such as the ophthalmoscope, the ophthalmometer, the tonometer, the Snellen visual acuity test, instruments for transillumination, the phoropter, perimeter, and slit lamp, were essential in allowing ophthalmology to "*differentiate itself from general surgery*," but other conditions were equally important. Public acceptance of specialized medicine was partly the work of individual ophthalmologists, but also a product of accumulated experience and knowledge that society gained from individual cases, technological innovations, the growth of medical institutions, the exchange of information within the medical profession, and advances in technique.

Rosen, George, Specialization of Medicine, Prologue, n.p.

According to Rosen, in the United States and Great Britain, the origin of special ophthalmic institutions preceded the appearance of ophthalmology. William Rothstein showed that doctors needed to observe hundreds of cases of eye disease and obtain first-hand knowledge about the effects of treatment on those cases before they could become fully competent to treat patients. It is now generally recognized that hospitals staffed by numbers of practitioners were necessary to the rise of specialization. Had there not been institutions to acknowledge the specialties and permit doctors to employ new technologies, the use of new devices might have been accepted more slowly. This in turn required a population large enough to produce cases for accurate description, analysis, and treatment, and these levels were usually to be found only in major cities. Rothstein concluded that institutional change preceded technological advance and that the rise of specialized medicine corresponded to the rise of cities and creation of medical centers there. His studies showed that at a minimum, at least 12,000 people who enjoyed a significant level of economic prosperity were needed to support specialized medicine, along with urban hospitals where the care of patients afflicted with eye disease could take place and doctors could demonstrate the value of the science to the profession. It is logical, therefore, that the Chinese facing their considerable population established an ophthalmic hospital as early as 1827.

Rosen, 33; Rothstein, 24, 44, 64; Chance, 8.

The emerging model suggests that at least six separate factors have aided in the evolution of medical specialties, of which only the first is purely scientific, and that ophthalmology did not mature in an area unless these factors were present. To test the model, this work will trace these six factors in the development of ophthalmology in South Texas by answering the following questions:

1) *Did a medically-valid body of knowledge and technique for use in practice, adapted to the needs of the patient, serve as the basis for a scientific approach to medical care in South Texas?*

2) *Were cities or urban populations large enough to educate and support specialists and supply a sufficient number and variety of cases important to facilitate learning by specialists?*

3) *Was the rise of large hospitals and medical institutions with training programs dedicated to the specialty important to establish professional standards and practices?*

4) *Were professional organizations capable of overcoming public skepticism, establishing communication between practitioners, and creating uniformity among practitioners fundamental to growth in South Texas?*

5) *Did institutions capable of carrying out research or scientific investigation to produce new knowledge help the profession adapt to new needs?*

6) *Did community involvement on the part of individual practitioners add to the stature of the medical profession and help specialists succeed?*

Starr, 2,3,54,60.

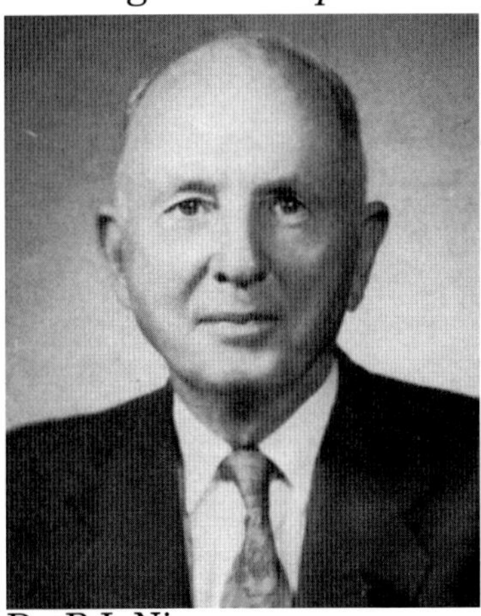

Dr. P. I. Nixon
The great Texas medical historian whose writings were an important resource for this book.

## UNIQUE ELEMENTS IN THE SOUTH TEXAS STORY

The principal objective of this study is to examine the process by which South Texas ophthalmology developed. In addition to scientific developments, it will focus on the social and cultural forces that operated on that development as well as key scientific advances. To date, few attempts have been made to describe or assess the development of ophthalmology in this region, and no full-length account of medicine in Texas as a whole or a regional such as South Texas has yet been written. For almost fifty years, three titles and a handful of articles have been nearly the only sources of information available. P.I. Nixon's Medical Story of Early Texas, Red's The Medicine Man in Texas, and Coleman's Aesculapius on the Colorado laid down the basic outlines of Texas medical history and compiled a list of early physicians that still serves as a key reference for scholars. It is not difficult to understand, therefore, why the section on Texas in Gorin's 1982 History of Ophthalmology makes no mention of any San Antonio institution or practitioner whatsoever. Little effort has been made to determine the degree to which frontier specialists simply recapitulated the experience of ophthalmologists in major cities or what effect frontier conditions had on the development of specialized medicine.

Gorin, 344

With today's sophisticated medical environment, it may be hard to appreciate the men who transformed rural frontier medical practice into modern cosmopolitan and scientific medicine. This book tells the story of some of those individuals and the events and changes that transformed the experience of early South Texas eye doctors into the work of modern ophthalmic professionals in the region today. Building on the existing literature, this study offers evidence that, although it constitutes a relatively short chapter in the chronology of ophthalmic history, the history of South Texas ophthalmology adds a significant dimension to our understanding of ophthalmological specialization. Although aspects of South Texas ophthalmological history mirror growth in other places, several elements in the region's development are unique. These unique elements range from links with the nation's efforts in space and close ties with military medicine to the impact of immigrants on growth of the field in particular towns. Influences described by the general paradigm do not account entirely for local influences, individual achievements, and unique forces that shaped the profession in the triangle of land that includes San Antonio and the Rio Grande Valley. Organizing a sizeable hinterland stretching from the Gulf Coast northward toward Austin, a string of events took San Antonio's medical development in different directions from that of other cities. The history of South Texas ophthalmology is a case study within a larger story, and to that degree this narrative is representative, illustrating how paradigms or patterns established elsewhere were repeated here. Successive generations of South Texas doctors produced the required configuration of hospitals, medical schools, residency programs, and research components necessary to make ophthalmology a mature field of medical specialization, yet "*some have estimated that Texas was perhaps at least twenty years behind other parts of the country*." Not only did the first significant Texas medical developments occur in South Texas, but ophthalmology's development here differed from that in other parts of Texas. If in many ways the regional story parallels the general picture of the growth of specialized medicine, therefore, to conjure up the Texas past is to hear a familiar story with a twist.

Gorin, 344;Dunlop, 2, 4, 64;
Ferris and Hoppe, 142.

George E. Arrington believed that ophthalmologists could benefit from knowing their history, or more specifically, that history revealed "*what constitutes ophthalmology and rational ophthalmological thought*." Based on a series of interviews conducted with elder San Antonio ophthalmologists and others who participated in the growth of its medical institutions, this narrative seeks to establish a broader context for individual stories and a fuller appreciation of individual achievements. In so doing, it constitutes the first resource of its kind. Although primarily intended for those interested in ophthalmological history, however, it also offers material of interest to those who study the American frontier, the history of science, military history, medical history, German immigration, space science, Texas history, and the growth of the professions in the United States.

University of Texas Health Science Center News Release,
"Burns Memorial Library Dedication," May 14, 1970.

Specific events made the appearance of ophthalmology in South Texas possible, each representing the culmination of numerous individuals' efforts that are part of the story of Texas as well as of Texas medicine. The first generation of frontier horse-and-buggy doctors ended traditional practice, adopted a scientific approach, and developed surgical techniques that improved people's ability to see unimpeded by diseases, physical disability, or injuries such as cataract, glaucoma, conjunctivitis, iritis, and trauma. Members of the second generation most of whom specialized in eye, ear, nose and throat, categorized and classified diseases to define and control them and began to trace the links between eye problems and disease conditions in other organs of the body. The observation that the public was slow to accept specialized medicine and quackery thrived almost until the turn of the century suggests the importance of professional organizations and professional standards. A third generation brought the first true ophthalmologists to the Texas frontier, carrying with them a sophisticated level of medical science that grew like a prairie sunflower. These individuals defined techniques for controlling different aspects of vision, established visual standards, and explored the possibility that vision enhancements could improve limitations and expand normal visual capacity. Their history and that of the region's medical institutions—medical societies, military and civilian hospitals, the first residency training programs allowing specialization in ophthalmology, the University of Texas Health Science Center, and early research centers have much to tell us about how science grows and what types of experience have contributed to the growth of medical specialization. Because many details are unique, the story of ophthalmology's appearance in South Texas offers an important chapter in the saga of American medical history and adds a significant dimension to our understanding of ophthalmological specialization as a whole. For Texans, it is also part of a heritage that binds them together through the sharing of a common past.

Cary, "EENT as a Specialty," n.p.

# CHAPTER 2

## SPANISH IMPERIALISM AND THE START OF MEDICAL SPECIALIZATION IN EUROPE AND AMERICA

*His years in training are hard, a marathon of work; his years in practice are hard, a marathon of service. His compensation is this: to solve in the degree that science and humanity may, the manifold problems of mortality.*

A.A. Ross, Stepping Stones

Familiar with the techniques of modern medicine and the extensive network of medical institutions that exist in South Texas today, it may be difficult to imagine a time when house calls were common and people in small towns enjoyed close personal relationships with their doctors. Many Texans may have forgotten how dedicated physicians transformed frontier medicine into modern scientific practice while the "*chili queens*" still sold their fiery product in the streets of San Antonio. An appreciation for the pace of medical advance in Texas can be gained quickly, however, by comparing San Antonio and Vienna in the early nineteenth century. In those years American doctors struggled to bring basic medical care to the western frontier at the same time physicians in Europe ushered medicine, and specifically ophthal-

# HISTORY OF OPHTHALMOLOGY IN SOUTH TEXAS

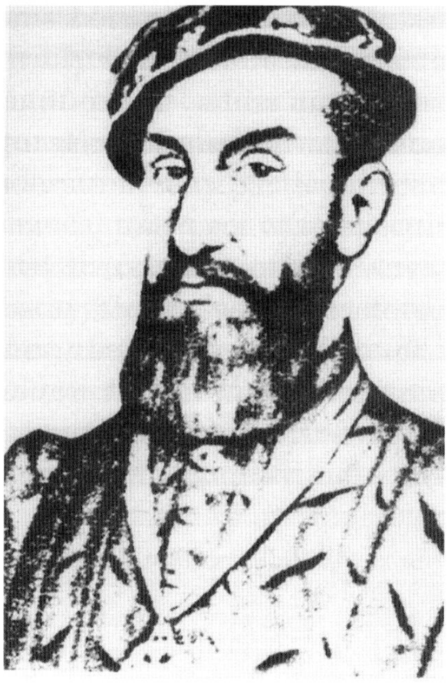

Spanish explorer Cabeza de Vaca (1528) was the first to describe the state of medicine in South Texas and specifically referenced eye disease, especially cataract.

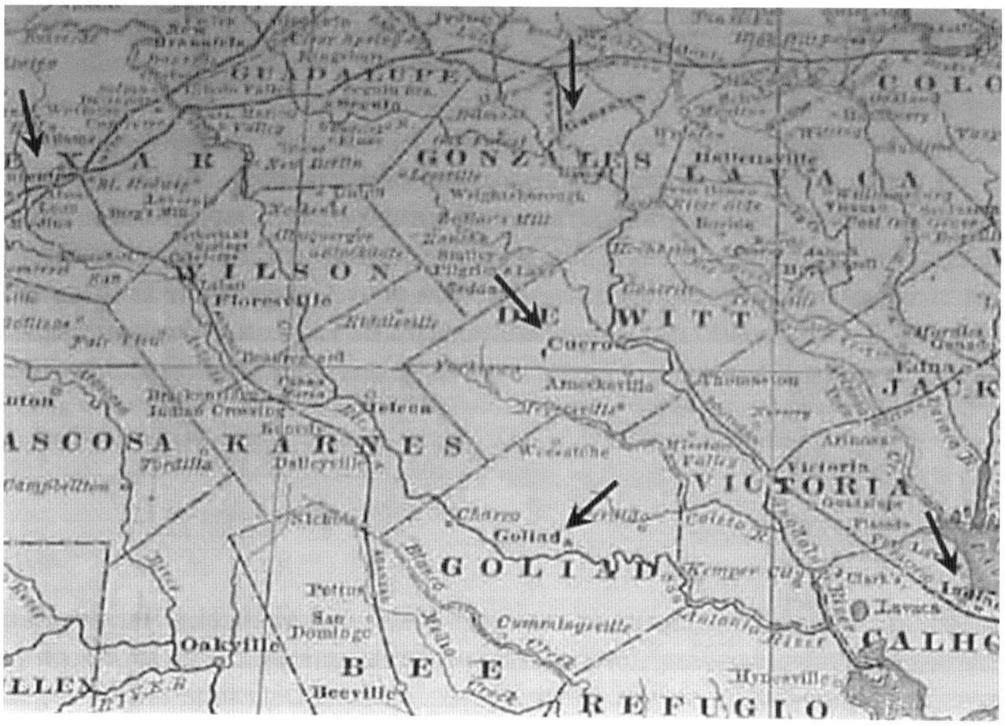


Detail map of South Texas with arrows indicating San Antonio (Bexar County), Gonzalez (Gonzalez County) , Goliad (Goliad County), Cuero (De Witt County), and Indianola (Calhoun County), each of which played an important role in bringing modern medicine to the area.

mology, into a golden age. Medical conditions in Texas remained primitive relatively briefly because immigration and communication between these places facilitated transmittal of powerful new ideas being developed in Europe. For achievements to find their way to such distant outposts as the Texas frontier, however, a foundation must first be laid for this important cultural transfer.

Before the arrival of Europeans, much of what would become today's Texas was an empty wilderness and the conditions of living primitive at best. Native American tribes that had inhabited the region possibly for centuries administered the only known medical treatments, including eye care. Unfortunately, although native peoples sometimes performed suturing and understood how to apply pressure to stop bleeding, many of those who roamed the prairies possessed only primitive medical knowledge. The authority for medical care in most tribes, a designated shaman, was an elderly man or woman who had undergone a spiritual experience or seen a vision and attempted to heal the tribe's ailments by contacting supernatural forces. Shamans also used herbal remedies and an array of ministrations such as cauterizing or blowing on affected areas, the laying on of hands, sweating and smoking, or ritually invoking the power of an object with religious significance. Such "*medicine men*" were accorded honors like those of the priests of ancient Greece whose religious and healing duties were indistinguishable. These individuals often enjoyed privileges in the community, including permission to possess several wives and obtain awards of food and other goods for satisfactory service. On the other hand, a medicine man who failed to find a cure often forfeited his life for an unsuccessful treatment. Native tribes also frequented natural sites believed to have healing powers, as evidenced by the remains of campsites left by bands of Coahuiltecan Indians at the healthgiving "*hot wells*" near the San Pedro and San Antonio Springs.

Nixon, Medical Story, 1-27;
Red, 14;
Newcomb, 29-57; Richardson, 1-19; Coleman, 3-9.

## THE RULE OF SPAIN

The region that eventually became South Texas did not remain in native hands for long, but would be conquered successively by different groups wanting to forge a niche in its history. The Spanish were the first to attempt conquest by pushing a line of settlement from Mexico through today's Texas, a strategy that made South Texas' role in both the state's development and that of its medical profession an early and essential one.

Although Americans have been taught that pioneers setting forth in waves of Conestoga wagons moved civilization westward from the Eastern Seaboard in a steady march of Progress, records show that European influence actually traveled along a South-North axis northward from Mexico and the Gulf Coast through the fertile but dry lands of the lower Rio Grande Valley. Similarly, medical specialization traveled along the waterways that flowed into the Gulf of Mexico and later followed the branching path of the railroads that opened up the Texas interior after the first military incursions. Professional medical care remained practically non-existent until 1830, because early settlers lacked the necessary infrastructure to support a medical establishment. Only when Spain relinquished its imperial designs on the region, and other Europeans collectively referred to as Anglos arrived, did the benefits of medical advances made in Vienna and other distant capitals, including the knowledge of ophthalmology, reach the frontier. Only Dallas, whose inhabitants hailed primarily from the Midwestern states and more northerly places, was an exception to the south-to-north pattern of growth. Most Dallas residents initially came from the Midwest rather than from the Deep South or along a line north through Galveston and Indianola.

New Handbook of Texas;
Richardson, 20-43.

Several European countries outfitted expeditions to explore the territory, but those who came on an errand of empire for the kings of Spain were the earliest. Spaniards bent on conquest, following the orders of their government to explore the region for gold and other resources, made the first attempts to create an empire in North America. Long before cowboys walked the dusty streets of frontier Texas towns, Spanish empire builders extended a line of missions and presidios (the Spanish word for a type of fort) north from Mexico, planting the roots of their powerful cultural heritage as in villages that sprang up around the missions. The Spanish believed that the combined efforts of missionaries and soldiers would eventually create permanent settlements and long-term political control, and evidence suggests that few professional physicians accompanied expeditions to New Spain's northern borderlands. In time, the Spanish attempt failed when the Mexican and Tejano people they sought to rule overthrew their would-be conquerors for control of the region.

New Handbook of Texas; Richardson, 43-58.

Among the most famous Spanish explorers was a man called Cabeza de Vaca, whose name meant "the head of a cow" and whose adventures reveal the general level of medicine available to men who made the treacherous journey. De Vaca came to South Texas as part of an early Spanish expedition in 1528. His party's plans changed swiftly, however, when their ship ran into a major storm on entering the Gulf of Mexico. The storm deposited de Vaca and a handful of survivors on the sands of Galveston Island on the Texas Gulf Coast, where they were taken in by Native-Americans who cared for them but then made the grateful travelers their prisoners and slaves. Conditions changed only when an epidemic broke out and their captors pressed them into service as doctors, withholding food until de Vaca and his companions agreed to act as healers. In The Medical Story of Early Texas, Dr. Pat Nixon reminds his readers that this was "*a role forced on them by pressure of desperate necessity, for none in the group were trained in the medical arts.*" Fortunately, the natives were indifferent to their doctors' lack of medical credentials, and De Vaca and his party succeeded in convincing the natives that they had achieved a cure.

"De Vaca, Cabeza," New Handbook of Texas;
Coleman, 6; Nixon, Medical Story, 27-36

For the next several years, de Vaca's party wandered across the region, witnessing the considerable skills of Native-American shamans in treating the sick in the various tribes they encountered along the way. Seven or eight years later after wandering for some time alone, Cabeza de Vaca found his way back to Mexico and recorded his experience in a book that became one of the most influential of the period. The Relacion, as he called it, described to the outside world a new and hitherto unknown territory that only increased Spanish enthusiasm to establish settlements in the region, and was eventually credited with sparking expeditions by Coronado and de Soto of Spain and LaSalle of France.

Richardson, 21.

From the standpoint of ophthalmology, one of the most interesting sections of the Relacion contains de Vaca's references to blindness and eye disease. In this section he states that his "*indian master, his wife, and his sons were all blind in one eye.*" "*The greater part were clouded of an eye,*" he noted, "*and others in like manner were entirely blind.*" A contemporary historian, Gonzalo Fernandez de Oviedo, who wrote about de Vaca's experience among the Texas natives, confirmed the idea that many were blind and "*great numbers were one-eyed from clouds.*" According to Dr. Pat Nixon, both accounts were likely to have been early descriptions of cataracts.

Red, 5-9; Nixon, Medical Story of Early Texas, 27-37

De Vaca also described the performance of a surgical operation that was likely to have been the first such medical care offered by a European in Texas. After successfully removing a large arrowhead lodged just above a man's heart, he was rewarded with a season of celebrations and dances by the grateful patient and his tribe. De Vaca also recounted the means he and other reluctant healers in his party used when faced with demands for care:

*"Our method was to bless the sick, breathing upon them, and recite a Pater-noster and an Ave-Maria, praying with all earnestness to God our Lord that he would give health and influence them to make us some good return. In his clemency he willed that all those for whom we supplicated, should tell the others that they were sound and in health, directly after we made the sign of the blessed cross over them. For this the Indians treated us kindly; they deprived themselves of food that they might give to us, and presented us with skins and some trifles".*

Nixon, Medical Story, 3

In the seventeenth and eighteenth centuries, Franciscan padres representing Spanish imperialist interests established missions for Native-Americans in East Texas and along the San Antonio River. These friars first made the association between location and health that led to the founding of the community called San Antonio de Bejar (later spelled Bexar), known today as San Antonio. A graceful river flowed near the mission from gushing springs in the wooded hills a few miles to the north, and the ribbon of milky green water that wound its way southward created a verdant valley capable of sustaining a sizeable community. The Spanish acknowledged the place as a natural one for healing as early as 1784 in a royal decree that regulated "*the use of medicinal baths and waters to the members of the army,"* and Spanish government officials acknowledged the value of the place by making San Antonio capital of the Spanish Province of Texas. From then until the present, the town maintained close associations with the idea of improving human health.

MacMillan, Esther, ed., 84-88; Nixon, Medical Story, 270-5

The first settlement at San Antonio began in 1718 when a community or *villa* sprang up around the local mission and its adjoining plazas. Sixteen families from the Spanish Canary Islands that arrived in 1731 quickly employed the native population as farmers. Soldiers were housed in the military presidio responsible for securing the safety of the settlers and clergy at the mission. With the appointment of a cabildo or governing body in August of 1731, the town became the first formally-organized municipality on land that would become the state of Texas.

"San Antonio," New Handbook of Texas

Unfortunately, the creation of a permanent settlement at San Antonio did little to improve medical conditions across the region. With scant medical knowledge, equipment or supplies, the Spanish missionary fathers and civilian settlers managed to improve the health of the tribes by introducing dietary and cultural changes, but frequently used medical remedies little more advanced than those of the tribal medicine men. They did succeed, however, in stopping the native peoples from grubbing for worms, ant eggs, lizards and agave bulbs as sources of nutrition, and in teaching them agriculture and animal husbandry. Despite this, however, local tribes continued their raids on the growing population of settlers for sustenance. The missionaries reported on the illnesses and diseases of their charges and described the medicine men they encountered as "sorcerers dealing in herbs," among which according to the San Antonio Institute of Texan Cultures were some used specifically to relieve eye problems.

Nixon, Medical Story of Early Texas, 42-44;
Red, 12-24; Richardson, 1-20;
Cyndi Gonzales Interview.

*Agua de sandia* or watermelon juice was used as an eyewash for sore eyes. Flor de San Juan, the flower of St. John which grows abundantly in dry sandy soil, was boiled in water and the flower water was used as an eyewash for swollen or infected eyes. The plentiful mesquite pods and leaves were made into a decoction to treat conjunctivitis or pinkeye, and later were found to be as effective on livestock as on children. Eyewashes were brewed from the stems and pods of the prickly pear cactus, anise seeds, stinkweed or camphorweed, and the flowers of the elderberry tree.

A sty was bathed with the milky juice of the squaw spurge, and pain in the eye was said to be eased by rubbing fat of opossum on the eyelid. More drastic, aggressive therapeutics were used to remove foreign objects from the orbit. A dry "frijole" or pinto bean was inserted next to the eyeball and the lid held closed. The bean was rotated around the eyeball with the aid of the fluid in the eye, until it washed out the foreign matter. Another method used the miniscule seed of red salvia. It was placed in the lower lid, and as it came in contact with moisture, it released a mucilaginous substance to which the foreign body adhered and could then be easily dislodged.

The population was spared the harsh methods of "heroic medicine" such as bleeding, cupping, and the administration of purgatives that flourished in Europe before physicians developed a scientific understanding of the body. While rejecting the shaman's remedies as evil "*superstition*," the Fathers probably borrowed some of their counterparts' traditional herbal decoctions to address the maladies of mission inhabitants and the soldiers who protected them.

Nixon, Medical Story of Early Texas, 42-26.

The Spanish did little to improve the quality of medical care across the region, however, largely because the colonists proved unable to maintain the settlements they established. When a number of East Texas missions failed in the 1730s, the effort at those sites was abandoned and their settlers and missionaries moved to new locations along the course of the San Antonio River. While this strengthened the growing community at San Antonio de Bejar, the Spanish introduced epidemic disease and caused injuries that led to the deaths of large numbers of native people, neither the missions nor the surrounding settlements could be considered bastions of good health. A succession of Spanish governors, responsible for the well-being of the citizenry but faced with limited resources, repeatedly petitioned the King of Spain for help to no avail. Eighteenth century correspondence between the governors and other Crown officials notes the absence of medical personnel in San Antonio and a persistent lack of even the most basic medical supplies. As the years unfolded, however, no settlement in

New Spain, including the provincial capital, could boast the services of a doctor. No trained European physician arrived in the territory, in fact, for another hundred years.

Nixon, Medical Story of Early Texas, 1-27;
Nixon, Century of Medicine, 8

Nonetheless, the creation of San Antonio and other key Texas townsites was Spain's most lasting legacy to the region. The mutual efforts of Spanish church and state in South Texas had established a population in mission settlements and soon would construct the region's first dispensary or hospital. A step in that direction was made with the arrival of San Antonio de Bejar's first physician in 1793, an event of considerable significance. The impoverished village at the time had little more than one hundred and fifty rude buildings made of stone, mud and wood, and was perhaps the most unremarkable capital city serving Spain in the new world. In that year, however, the townspeople and their governor gratefully welcomed Dr. Augustin Guillermo de Spangerberg, alternatively Agustin Guillermo de Espangemberg or Spangemberg, a twenty-eight year old German and English-speaking doctor who was likely the first trained non-Hispanic physician in Texas. The spelling of his name indicates that Spangerberg may have changed his name to suit the Spanish culture around him or possibly that he had some Spanish background. The new doctor had spent four years in New York State and two years at Lewisberg in the "capital of old Virginia." Apparently, his reasons for making the long trip were personal—he had come to the frontier looking for a brother—but for the local population his medical skills were of greater importance.

"Spangerberg, Augustin Guillermo de," New Handbook of Texas

Unfortunately, San Antonio's primitive economy and lack of any type of medical institution left it incapable of supporting the services of a professional, and Spangerberg left before he could significantly improve medical care in the community. When some of the new doctor's patients complained to the governor about the quality of their medical treatment, he replied that "*perhaps the reason his (Spangerberg's) patients did not like him was to evade the payment of his bills.*" Whatever the case, the doctor's request for a passport was honored and he departed for Coahuila in Mexico, leaving San Antonio once again bereft of medical services. According to the Bexar Archives,

Spangerberg had been *"a native of Strassburg in the Province of Alsace"* who studied at the College of Guetings, or the University of Gottingen, before coming to the United States. As such, he foreshadowed the coming of other physicians trained in Germany who would have a more positive influence on the region.

"Spangerberg," New Handbook of Texas

In the years that followed, official pleas for relief resumed. Records show that a series of Spanish doctors worked in San Antonio for a salary of between eight and thirty pesos a month. Little is known, however, about the background and training of Dr. Alfonso Reyes who practiced there, or that of the town's first Mexican doctor, Dr. Don Jose Joaquin Villaverde. French colonial efforts also brought several surgeons into the area accompanying military troops, but their names were not recorded by the Spanish who continued to dominate the region. Lack of royal response to the dispiriting medical situation in New Spain was probably less a matter of limited resources than bureaucratic fumbling and the Crown's fundamental lack of concern for the distant outpost. In 1795, however, the Spanish city council at San Fernando de Bexar did entertain sufficient interest in local medical conditions to license physicians and apothecaries.

Nixon, Century of Medicine in San Antonio, 8, 25;
Nixon, Medical Story of Early Texas, 81-90;
Ferris and Hoppe, 3, 190; Red, 22.

Not until 1803 did an event occur that produced significant change in San Antonio's medical circumstances. In that year, a daring project began to protect the colonists from the horrors of smallpox based on Jenner's discovery of the importance of vaccination with *"cowpox"* in 1798. King Charles IV sent a ship carrying twenty-two children described as a "living chain" of smallpox, but who were vaccinated successively during the voyage by a medical team who made the trip. In April 1806 San Antonio de Bejar received a vial of the vaccine fluid and a paperful of smallpox scabs from the passengers. Spanish doctors later vaccinated the local Native-American population, but the individual who inoculated twelve children in the community was destined to become its newest doctor. Dr. Federico Zervan, who lived in New Orleans from about 1790 to 1805, was described as *"a professor of surgery and medicine,"* and may have been the most qualified medical practitioner to serve the community in its short history. This was particularly true since in 1807, when Lieutenant Zebulon M. Pike visited San Antonio, the place could still be described as "*a city of perhaps two thousand souls, most of whom reside in miserable mud-daubed, grass-roofed houses.*"

Dunlop, 51ff.; Nixon, Medical Story, 56, 70-71; Red 15-17

Zervan's achievement was to significantly improve local medicine by administering San Antonio de Bejar's first institution dedicated entirely to medical care, a newly-established provisional infirmary housed in the old mission San Antonio de Valero, later known as the Alamo. Today, this hospital holds the distinction of being considered the first such institution in Texas. There Zervan employed a "*practitioner*" and pharmacist named Lazaro Orranti as his assistant, along with male nurses to tend the patients and women to do the cooking. Seriously ill or injured patients up to this time were frequently moved to hospitals in Mexico, but Zervan's presence gave the northern region its own hospital. This was no minor accomplishment, although the facility was ill equipped, crowded, and provided only rudimentary care for soldiers and villagers. As the first medical institution of its kind, the small hospital represented a major advance for medicine in the region.

Charles Ramsdell, 27;
Red, 18-19;
Nixon, Medical Story, 68;
Dunlop, 51ff.;
Ferris and Hoppe, 202;
Ross, A.A., 70-75;
"Zervan, Federico," New Handbook of Texas.

While Zervan documented no specific reports of eye disease or injury, such cases most certainly would have been a part of his practice. The following list of medical supplies that arrived at the infirmary by pack mule gives some insight into the kinds of equipment and curatives he most likely used for treating patients:

*Senna, sugar candy, cochineal, rhubarb, epsom salts, Jesuit's bark (cinchona officinalis), incense, cream of tartar, cantharis (Spanish fly-pulverized green blister beetle), American ipecac, opium, borax, catholic extract, three dozen rubber bougies, one rubber catheter, tarter emetic, wine, spirits of scurvy-grass, olive oil, frog cordial with mercury, sim-*

*ple cordial, divine cordial, one box of surgical instruments for operations for trepan, 12 pointed Spanish lances, thin catgut, two large syringes, Hispanic pharmacopoeia, active mercury, corrosive sublimate, sweet mercury, white arsenic, black bromide, four American cupping glasses.*

Ferris and Hoppe, 5; Nixon, Century of Medicine in San Antonio, 25

Although Zervan successfully ran his enterprise for two years, personal financial difficulties and those of the hospital eventually ruined his reputation, forced him to flee to Mexico, and brought the community's first permanent medical institution to an untimely end. The doctor's sudden departure from the city in 1807 was clouded by disputes with several townspeople, including a civil suit by the priest with whom he boarded and gambled who demanded payment of grievously overdue accounts. When Zervan left, Dr. Jayme Gurza and later Dr. Francisco Farina took over the infirmary, but by 1814 the Alamo hospital had ceased to function. Other practitioners in the Spanish province during these tumultuous years stayed for only short periods of time, and official letters describing the wretched health of local inhabitants and pleading for assistance continued to flow to various authorities. In the closing days of Spanish rule, Governor Don Antonio Cordero issued orders to citizens at San Antonio concerning general sanitary measures and Don Jose Joaquin Villaverde accepted a contract from the city to serve as physician for the community, but conditions remained largely unchanged.

"Health and Medicine," New Handbook of Texas;
Richardson, 36.

The next stimulus for medical change would come from a series of political events. Doctors might have reached the Texas frontier more swiftly had the Spanish empire builders succeeded, but by 1810 Spain's efforts had failed. As Spanish power declined, numbers of English, German and other European settlers largely from states in the American South began to filter in from the north and settle in the region. Spanish authorities, recognizing that their carefully planned mission-presidio system had failed to create settlements, now realized that Americans were willing to become Spanish citizens in exchange for the right to settle in New Spain. What they did not know was that when the Spanish government opened lands in the northern borderlands to Anglo-American (non-Hispanic and non Native-American) settlers, a more lasting medical influence would at last enter the region.

Richardson, 53-69

First among Anglo "*empresarios*" or Spanish government representatives who obtained permission to organize settlements of American colonists in Texas was Moses Austin, a Missouri businessman seeking to revive his floundering fortunes. Austin was successful in negotiating with the Mexican officials, and in 1820 received a petition to settle three hundred families on 200,000 acres between the Brazos and Colorado Rivers. Unfortunately, the entrepreneur died before he could organize the colony that bore his name. Rather, it was his twenty-eight-year-old son, Stephen F. Austin, who took responsibility for the empresario contract, gathered a group of Americans looking for a place to make a fresh start, and led them in December 1821 from New Orleans into Texas to fulfill his father's ambitions. The younger Austin had been living at New Orleans and studying law with a former U.S. Congressman and member of the Kentucky legislature, and had qualities that made him a natural leader for the settlers.

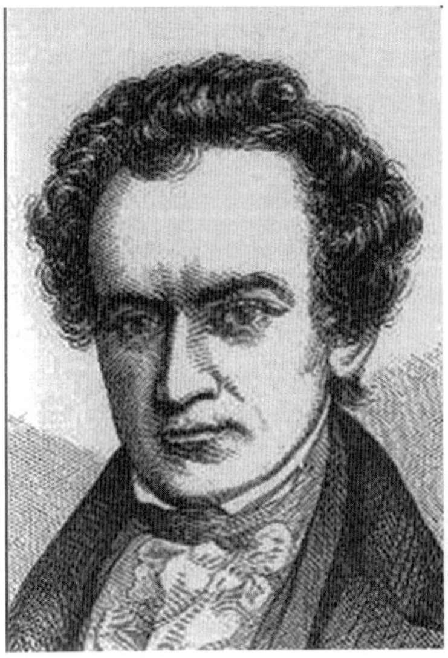
Stephen Fuller Austin, following his father´s initiative, introduced the first Anglos to South Texas, including the first physicians.

"Moses Austin," and "Stephen F. Austin," New Handbook of Texas.

Under Stephen F. Austin's direction, the Austin Colony introduced the first Anglos to successfully establish a permanent settlement in South Texas. By the time these colonists set out, however, a new and independent Mexico had emerged from the Spanish enterprise. Hardship and discontent had slowly generated a spirit of revolution against Spanish rule, and eleven years after the death of the patriot Father Hidalgo the Mexican people overthrew their conquerors and established a new government in Mexico City. Among its first official acts, the new Mexican government adopted Spain's land policy to make up for Mexican manpower and resources depleted by years of conflict, thereby allowing Austin the opportunity to carry out his plan. Mexican officials adopted the policy of awarding land grants to non-Spanish settlers to populate the region and farm the fertile river valleys of the Coastal Plain. Henceforth, control of the region would be enjoyed by people whose heritage and tradition replaced that of Spain with closer ties to emerging medical centers in England, Germany, and Vienna.

Nixon, Medical Story, 68, 146-7;
"Health and Medicine," New Handbook of Texas;
Red, 26-33

At least one physician accompanied the "*Old Three Hundred*," as members of the Austin Colony came to be known in Texas history, and other doctors swiftly found their way to its principal town, San Felipe de Austin, and other parts of the region. By 1830 the Austin settlement had at least three doctors—Dr. Francis F. Wells, Dr. James B. Miller, and Dr. Robert Peebles—in addition to women who served as midwives and the wives of plantation owners who provided medical care for slaves. Austin Colony surveyor Reuben Hornsby, whose job was to measure out land grants, later founded a dynasty of ophthalmologists through his descendants in the Mims family at San Antonio. By 1832, moreover, the Austin colonists created San Antonio's second Board of Health, largely to deal with epidemics.

Dr. James Mims Interview; Nixon, Medical Story of Early Texas, 146-7, 153-9

Because most settlers had little dispensable income, full-time physicians in the early Texas colonies found it necessary to farm or engage in trade or merchandising to supplement their incomes. Dr. Robert Peebles helped to place the medical profession in the Austin colony on a sound footing when he was appointed to a Board of Physicians there with authority to "*examine the qualifications of those persons who may wish to practice, and to issue to them the corresponding certificate of examination*." Given the difficulty of establishing a successful medical practice, however, he also trafficked in lucrative land speculations as the colony's land commissioner while practicing medicine. While his interest in improving medical standards won him some public appreciation, Dr. Peebles' dabbling in land transactions was not held in high esteem by his fellow Texans. He eventually fell from favor when one questionable deal awarded him and two copartners with a 400-league land grant, or an area roughly twice the size of Rhode Island.

Nixon, Medical Man in Texas; Barker, Eugene C., 302;
Wharton, Clarence R., 117;
Ferris and Hoppe, 192

By the 1830s, the Austin and its surrounding colonies flourished, doctors practiced, and basic health and medical regulations had been established. Progress was made, but conditions in South Texas contrasted sharply with those in Europe. European influence in creating specialized medical facilities, new forms of medical training, and the first specialists was a product of the same period, and patterns established in ophthalmology there soon would be followed a half a world away.

## VIENNA AND THE BEGINNINGS OF OPHTHALMOLOGY

While Texas temporarily remained on the edge of civilization, physicians in European cities were in the process of developing the paradigms and prototypes needed to create permanent medical institutions, professional medical practice, research and training programs, and professional societies to organize the control of medical practice. Austrian doctors invented the idea of medical specialization, and German and English physicians set up medical standards powerful enough to influence medicine the world over. By the 1830s, European doctors developed a new type of medical practice grounded in science that allowed them to end the use of techniques employed since the Middle Ages and stop the scourge of epidemics that regularly assaulted the great cities. The importance of these changes for Texas was that the distance between Europe and the frontier ultimately proved to be insignificant. The first Anglo colonies in Texas and the birth of ophthalmology in Europe nearly coincided, with the result that the practice of specialized medicine took only a generation to reach the frontier.

History shows that the organization of European hospitals and ophthalmic institutions preceded the appearance of actual ophthalmologists by several decades. In the early nineteenth century as South Texas struggled under the declining power of Spanish rule, European doctors established the first medical institutions dedicated to the treatment of particular types of disease or injury. The idea of hospitals limited in this way first appeared in 1805 in England after the population, and especially English soldiers, experienced an epidemic of purulent ophthalmia. Dr. John Cunningham Saunders, an English surgeon, responded to the event by introducing the "concept of a special ophthalmic hospital" in the form of the London Eye Infirmary for Curing Diseases of the Eye and Ear, an institution that two years later limited its work to ophthalmology and took the name of the Royal London Ophthalmic Hospital. Eventually, this hospital became the site of a school of ophthalmology known as Moorfields Hospital and went on to influence the field for generations.

Lesky, 33, 39; Chance, 152-53

For most of the nineteenth century, however, Vienna was Europe's most advanced cultural, scientific, and medical center. Before the rise of either Paris or London, the Austrian capital at the center of the Habsburg Empire was the intellectual and social capital of the world and a place where people congregated who excelled in almost every field. One writer saw the Vienna rebuilt by Francis Joseph between 1858 and 1888 as symbolized by her sixty-foot-wide, tree-lined Ringstrasse boulevard and monumental Imperial Palace, opera, theater, and museums and "*synonymous with Strauss waltzes, charming cafes, tantalizing pastries, and a certain carefree, all-embracing hedonism.*" In these years, Vienna became a gathering place for leaders in science, music, the arts and literature, including Sigmund Freud, musicians Gustav Mahler and Anton Bruckner, writer Karl Kraus, and modernist architect Adolf Loos. Austria's principal university as well as its creative circles made the city a "*matrix of cultural creation*" with a "*supranational, cosmopolitan consciousness.*" As one scholar put it, "*any of the city's cultural leaders could make the acquaintance of any other without difficulty.*" According to historian Victor Lesky, the Viennese metropolis also became the "*place to which the sick flocked from everywhere*;" by the turn of the century, "*Vienna was the medical center of the world.*"

Janik, Allan and Stephen Toulmin, 18, 33-35, 41

The medical paradigms that emerged in Vienna made clear the importance of both population density and high levels of professional development. Large cities were long known as "*devourers of population,*" especially children and the poor who congregated in the great cities of Europe. The necessity to stabilize the growing population in major cities such as Vienna required public health efforts and a high level of medical organization possible only in permanent medical institutions. Urban living fostered health problems of all kinds, including many that affected the eyes, and cities were the only places with a large enough number of cases to allow physicians to concentrate on and describe specific types of diseases. As Dr. Edward Reynolds of the Massachusetts Eye and Ear Infirmary wrote: "*Whoever would study the diseases of the eyes, must pass by the houses of the affluent, and enter those of the poor.*" "*A large proportion of all the accidents to which the eye is liable, is to be found, not in the office of the professional man, or the counting house of the merchant, but in the workshop of the poor but industrious mechanic.*" In other words, large cities with hospitals where doctors might observe eye disease and injury among the poor offered conditions roughly equivalent to those found in a modern research laboratory.

Lesky, 59

In caring for injuries and eye diseases, Austrian physicians enjoyed the first medical institution that fostered the creation of a tradition of research and introduced professional standards. In 1812 the Emperor of Austria established the first department of its kind to restrict its activity entirely to medical treatment of the eyes at the General Hospital of Vienna by special decree. This act alone marked the beginning of ophthalmology as an independent scientific specialty, but the Viennese reinforced the distinction by creating the world's first chair and clinic dedicated solely to ophthalmology as well. Because of these events, specialized medicine radiated outward from a Viennese hub. Here, for the first time, doctors demonstrated to the

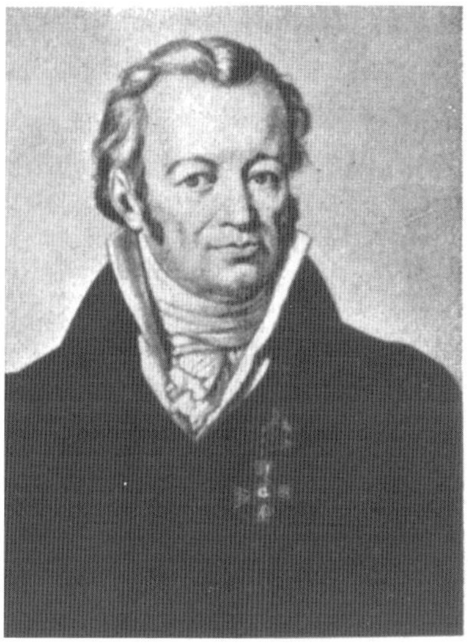

G. Joseph Beer, early chief at Vienna, who taught many "giants" in ophthalmology, including Carl Ferdinand von Graefe

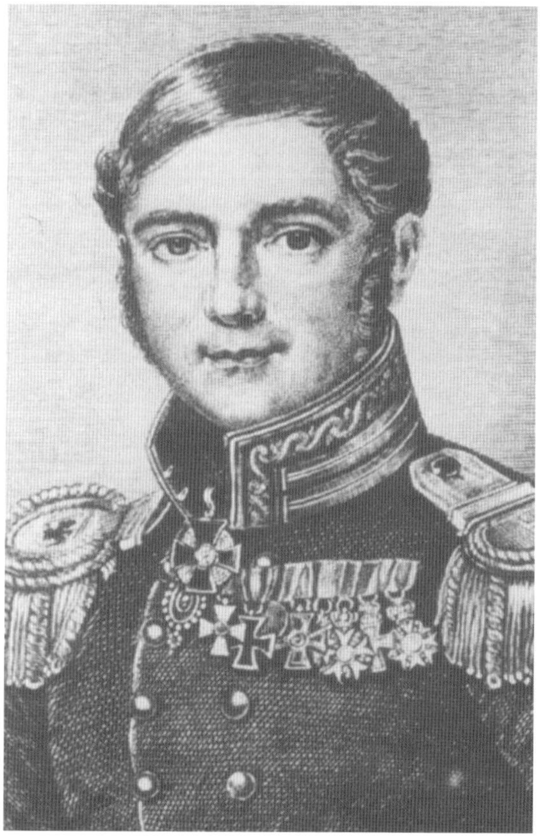

Carl Ferdinand von Graefe (1787-1840), father of Albrecht von Graefe, both of whom taught many Americans traveling to Europe for their ophthalmic education.
*(Hirscberg, History of Ophthalmology, vol.5)*

profession the value of medical practice limited to a particular part of the body. The existence of multiple hospitals, including some dedicated entirely to the eyes, also created the medical infrastructure needed to generate a new type of medical training.

Janik and Toulmin, 81

Before medical schools offered internship and residency programs, European physicians relied on "*preceptorships*" to train new members of their profession. In this system, doctors drew on a practice common to the trades and one of the earliest forms of educational training. Preceptorships were a variation on an idea used by trade guilds in the Middle Ages to teach young men a craft by having them serve as apprentices to the masters of a guild. This simple method conveyed a master craftsman's skills by the process of "*learning on the job*" or "*learning by doing*," and gave novices experience in a controlled setting. The apprenticeship system also allowed the profession to regulate the number of its practitioners. Young boys developed from apprentice to journeyman to master by exchanging, usually in a family context, labor and effort for training and care.

Medical preceptorships, like apprenticeships, helped physicians to establish their authority and extend their influence. A preceptorship achieved the equivalent of integration in a business enterprise by expanding a doctor's influence in one direction to shape the knowledge of his profession and in another direction to shape the experience of the next generation. Medical students typically obtained formal permission to work with a preceptor to gain hands-on experience in a one-to-one learning situation. Aspiring young doctors changed bandages, kept records, and swept out the office of their mentors and teachers. Unfortunately, as many of them discovered, no standard requirements existed either for their training or for entering the profession. As a consequence, the quality of medical education varied drastically; some doctors were well-trained, but others were exploited to do the labor the physician chose not to do himself with no chance to perform operations or acquire necessary skills. The first preceptorships in the United States typically included two segments of two or three years during which the young man "*read medicine*" and worked as an assistant to his mentor.

Ferris and Hoppe, 35; Nixon, Medical Story, 280

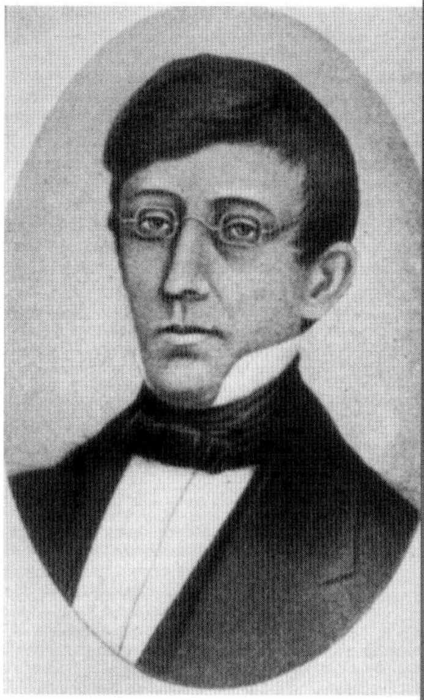

Georg Frick (1793-1870)
The first American ophthalmologist to study in Vienna under G.Joseph Beer and the first American to write a textbook in ophthalmology.

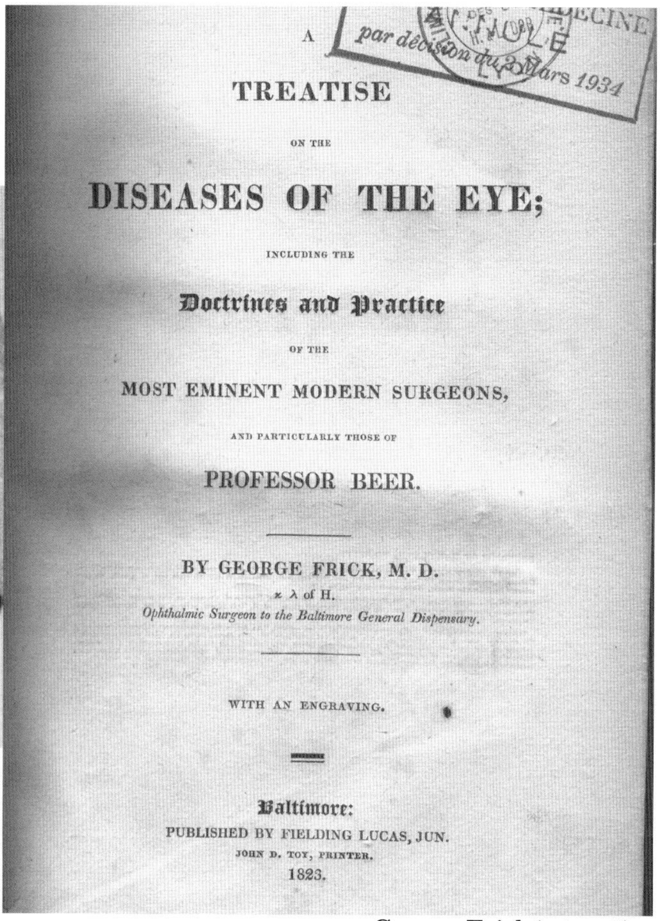

A
TREATISE
ON THE
DISEASES OF THE EYE;
INCLUDING THE
Doctrines and Practice
OF THE
MOST EMINENT MODERN SURGEONS,
AND PARTICULARLY THOSE OF
PROFESSOR BEER.

BY GEORGE FRICK, M. D.
Ophthalmic Surgeon to the Baltimore General Dispensary.

WITH AN ENGRAVING.

Baltimore:
PUBLISHED BY FIELDING LUCAS, JUN.
JOHN D. TOY, PRINTER.
1823.

George Frick´s treatise
(Wayenborgh Collection)

Ophthalmologists in the Vienna Eye Department achieved another innovation by organizing the first classes to replace the preceptorship with formal training plus an equivalent of grand rounds. Describing the famous classes of Dr. Ferdinand Arlt at the new eye clinic, an observer said, "*Outpatients came to the lecture hall. . . . where the teacher sat on a three-legged stool surrounded by 100 students and a mass of patients. The diseased eye itself provided the direct means whereby Arlt taught the beginner what to observe and how to diagnose.*" One of Director and Professor Extraordinary George Joseph Beer's early students was Carl Ferdinand von Graefe, one of the most important contributors to the emerging specialty field of ophthalmology. At institutions where specialists could congregate and learn, a generation of Viennese medical giants was soon training physicians from all countries, including the United States.

Janik and Toulmin, 81, 96;
Chance, 59

Although another half century would pass before these important medical developments reached Texas, cultural transfer of European advances to the United States took less than a generation. Americans had maintained their contact with European centers of learning despite the distancing of the American Revolution, and now, hearing of advances in Vienna, a few courageous American physicians decided to complete their medical training by going abroad. While Spain still controlled South Texas, two graduates of the New York College of Physicians and Surgeons went to Europe in 1816 to "*improve themselves in the knowledge of the profession of their choice*." The highlight of their program was their study of the "*nature and treatment of eye diseases*" at the London Eye Infirmary founded by John Saunders. Dr. George Frick received his medical license in 1811 and became the first American in 1817 to study in Vienna, where he heard lectures, studied eye diseases, and attended clinics given by George Beer. American physicians also swiftly adapted European ideas and began to improvise on them to fit the needs of their patients at home. Frick established an American tradition of medical training until World War II, and not only became an ophthalmologist but later wrote the first American text on ophthalmology

Scheie and Albert;
Bonner, 67-75;
Rosen, 33;
Chance, 60

Another famous early American physician, Philadelphia's Dr. Samuel David Gross (1805-1886) who appears in Eastman's famous painting entitled the "*Gross Clinic*" standing at an operating table in a surgical amphitheater surrounded by a cluster of doctors, also employed a style of educational training and demonstration he had learned from European ophthalmologists. Although the painting is most often cited in connection with the history of American art, it also represents a significant moment in American ophthalmological history. Gross wrote his doctoral thesis on the nature and treatment of cataract and went on to practice ophthalmology. In 1842 he published an article on the operation for strabismus in the Western Journal of Medicine and Surgery and in 1857 he served as a delegate to the First International Congress of Ophthalmology in Brussels.

Chance, Burton, 81-83.

Although it took three and a half days to reach Philadelphia from Houston until the late nineteenth century, Americans established several medical institutions specializing in eye care before 1830. American cities, and particularly those in contact with Europe, were key to the growth of ophthalmology. Dr. Elisha North set up the New London Eye Infirmary in 1817 in Connecticut, and a few pioneering and path-breaking American eye infirmaries opened in the early 1800s in other major cities. North's Infirmary ceased to operate around 1830 and exerted little influence on the development of ophthalmology, but holds the distinction of being the first such institution and further proof that the appearance of specialized hospitals historically preceded that of specialists.

Vail, 13-17;
Silverthorne, 183-4;
Rosen, 33

In keeping with the idea that concentrations of population were important to the rise of specialized medicine—first discussed in Rosen's 1939 study claiming that a population of at least 25,000 was necessary to support specialization—other ophthalmic hospitals and dispensaries grew up in the 1820s and 1830s at Philadelphia, Boston, and Baltimore, where larger numbers of people had the economic means necessary to pay for specialized medicine. The largest nineteenth-century American metropolis, New York City, gained its first permanent eye disease hospital, the New York Eye and Ear Infirmary, in 1820 on its way to achieving a population of over 300,000 people in 1840. Intended to serve the poor who suffered from eye diseases, this institution was founded by two physicians trained at the London Eye Infirmary who obviously found a model for their institution overseas. European innovations in medical education were added to the American medical agenda when the New York Eye and Ear Infirmary began training the first American ophthalmologists. The successful New York experiment also gave rise to the Massachusetts Eye and Ear Infirmary in Boston. Acknowledging that the idea behind this institution ran back all the way to Vienna, co-founder Dr. Edward Reynolds said, "*As the London Eye Infirmary owes its origin to the Institution at Vienna, so the Massachusetts Infirmary, where we are this day assembled, must claim its parentage from that.*" Later, Reynolds became a prime mover in creating the American Ophthalmological Society, the first professional medical organization of its kind in the United States.

Albert and Scheie, 34-5, 46, 52;
Rosen, 33;
Vail, 13-17.

European ideas took longer to arrive in states west of the Atlantic Seaboard, but were felt in a remarkably short time. After visiting the Pennsylvania Infirmary in mid-1820s, Daniel Drake of Kentucky and Ohio founded the Cincinnati Eye Infirmary that lasted from 1827 to 1839. Although differences between medicine in Vienna, the eastern United States, and Texas remained extreme, however, Texas medicine in a few decades would catch up and begin to overtake its counterparts to the east. The first wave of cultural transfer had begun when the first American doctors went abroad for training. A similar vehicle would accomplish the transfer of medical specialization from Europe to Anglo settlements in the former Spanish Southwest. It was only a matter of time.

(Albert and Scheie, 34-5, 46, 52).

## CHAPTER 3

# ANGLO DOCTORS AND THE ROLE OF THE MILITARY, 1810-1850

*But the bravest are surely those who have the clearest vision of what is before them, glory and danger alike, and yet notwithstanding go out to meet it.*

Thucydides, Funeral Oration of Pericles

If partly influenced by events in Europe, the origins of ophthalmology in South Texas were also a product of links between medical and military efforts going back to the days of the Texas Republic. Military-medical associations have been important in South Texas since troops first came into the region to secure the frontier for settlement. Conflict created the Republic of Texas, and a military presence was needed to sustain the state of Texas even after settlers voted to annex themselves to the United States. In fact, so strong were military-medical connections that they constitute one of the distinctive features of the region's medical history. Civilian medical institutions, professional medical organizations, and eventually the first residency training programs grew up in close proximity to, and strongly influenced by, their military counterparts. Remarkably, military activity also sparked changes that accelerated the cultural transfer of specialized medicine to the frontier.

Positive links between medicine and warfare go back to the ancient Greek word for physician, "Iatro's," that refers to both a healer and an "extractor of arrows." Texas medical historian Pat Ireland Nixon acknowledged the necessary relationship between medical and military professionals as follows:

> *A soldier fights his fellow man and hastens death; a doctor fights disease and delays death.*
> *A soldier fights for the extension of national boundaries;*
> *a doctor recognizes no national boundaries;*
> *The world long exalts the soldier; it soon forgets the doctor.*
>
> Nixon, Century of Medicine, viii, 12

The historical relationship between war and medicine, however, is even more complex. Despite their seemingly different objectives, doctors who support military efforts often produce significant advances in promoting human health. War employs healers to relieve the suffering of the sick and injured, but military doctors in the process often learn as they bandage wounds, amputate damaged limbs, and administer everything from opium to ipecac to relieve fever and pain to produce new knowledge, promote longevity, and preserve life. Because they must work outside organized hospital settings, military doctors often have been forced to invent innovative treatments and practices. South Texas military operations that established links between military and civilian medicine also stimulated medical developments, including the creation of the foundation for a tradition of research. At the same time, war brought into the region doctors trained at some of the world's finest medical centers. P.I. Nixon said it best. "From the time...when there was a small government hospital on Houston Street...there has been an intimate relationship between the medical profession of San Antonio and army surgeons at Fort Sam Houston and outlying posts." The presence of military doctors goes back to at least 1805, when the Spanish Governor, Manuel Antonio Cordero y Bustamante, designated that a room in the San Antonio de Valero mission be used as a military infirmary.

Naythons, Introduction; Nixon, Century of Medicine in San Antonio, 203, 311-12; McBride, 1; Nixon, Medical Story, 121, 125; "Health and Medicine," New Handbook of Texas

## EVENTS LEADING UP TO THE TEXAS REVOLUTION

Geography made South Texas a site of repeated military conflict and a place where military doctors were needed almost from the moment when outsiders first ventured into the region. While the Spanish pursued their imperial interests, the Rio Grande River that runs today between the United States and Mexico formed a natural boundary that left the Rio Grande Valley a no man's land to which no nation held certain claim. The borderland was a tinderbox where numerous disputes among foreign governments erupted over rights to the land. Soldiers who accompanied the Franciscan friars setting up missions along the San Antonio River were only the first to pursue some sort of military activity in South Texas, and "*doctor-soldiers*," or military surgeons, were stationed with coastal garrisons prior to the arrival of the first settlers.

"Health and Medicine," New Handbook of Texas;
Dunlop, 54, 70-88;
Nixon, Century of Medicine, 8, 87-88, 311.

Beginning in 1810—over ten years before the first Anglo colonists set out for the region with Stephen F. Austin—hostilities developed in New Spain (as the Spanish settlements in Texas were called) leading up to Mexico's revolt against the Spanish government. A volatile political situation gripped the country, and the growing political instability of Spanish rule in Mexico caused France, the United States, and other European countries to consider the possibility of establishing an interest in the territory. Among Americans who first came to vie for dominance in the region was a physician, Dr. James Long, who led a filibustering expedition to overthrow the Spanish and create "*a free and independent republic*" for Anglo settlers in Texas. Although Long's efforts failed, his wife Jane came to be known as the "*Mother of Texas*" for spending a harsh and lonely winter at Bolivar Point on the Gulf Coast awaiting her husband's return. After his death, Jane Long supported early Texas leaders in the fight for freedom for the rest of her life. Mexico achieved her independence from Spain in 1821 after ten years of struggle, but the ascendant nation suffered from depleted resources and a population devastated by the conflict. Change in the government at Mexico City brought meager relief from the problems that plagued the northern borderlands under Spanish control, including their lack of qualified medical practitioners. Mexican political instability further exacerbated these problems, and prevented all but a handful of doctors from reaching the old Spanish settlements.

Dunlop, 54, 70-88;
Nixon, Medical Story, 80-90, 114-6, 142;
Red, 12-25;
"Dr. James Long," New Handbook of Texas;
Nixon, Century of Medicine, 8, 87, 88, 311

Only six months after declaring its independence from Spain, the Mexican government declared Don Jose Joaquin Villaverde's credentials inadequate and nullified his appointment as San Antonio city physician, leaving the region once more without the benefit of a practitioner to care for friends and families when illness or injury struck. As the Anglo colonies expanded, San Antonio retained its Hispanic population but went through successive phases of ruin and revival, beginning with a devastating flood in 1819 that floated a good bit of the village into the river that bears its name. Mexican independence temporarily improved the city's fortunes, but various parties in the contest for freedom who sought refuge in the outpost made it a hotbed of intrigue and conspiracy and, in subsequent years, Mexican Revolutionary and Spanish Royal forces alternately attacked and occupied the community.

"Health and Medicine," New Handbook of Texas

Although a new Mexican governor, Colonel Jose Felix Trespalacious, marched into San Antonio's Military Plaza in 1822 to visit the capital city of the province, Mexico needed to consolidate its power to build its strength and the town's days as a capital city were numbered. The memory of years of Spanish and Mexican rule lingers today in San Antonio's almost two-hundred-and-fifty-year-old Spanish Governor's Palace, but the occasions on which the governor and his lady presented visiting officials with delightful entertainments and gracious hospitality were over. With the adoption of the Mexican Constitution of 1824, the provinces of Coahuila and Texas were combined into a single political unit and officials transferred governmental functions at San Antonio to Saltillo.

"San Antonio," New Handbook of Texas.

Almost 5,000 people had lived on the Spanish frontier in 1800 and almost 9,000 people resided there in 1834, but as late as 1828 no hospital existed in San Antonio or the surrounding countryside. If the comings and goings of explosive factions discouraged political stability, medical stability suffered from droughts, epidemics, Native-American raids, and a shortage of doctors despite the fact that the Mexican government regulated the practice of medicine in both San Antonio and the Anglo colonies. Minutes of the municipality or ayuntamiento of San Felipe de Austin from 1828 to 1832 show that physicians and apothecaries were required to present a diploma or certificate from some scientific authority in order to exercise their professions. Other records show that a petition was presented to the court in the municipality of Nacogdoches in 1835 asking that a law to regulate the practice of medicine be enacted there. Nonetheless, many settlers died with every outbreak of disease from 1821 to 1836. A particularly devastating outbreak of cholera afflicted San Antonio in 1834 and proud braves raided the community almost at will, riding their mounts insolently through the streets wearing their victim's clothing.

Nixon, Medical Story

While the region remained under the Mexican flag, conditions changed only when waves of Anglo newcomers arrived who made San Antonio's ancient plazas teem again. Despite frontier conditions, tough-minded pioneers following in the footsteps of the Austin colonists left their pasts behind and laid claim to their future with the abrupt announcement "*G.T.T.*" or "*Gone to Texas!*" Americans in a position to answer Mexico's need for manpower took advantage of her liberal land policies and flooded into the region, bringing with them a number of doctors willing to join their enterprise. Soon, activity bustled along the streets as Mexican settlers and the new immigrants passed through on their way to land where they hoped to establish farms or ranches. The San Antonio population once again climbed to over two thousand residents—the number Lt. Zebulon Pike had reported 28 years earlier on his visit to the community—and the stable conditions translated into substantial housing improvements that made stone and adobe residences increasingly more common.

Nixon, Medical Story

Many of the first "Anglo" physicians who brought the arts of healing into the region spent part of their time as military surgeons, and most of the handful of general practitioners who came as settlers soon found themselves involved as either surgeons, soldiers, or soldiers of fortune in ensuing conflicts. For years, every settler served a quasi-military and quasi-medical role to protect and heal as the need arose. At least one doctor was among the empresarios who founded colonies along the South Texas river valleys. Dr. John Cameron, who had become a Mexican citizen to obtain his empresario contract, established one such settlement in 1827. By the 1830s, so successful were the Anglo settlements that the colonists began to entertain the thought of separating from the Mexican government. Five years later, the physicians among them would serve with distinction as soldiers, civic leaders, and statesmen when the colonies decided to relinquish their affiliation with their Mexican hosts and create a republic of their own.

"Zebulon Pike," "San Antonio,""Austin Colony," New Handbook of Texas;
Richardson, 80-98;
Ross, 70-75

Separate interests placed the emerging Mexican government and the Anglo colonies on a collision course, but the catalyst for military action was brewed in the Mexican capital. As Mexican leaders struggled to set up a working government after 1821, the country endured severe political convulsions under the administrations of eleven different presidents. Such a vacuum of leadership had been created by 1835 that shifting political developments in Mexico City enabled a ruthless man, General Antonio Lopez de Santa Anna, to fulfill the ambitions he had developed as a Mexican soldier and become a self-proclaimed dictator who publicly referred to himself as the "*Napoleon of the West*." Elected President in 1833, the opportunist destroyed the federal system of government by issuing the Seven Laws Act that effectively invalidated the country's liberal Constitution of 1824, an act set in motion events leading to the revolutionary battle that made San Antonio a name known around the world. As reports of Santa Anna's preemptory decisions filtered into Texas, respect for Mexican authority rapidly deteriorated among the Anglo colonists and their feelings of betrayal exploded into a torch for liberty known as the Texas Revolution.

Richardson, 498-125;
"Antonio Lopez de Santa Anna," New Handbook of Texas.

## THE TEXAS REVOLUTION

By the fall of 1835, Anglo colonists and others who had settled in Mexican municipalities along the Gulf Coast braced for conflict. Stephen F. Austin's efforts to negotiate autonomy on behalf of the colonies failed, and the Mexican government now saw the settlements as more American than Spanish and a potential threat to Mexican sovereignty. As tensions mounted, General Martin Perfecto de Cos, a brother-in-law of Santa Anna who commanded twelve hundred Mexican soldiers in the region, was sent to fortify San Antonio and put down the rebels. Because San Antonio still constituted the heart of Mexican Texas, a segment of her population welcomed the presence of official Mexico. While some of the town's Anglo population fled, however, a number joined gatherings of volunteer troops that met in the ruins of the ancient Spanish missions on the outskirts of the town to form the beginnings of a military force for the settlers.

Nixon, Medical Story, 176-78; Richardson, 98-125.

In the ensuing months, these colonists began to think of themselves as a Texan or "*Texian*" army. Ignoring orders to retreat to Gonzales where a skirmish over the surrender of a cannon further incited them to war, men in the new army prepared to fight for their homes. When the firebrand, Ben Milam, called them to action, this small military force launched an early morning assault on General Cos at San Antonio on December 5, 1835. A street-by-street, house-to-house, hot and bloody battle began that ended five days later when Cos surrendered what was left of his army and signed articles of capitulation, leaving much of the town in shambles. The incident precipitated a more substantial reply, however, when news of the defeat reached the Mexican interior.

Richardson, 98-125.

Although those remaining in San Antonio quickly went to work to overcome hardships left by the battle, the relative period of calm they would enjoy was shortlived. Enraged by his loss of the town, Santa Anna decided to avenge the personal disgrace he had sustained in his brother-in-law's failure. Disregarding winter weather that meant a lack of forage for his animals and extreme conditions for

Mexican troops, the dictator decided to push north immediately to confront the rebellious settlers. Mexican loyalists in San Antonio remained on hand to herald the general's arrival in the Main Plaza a few weeks later, but news of Santa Anna's approach only strengthened the resolve of others to resist the Mexican forces.

Richardson, 98-125; "Texas Revolution," New Handbook of Texas.

On March 1, 1836, at a convention held at Washington-on-the-Brazos, seven physicians signed the Texas Declaration of Independence in recognition that ties with Mexico had been broken. Soon thereafter, as Santa Anna approached, a group of Texas patriots and the families of local soldiers took refuge in the ruins of the San Antonio mission that had come to be known as the Alamo. The volunteer army now included reinforcements who had arrived since word of the December victory reached the United States, including David Crockett and his band of volunteers from Tennessee. For thirteen days, Santa Anna held court on the Plaza while his cannon held the mission-turned-fort under siege. His final charge swept over the stone walls in the cloudy mist of dawn on March 6, accompanied by the Mexican band playing the "*Deguello*"—a traditional Spanish song of "*no quarter.*" When it was over, every Texas defender lay dead and San Antonio had been reduced to a dismally subdued village.

"Battle of the Alamo," New Handbook of Texas.

No organized medical support was made available to the men who fought at the Alamo, but a number of physicians were caught up in the fervor to create an autonomous Texas and took part in battles of the Texas Revolution as both soldiers and physicians. Six doctors, including John Hubbard Forsyth, William D. Howell, Edward F. Mitchusson, John Purdy Reynolds, John W. Thomson, and the surgeon-in-charge, Amos Pollard, were among the over one hundred eighty men who died during the chilly, pre-dawn Mexican attack on the Alamo. Joseph H. Barnard later estimated that more than 500 Mexican soldiers required treatment after the battle, but found that disgracefully poor medical care was provided for the Mexican wounded. Aid came two weeks later only after more than four hundred Texans were taken prisoner at Goliad—a town whose name was an anagram of "Hidalgo" (the priest who led the Mexican revolt against Spain)—and then savagely massacred on Palm Sunday, March 27.

Eight Texan surgeons who participated in the Goliad campaign were spared the slaughter there to return and care for wounded Mexican soldiers who remained at the Alamo. Their written accounts are the source from which much of the horror of the battle has come to be known. According to accounts of two of these physicians, Drs. John Shackelford and Joseph H. Barnard, who described the ghastly medical conditions they found in San Antonio, almost every man was still carrying the lead he had received the morning of the assault. Surprisingly, the two doctors recorded that they were shown respect and courtesy from both the townspeople and the Mexican officers and soldiers. In addition to caring for the Mexican soldiers, they also treated civilians.

"Battle of the Alamo," New Handbook of Texas"."Texas Revolution,"
New Handbook of Texas;
Richardson, 98-125.

For the surviving ragtag citizen-soldiers of General Sam Houston's army who now identified themselves with Texas as they went to face the Mexican forces, the terrible accounts of crushing defeat at Goliad and San Antonio determined their will in the final encounter of the Texas Revolution on a flat plain near the San Jacinto River. Sam Houston's decision to attack on a quiet Sunday afternoon while Santa Anna and his troops were at siesta enabled the Texans to rout the Mexican army in a fight that lasted only eighteen minutes. Thereafter, all ties to Mexico officially were broken on April 21, 1836, when a new and separate nation known as the Republic of Texas became a reality. Remarkably, as the smoke cleared, doctors treating the Texans at San Jacinto discovered only twenty-three wounded. Among them, Sam Houston, whose right leg had been fractured by a gunshot, was treated by Dr. Alexander W. Ewing. Sixteen surgeons were on hand to treat the survivors of the historic event, and only one of their number, Dr. Junius William Mottley, died of his wounds.

"Health and Medicine, Handbook of Texas.

## THE REPUBLIC OF TEXAS, 1836-1846

During the ten arduous years during which the Republic of Texas endured, a majority of the Lone Star population and most of its practicing physicians remained concentrated in what today constitutes northern and eastern parts of the state. In 1839, however, officials established the capital of the Republic at Austin on what was then the vulnerable edge of the western frontier, a point on the upper banks of the Colorado River close to the center of today's Texas. According to several disgruntled Congressmen, irritated with the Austin location, it was a place where "*Indians stalked through the streets with impunity and a fellow could easily get knocked over and lose his hair!*" The fact that Great Britain, Belgium, France, Holland and the United States officially recognized the new Republic of Texas suggests that a powerful new nation had emerged, but in reality the Lone Star Republic was still a group of scattered settlements along the frontier. The entire Republic had a population of less than forty-thousand non-Native American people when independence was declared. Due to these precarious beginnings, Texans would forever take pride in the idea that their military prowess that had prevailed against all odds.

Richardson, 125-50.

Residents and officials of the new Republic of Texas soon realized that their survival was not yet assured and that military support would continue to be needed. Cotton planters who had come from Southern States and settled along the parallel river valleys that ran into the Gulf of Mexico remained dependent in colonial fashion on goods manufactured in the Northeast. Many other settlers lived at subsistence levels. Facing the need to increase the population and strengthen the new Republic, the Lone Star government decided to stimulate immigration by adopting the Mexican empresario, or contractor system and passing a Headright Ordinance. Headrights, with some variations, were awards of sizeable parcels of land to those who agreed to become permanent residents. The success of cheap land in attracting desperately-needed colonists to Texas is witnessed by the fact that when the Republic joined the United States ten years later, the population had more than tripled to almost 125,000 people. From a medical standpoint, however, the vulnerable Republic's ongoing need for military readiness meant that, for many, military doctors and military forts would continue to be the sole source of medical care for years to come.

Richardson, 125-50.

Many physicians who practiced in the Republic or during the early years of statehood were men who had served in the military and who, for the most part, practiced without the benefit of professional standards, organizations, or hospitals. County and town records record the esteem in which area residents held their physicians. Hill County takes its name from Dr. George Hill, who had a medical degree and served as an official of the Lone Star Republic, and Throckmorton County from Dr. William E. Throckmorton. Jones County and the town of Anson are named for Dr. Anson Jones, and Brenham for Dr. Richard Fox Brenham. Starr County takes its name from Dr. James H. Starr, Archer County from Dr. Branch T. Archer, and Baylor County from Dr. H.W. Baylor, who participated in military battles against the Indians and served as a surgeon with the Texas Rangers in the Mexican War. Motley County shortened the name of Dr. Junius William Mottley, a post surgeon at Goliad and aide-de-camp to General Thomas J. Rusk who died in the battle of San Jacinto. Other counties named for physicians include Irion County for Dr. Robert Anderson Irion; Shackleford County for John (Jack) Shackleford, an eyewitness at the Goliad Massacre; and Zavala County for Dr. Lorenzo de Zavala, a signer of the Texas Declaration of Independence.

Ferris and Hoppe, 230-33.

To measure the level of these accomplishments it is helpful to remember that while Texas was a Republic, conditions in the United States were comparatively more advanced. The Wills Eye Hospital had been founded in Pennsylvania in 1832 along with a number of other specialized medical facilities in the eastern United States. In his book A Century of Medicine in San Antonio, Dr. Pat I. Nixon describes medicine in the Texas Republic as far more limited, yet recognizes that it was nonetheless an important achievement given conditions there:

> *The political and economic state of the republic was at all times unsettled and at certain times precarious. The ever present menace of Mexican invasion and Indian depredation kept the problem of individual and family security uppermost. In such surroundings medicine was not calculated to grow and develop, however much its devotees were addicted to the science or even to the art of medicine. For the physicians of this period to have consolidated the medical gains of the previous generation was no small accomplishment; this they did.*

Nixon, Century of Medicine, 140.

Less than ten years after the Battle of San Jacinto, newspaper reports of one sensational event prove that at least one doctor in South Texas was engaged in some sort of scientific research. When several

Native Americans died in a fight outside San Antonio in 1840, a local doctor named Weideman—who was apparently studying the human anatomy—cooked the bodies to obtain their skeletons. Reports reached the paper when residents complained of the pollution caused when the doctor flushed the remains of the victims into the local Acequia. Four years later, the Congress of the Republic in 1844 awarded a franchise to Hermann University in Houston with medicine as part of its curriculum. This institution failed due to poor economic conditions, lack of funds, Indian uprisings, and new Mexican invasion, but represents a first step in the development of medical training in the region.

Faculty and Staff, University of Texas Medical Branch, Galveston, 4.

Of greater importance in 1844 was the arrival of a Scottish physician, Dr. George Cupples, who was among the first to practice some type of specialized medicine in the struggling Republic. Dr. Cupples was not only one of Texas' most colorful practitioners, but one who had received advanced medical training before coming to the frontier. The son of a British navy surgeon, Cupples had been a staff assistant-surgeon in the Spanish service of the British auxiliary legion for two years before entering the University of Edinburgh, Scotland, where he graduated in 1838. He then studied "on specialties," a term used for training that likely included a component of ophthalmology, at several London hospitals and the University of Paris from 1839 to 1843 in order to accept an official position at a hospital in France. Instead, he came to Texas when his wife's or his wife's sister's health failed, arriving in time to serve as a surgeon in the Mexican war. In San Antonio, where he settled, Cupples went on to become one of the community's most distinguished early practitioners.

Hubbell, 144; Encyclopedia of the New West, 340

And what of San Antonio throughout these turbulent years? Creation of the Republic of Texas did little to revive the town's immediate prospects, and sadly, incidences of hostility continued. This would not be the first nor the last time the town would court destruction, and violence never seemed far away. The Mexican army had retreated across the Rio Grande River, but the border remained in contention and not all of the region's residents immediately returned to their homes. Some citizens refused to accept the Republic's authority, viewed the entire revolution as an act of treason, and followed the defeated army into Mexico. Other inhabitants did not return to their homes until the United States flag flew over Texas in 1846. Ultimately, Mexico never officially acknowledged Texas' independence and those who believed San Antonio was too close to Mexico to be truly safe, both in distance and inclination, proved to be accurate.

Richardson, 125-50;
Daughters of the Republic of Texas Archives.

In the waning days of the Republic, San Antonio heard the cadence of marching feet twice in 1842 when Mexican soldiers reoccupied the town. On these occasions as before, many citizens, but especially women and children, deserted the town ahead of the advancing armies. In the last invasion, conducted by the Mexican commander, General Woll, San Antonio was devastated once more, and much of its resources spoiled or ravaged. Fluctuations in the population uprooted any possibility of real development and the loss of resources lowered what little quality of life residents had managed to achieve. The Mexican army retreated before Texas could rally a serious defense, but a number of the Republic's captured leaders spent months languishing in Mexico's Perote Castle dungeon and this final conflict reduced the San Antonio population to around six hundred people. As a result, the town remained a Headquarters of the Military Department in Texas with three military doctors in 1845, including a Surgeon Major, a Captain who served as Assistant Surgeon, and an Acting Assistant Surgeon who offered medical service on a contract basis. In the waning days of the Republic it seemed the proud old city was just taking time to catch its breath.

"General Adrian Woll," New Handbook of Texas

## TEXAS STATEHOOD AND THE CONTINUED IMPORTANCE OF MILITARY MEDICINE

The Lone Star Republic lasted for ten years, but by 1845 Texans recognized that they were at the mercy of larger governments and could prosper best by joining forces with the United States. While Sam Houston finally won the vote that annexed Texas to the United States, it was a doctor who proclaimed that statehood had been achieved.

Among those who had served in the Texas Revolution, Dr. Anson Jones fought at the Battle of San Jacinto and then laid aside his medical practice to devote himself to appointed or elected political office. It was Jones who not only had the honor of being the last President of the Republic of Texas, but who furled the Lone Star flag on February 19, 1846, and raised the Stars and Stripes with the announcement that "*The Republic of Texas is no more.*"

Richardson, 150-75

When Texas became the twenty-eighth state in the Union, San Antonians celebrated thunderously and the clamor seemed to stir fresh breezes of hope. Conditions in the town a year later when German geologist Dr. Ferdinand Roemer visited in 1846, however, could only be described as dismal. "*The entire place gave the impression of decay*" rather than more "*brilliant days.*" Many of those who walked along the avenues no doubt would have found Dr. Roemer's comments to be a generous understatement. Once the center of Spanish Texas, San Antonio was now a nearly deserted hull, empty of all but the most resolute souls. Along with the fires that had ravished the Alamo, subsequent events had left the town in chaos and confusion. In little more than a decade after retreating Mexican troops left the town to its last six hundred residents, however, San Antonio would achieve a remarkable recovery despite its relative isolation from the rest of the United States. By 1860, the population that numbered just under 3,500 would more than double in size.

"San Antonio," New Handbook of Texas.

The new state of Texas did not enact further laws to regulate medical practice for about a quarter of a century. With no city yet large enough to support more than a few physicians or hospital facilities and most of the Anglo colonies still sparsely settled, military doctors remained a valuable asset and continued in many cases to provide the only available medical resource for soldiers and settlers alike. The first doctor at Victoria after the county was created in 1836, for example, was Dr. J.B.P. January, a Kentucky native who had been a soldier and a surgeon in the Texas Army and who would later treat soldiers in both the Mexican and Civil Wars.

Ferris and Hoppe, 191.

When Texas achieved statehood, the U.S. government took responsibility for the frontier by establishing federal troops at San Antonio and other key sites, thereby increasing the presence of military doctors. Federal military forces supported an expanding line of settlement that alternately advanced and retreated until the late nineteenth century due to ongoing Indian depredations. For years, hostile Comanches who used expert horsemanship and knowledge of the terrain continued their custom of surprise attacks on white settlements during the full moon, making South and West Texas among the last parts of the U.S. frontier to close. Some of the nation's best military men found their way to Texas in this period as a result, including West Point graduate Robert E. Lee who helped to establish fortifications against Native Americans following game across the region. In many cases, the first hospital in newly opened parts of Texas was a military post hospital. Medical reports regularly received from doctors at Fort Ewell, Fort Merrill and Ringold Barracks, Fort Brown, Fort McIntosh, Fort Belknap, Fort McKavett, Fort Worth, Camp J.E. Johnston and other posts document the beginnings of a more organized medical effort. This was true in Austin as late as 1867, where records show that a military hospital opened under an individual simply known as Dr. Kirk.

"Health and Medicine," Handbook of Texas;
Ferris and Hoppe, 181, 191;
Grimes, Roy, ed., 530

The mortality rate for soldiers who garrisoned frontier forts in Texas from 1849 to 1859 was about 3.5%. Living conditions were described as miserable, and diseases numbering as high as 66,846 cases reported among 20,393 soldiers. Soldiers consumed large amounts of alcohol and suffered from wounds and injuries causing most military forts to designate space for a hospital and require the services of a doctor. Although many military doctors and soldiers who served as lay surgeons could be only loosely called physicians, however, military medicine no doubt introduced more doctors to the region than the pioneer settlements alone could have attracted. While tending the injured and attempting to preserve soldiers' health, these men often worked as everything from chaplains and mapmakers to veterinarians and counselors. Without medical standards or institutions for support, they tended to rely on improvisation as much as accepted practice and, in most cases, practiced alone for the majority of their careers. Nonetheless, their influence constituted an important cultural force and their rich experience no doubt enabled them to produce new knowledge and considerable skill in surgical techniques depending on the amount of time they spent in practice.

"Health and Medicine," New Handbook of Texas;
Nixon, Medical Story of Texas, 388;
Ferris and Hoppe, 205.

## THE MEXICAN-AMERICAN WAR

Unfortunately, protecting the frontier was not the only military activity required after the coming of the Stars and Stripes. In 1845 military supply wagons rumbled once again into San Antonio as South Texas was caught up in efforts needed to secure the borders of the new state. After pronouncing the annexation of Texas by the United States an act of hostility, the Mexican foreign minister called for a formal declaration that led to the start of the Mexican-American War. Anticipating the conflict, troops gathered at Fort Jesup in western Louisiana for transfer by boat to Aransas Bay on the Texas coast while Mexican troops formed at Matamoros. At the same time, the U.S. Army designated the Post of San Antonio a military supply depot and refurbished the ruins of the Alamo for use as a quartermaster's depot because of its location at a strategic point along the supply line to the federal troops. A year later in 1846 the town's military role further expanded when General John Ellis Wood arrived to train 1400 volunteers to join General Taylor in Mexico at San Antonio's San Pedro Park. Henceforth, after resuming the role of military headquarters it had served as part of Spain's mission-presidio system, San Antonio would serve as a military center with military doctors a permanent feature of her identity until the present day.

McBride, 2; New Handbook of Texas

When Texas was admitted to the Union, the Vance building on Houston Street in San Antonio at the site of today's Gunter Hotel was made into quarters for the U.S. Army. Barracks extended around a quadrangle at the rear of the lot on Travis and St. Mary's Streets.

Here doctors provided services to military personnel and their families, beginning a tradition that continues today at area military installations. As war broke out with Mexico, however, other medical facilities were needed. Although no fighting took place in San Antonio itself, the city served as a base of operations from which to maneuver in the ensuing struggle and was called on to provide medical support for soldiers on the battle lines. According to one observer, "*There were large hospitals established at San Antonio as the army advanced from Puebla between August 7 and 10.*" A hospital operated at Point Isabel or Corpus Christi on the Gulf Coast and, after the Battles of Contreras and Churubusco, wounded Mexicans filled general hospitals at San Agustin and San Antonio. Although they had numbers of their own surgeons to attend them, the observer wrote, the Mexicans "*showed a decided preference for our officers.*"

Nixon, Medical Story, 387-9;
Ferris and Hoppe, 117;
U.S. Surgeon General's Office, Historical Notes Concerning the Medical Department of the U.S. Army from 1775 to 1873, 180, 189

Among San Antonio practitioners who served in the Mexican War was Dr. George Cupples, who had been in Texas only a short time before he joined Hay's second regiment of cavalry as a surgeon. Another was Dr. Thomas R. Cocke, a Kentucky native who attended the University of Virginia and received a medical degree in 1838 from Jefferson Medical College in Philadelphia. Cocke came to Texas when it achieved statehood in 1846, and established a practice at Victoria while many local homes were still made of split logs. He then practiced locally until the Mexican War when he found himself in charge of a temporary U. S. Army hospital, caring for sick and injured men from the regiments of Kentucky, Tennessee and Illinois on their way to Mexico.

Encyclopedia of the New West, n.p.

Seen in retrospect, the Mexican-American War foreshadows the mutually advantageous relationship that would develop between military and civilian medical interests in South Texas. Despite hostile forces and difficult conditions, the medical profession gradually succeeded in becoming part of frontier society. As frontier settlement progressed, physicians not only accompanied wagon trains, worked at mining camps, and tended riverboat travelers and cowboys grappling with the vastness of the continent, but supported the soldiers who protected these advances. With cattlemen, farmers and adventurers now came "*saddle-bag*" doctors who limited their equipment to what could be carried on horseback and more wealthy physicians who traveled to their patients in horse and carriage. For years, the typical medical practice made doctors itinerant, requiring long trips miles from home on horseback to reach patients. Few doctors enjoyed offices at a fixed location where they might employ the latest technology. The practice of making house calls precluded sophisticated diagnostic equipment and treatment. Physicians set up their practices, assumed roles in their communities, and responded to demands for care from both Anglos and the local Hispanic and Native-American communities where they lived. In addition to delivering babies, most of these men provided care for eye injury and disease.

Ferris and Hoppe, 81 ff, 191.

The military medical tradition established in South Texas in the days of the Texas Revolution must be considered a key force in creating a foundation for the medical profession and strengthening its influence in the region. Although the arrival of ophthalmologists awaited the closing of the frontier, some precedents needed for specialized medicine to take hold were established in a military context long before they came. Immigration, further wars, and discoveries made a world away, however, would be necessary to further transform medical practice, add a new dimension to the region's Spanish culture, and expand the progress of medicine in South Texas.

## CHAPTER 4

# URBANIZATION, IMMIGRATION, AND THE CIVIL WAR, 1846-1865

*The Hospital is the only proper College in which to rear a true disciple of Aesculapius.*

Abernethy (quoted in Osler, Aequanimitas)

*The most essential part of a student's instruction is obtained, as I believe, not in the lecture room, but at the bedside.*

Oliver Wendell Holmes, "Introductory Lecture," 1867

In the antebellum years leading up to the Civil War, San Antonio was an important stop along commercial routes that began in Mexico and stretched across South Texas to Louisiana and the north. Ten to fourteen oxen hitched to enormous wooden-wheeled carts hauling tons of freight inched their way along the Chihuahua Trail that ran through the city, making it a major crossroads for trade. Skilled teamsters drove the teams as they snaked to and from Mexico in long trains, bringing exotic goods from ports along the Gulf Coast to local store shelves and creating the vitality and cosmopolitan atmosphere that still exists in the city today. Along with immigrants from other nations and travelers stopping briefly along stage lines that carried the transcontinental mail, swarms of "Forty-Niners" also passed through San Antonio headed to the gold fields of California. Growing opportunity for new enterprise helped to boost the population and produced other changes in the town's infrastructure. In 1848 San Antonio's first newspaper, The Western Texan, linked the community to a wider world. At the same time, a new courthouse and jail on Military Plaza strengthened the law's presence and schools and churches of several denominations enriched the quality of local life and culture. Health care improved after the cholera epidemic of 1849 stimulated local interest in public health and eventually prompted the city government in 1854 to establish the office of a City Physician. Together, these events hastened the building of a community large enough to support medical specialists.

Herff, 45; Nixon, Century of Medicine, 176, 179, 184

While South Texans were occupied with these activities, however, the corresponding period in Europe saw enormous gains in medicine, and specifically in ophthalmology. It was during this period that Hermann Ludwig Ferdinand von Helmholtz (1821-1894) did the work that led to his invention of the device that enabled ophthalmologists to differentiate themselves from the rest of medicine. The ophthalmoscope, according to scholars, led to European achievements in ophthalmology between 1850 and 1870 that were "so fundamental. . . . that they electrified the world of science and revolutionized the treatment of eye diseases." In Texas, the birth of the ophthalmoscope in 1851, however, coincided with an influx of European immigrants who helped to create the urbanization necessary to set up permanent medical institutions that could support ophthalmologists and other specialists. Among those who came, German immigrant physicians such as Dr. Ferdinand Herff at San Antonio improved the level of available medical care and established the standards necessary for medical specialization to take root, while others who arrived at the ports of Galveston and Indianola formed a human conduit through which the ophthalmoscope eventually reached the frontier.

Albert and Scheie, 1-20;
Rucker, 1-5;
Nixon, Medical Story of Early Texas, 414-421

Using the yardstick proposed by scholar George Rosen that medical development required the rise of cities or, more specifically, that at least 12,000 inhabitants were needed to support medical spe-

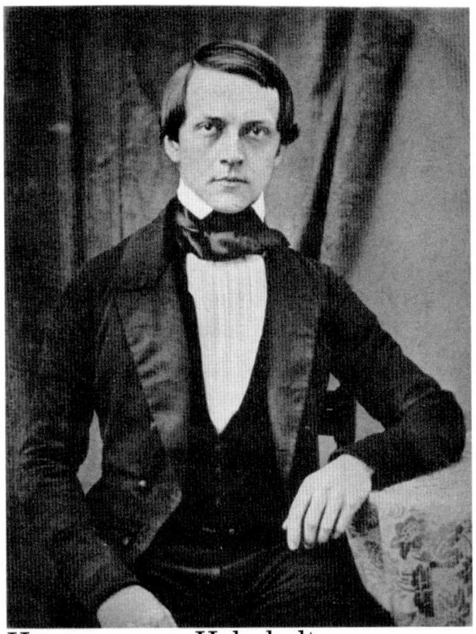

Hermann von Helmholtz
as a young man

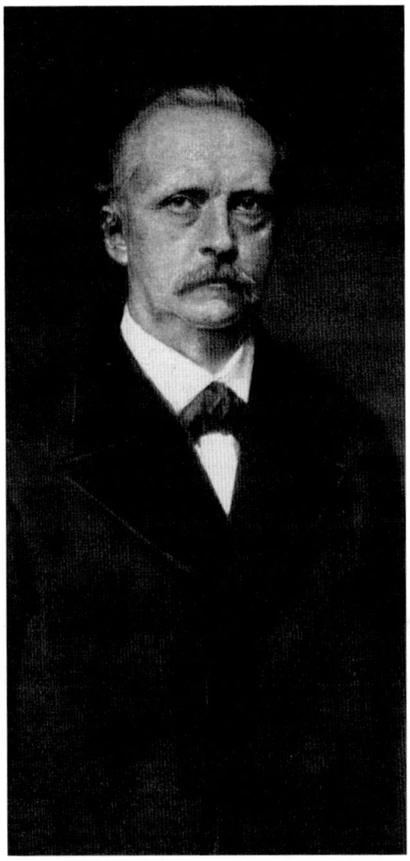

Hermann von Helmholtz
(after a portrait by
Franz von Isenbach in 1876)

cialists in individual communities, one might anticipate that ophthalmologists succeeded in South Texas only after the region attained levels of population that fit the paradigm. History shows, in fact, that permanent settlements with sizeable and stable populations were as important here as they had been in Europe and the eastern United States. The first was Galveston, whose port of entry enabled it to reach the required number of residents and to become the region's first important medical center and the place from which immigrant physicians fanned out across the state. Although San Antonio did not acquire the necessary 12,000 inhabitants until after 1870, the town and its surrounding area attracted health seekers to its climate and mineral springs almost from the time Anglo settlers arrived. Once established in the public mind, the association between the place and the idea of health improved the local climate for medicine. Unfortunately, the Civil War interrupted the process of cultural transfer from Europe, pushed the line of frontier settlement backward, cut off the flow of immigrants temporarily, and halted South Texas medical development for a generation. Had not the Civil War interrupted the pace of change, medicine would have progressed faster, but this war, like its predecessors, ultimately proved beneficial to the growth of specialized medicine and advances in ophthalmology.

Wygant, 25-30, 120;
Rosen, George, Specialization of Medicine,
with Particular Reference to Ophthalmology.

## THE OPHTHALMOSCOPE DEFINES OPHTHALMOLOGY

The most important nineteenth century influence on the growth of ophthalmology worldwide appeared in Europe as a new technology. Hermann Ludwig Ferdinand von Helmholtz (1821-94)--a military surgeon who spent five years in the Prussian army before becoming a professor of physiology--devised the world's first ophthalmoscope in 1851. By holding the instrument in front of a patient's face and shining its light directly into one of their eyes, Helmholtz visualized the interior fundus of the human eye and acquired a technique to directly view numerous manifestations of systemic disease for the first time in history. Before his invention, eye doctors had learned how to distinguish the blindness caused by glaucoma from that produced by cataracts, but in 1850 the only instruments they had to aid in diagnosis were magnifying glasses that improved natural vision, but provided little more than external and superficial information about the eye. Because the ophthalmoscope expanded the traditional treatment of eye diseases beyond surgery to considerations of fundal pathology, however, this new technology had the powerful effect of separating ophthalmology from the rest of medicine. Use of the new device, in essence, made ophthalmology a specialty by introducing a deeper level of knowledge about the human eye than existed about other subjects of medical practice. Finally, Helmholtz's ophthalmoscope served as the foundation from which a long list of related technology was devised, a "*succession of new and more refined diagnostic methods and instruments, including the ophthalmometer, the tonometer, visual test types, instruments for transillumination, the phorometer, the perimeter, and the slip lamp corneal microscope.*"

Koenigsberger, 29-58; Chance, 66-80; Rucker; Rosen, 24, Hubbell.

Any technology represents the effort of many contributors, and the ophthalmoscope was no exception. Although it was von Helmholtz' creation, the new device represented the accumulated scientific knowledge of numbers of practitioners who could not yet call themselves ophthalmologists. Among this group were Albrecht von Graefe--an aristocratic physician living on a grand estate called Finkenherd in Berlin's Zoological Garden--and a host of others working at European centers of medical research and education such as Franciscus Cornelis Donders, who was the first to describe refraction. Albrecht von Graefe's relative, Friedrich W.E.A. von Graefe (1828-1870), produced applications of the ophthalmoscope in his Berlin clinical practice that revolutionized the field in ten years. In 1857 he devised the operation known as iridectomy that created a hole in the iris to relieve acute glaucoma, and later he wrote publications on diseases of the eye, refraction, physiological optics, and cataract. With von Helmholtz' instrument, the first generation of European ophthalmologists learned to "*state the visual acuity of each eye and of both eyes, and to express the relative, or proportionate, acuity of either eye as compared not only with its fellow, but also with the average acuity of a number of normal eyes*." Donders and Helmholtz achieved success of such magnitude in a single generation that people became convinced that everything to be known about the human eye had been learned already! Subsequently, Herman Snellen perfected the eye chart and the operation known as tenotomy that relieved the condition of strabismus or crossed-eyes, but this was only the beginning. According to medical historians, once von Helmholtz had brought "mathematical stability" to the science, it was possible for Drs. Arlt, Jaeger, and other European physicians to make the progress needed to allow ophthalmic specialization to leap from Vienna to the other capitals of Europe and, ultimately, to South Texas. (A further base from which ophthalmology took the form of Europe's knowledge of optics, which was greater than that of any other part of the world. Benjamin Franklin, who invented bifocals, had them produced in Europe because of the expertise to be found there).

Chance, 60, 156;
Rucker;
Hubbell;
Bonner, 70;
Albert and Scheie, viii-x;
Arrington, 10-15;
Soresby, 79

## HEALTH-SEEKERS IN TEXAS

It is a coincidence of history that, as eye specialists in European capitals with permanent eye hospitals accumulated a growing body of ophthalmic knowledge and experience, waves of immigration to Texas, beginning in the early 1800s, helped to transfer that knowledge along with use of the ophthalmoscope to their counterparts in frontier South Texas. For their new ideas to take hold, however, professional conditions would have to improve considerably. Following Rosen's model, the region did not attract the level of population needed for permanent medical institutions until after the Civil War, but a step in that direction was made when people outside of Texas became aware of and interested in the healthful conditions to be found in the South Texas region. If distance from major American cities cushioned it from the impact of many social and cultural developments, the attractiveness of South Texas to "*health-seekers*" helped San Antonio and its surrounding communities to build some of the basic medical infrastructure they so desperately needed. Until the cause of tuberculosis was discovered in 1900, in fact, most states in the American West and Southwest drew consumptives and healthseekers.

Jones, 103-115

Reports associated South Texas with healthfulness as early as Mexican Independence in 1821. Fur traders, Santa Fe merchants, and other early travelers in the region attested to the powers of the landscape, and the idea grew exponentially after the Mexican War. Stories spread that Texas was so healthy that its residents had to leave to find places where they could die. One purpose of the annual volume of the Texas Almanac, first issued by the Galveston News in 1858, was to attract settlers and others seeking a healthful climate. Listing the resources to be found in individual Texas counties, the publication gave particular attention to the fertility of South Texas soils and local "*conditions relating to health.*" Advertisements designed to attract health-seekers no doubt caused many a physician to establish his practice with that fact in mind. Ferdinand Roemer, who settled in one of the German communities to the north, reported that "*the region around San Antonio*" had "*the reputation of being very healthful*" and observed that the climate was "*delightful, and a real winter is unknown*." Conditions that would later draw snowbirds to the region attracted nineteenth century physicians and those seeking treatment to visit and, in many cases, settle in South Texas.

Others qualified their support of the region's healthful properties by noting that conditions improved the further one receded from the Gulf, where swampy conditions frequently bred diseases such as malaria.

Roemer, 135;
Rosen, 30;
Jones, 66, 85, 103-115.

Among prominent leaders of early Texas who were considered "*invalids*" when they came were David G. Burnet, Benjamin R. Milam, Erastus (Deaf) Smith, Mirabeau B. Lamar, Anson Jones and Samuel Maverick. Frederick Law Olmsted brought his consumptive brother on his famous saddle trip through Texas in 1856. Dr. Sherman Goodwin, a foster brother of General W.T. Sherman, took his family to Victoria in 1849, and there recovered from tuberculosis and practiced medicine until his death in 1884. The idea that South Texas had healing powers spread to Germany when Viktor Bracht, who lived near New Braunfels, described "*thousands of his countrymen who had settled in the central Texas hill country*" after the revolution in their homeland. Bracht wrote: "*The experiences of many German physicians have confirmed the truth of earlier reports about the climate. In truth, the healthfulness and pleasantness of the climate of this entire region far surpasses that of the northern, western, and even southern parts of the United States.*" This information, added to reports of inexpensive land for farming, helped to encourage the important wave of German immigrants that brought some of the first European physicians to the region.

Bryan, 55;
Bracht, 13;
Jones, 65, 103-115.

By 1850 a dozen towns within a hundred-mile radius of San Antonio--all accessible from the Alamo city by rail or stage line--had acquired reputations as health centers, and the notion of therapeutic travel to "nature's sanatorium" attracted growing numbers of healthseekers to the area's "salubrious climate." Few were cured, but the practice established a connection between health and San Antonio, and this in turn created support for the construction of medical institutions. The custom of healthseeking embodied in hundreds of the chronically ill who settled permanently near the town encouraged San Antonians to build spas and sanitariums at sites near mineral springs such as the 80-room Hot Sulphur Wells Hotel and bathhouse and housing for the invalids who flocked to Mineral Wells. The incoming traffic of health seekers grew until the Civil War, stopped briefly, and then resumed after 1877 as railroad service regularly brought health seekers to San Antonio until the turn of the century. These developments foreshadowed the importance of the city's current health industry, but were insufficient to produce the kinds of centralized medical facilities needed for ophthalmology to take root. As a result, other forces enabled Galveston to precede San Antonio as the region's principal medical center and the site of some of its first permanent medical facilities.

The absence of many great resort hotels in the area today is attributed to the fact that the invalid traffic was largely made up of people of fairly modest means.

"Health and Medicine," New Handbook of Texas;
Jones, 49, 64-71, 103-115, 137-9, 169-72;
Littlejohn, 588.

## THE IMPORTANCE OF GALVESTON

To understand medical history in South Texas, it is necessary to recognize the role of each of a unique constellation of major cities within a single state. The order in which Texas cities developed explains why doctors chose to practice where they did and accounts to a large degree for why certain cities became medical centers. While most other states produced a single major metropolis, not one but five or six major cities developed in Texas, including Houston, Dallas, San Antonio, El Paso, Austin, and a few early towns that flourished for a time but eventually became ghost towns or disappeared, including the coastal town of Indianola. The growth of Texas cities was particularly difficult to accomplish because of her vast territory and the limited transportation available in many parts of the state, and little urban development succeeded until after the Civil War. Then, frontier towns became cities by organizing a segment of the region or serving as central shipping points through which goods ranging from cattle to minerals and farm crops flowed out to the wider commerce of the nation and the world. The process of urbanization in Texas was not completed until well into the twentieth century, which explains why the first physicians to limit their practices entirely to ophthalmology did not arrive in South Texas until the late nineteenth century.

Ferris and Hoppe, 142

In brief, the history of Texas cities may be summarized as follows. Dallas emerged from a long competition with Fort Worth as the dominant economic center in North Texas when refrigerated railcars ended the twenty-year custom of cowboys driving cattle to the railheads known as "*cattle trailing*." In West Texas, El Paso organized the state's desert regions on the farthest edge of the frontier. In the triangle of land rising northward from the Rio Grande Valley and northern Mexico to the edge of the Hill Country that defines South Texas, however, the port cities of Houston, Galveston, and Indianola as well as San Antonio alternately served as key cities in the region. Houston ultimately eclipsed Indianola when the latter community was hit by a powerful hurricane that destroyed it after serving briefly as a center for immigration and shipping, and eventually overshadowed Galveston as well. Houston became the state's premier city for several key reasons: entrepreneurs made it a terminus for the railroads; a gathering point for resources from the fertile river valleys near the Gulf and the thick pine forests of East Texas; the site of clusters of businesses that manufactured, processed or distributed those resources to northern markets; and a financial center for the oil industry.

New Handbook of Texas;
Richardson, 315-17

Before the rise of Houston, however, Galveston's fine port made it a center for all types of water transport which were then the principal means of moving freight across the region. It was also the principal gate of entry through which immigrants poured into the Lone Star State, and so attracted a substantial population earlier than Houston. Before the Galveston Hospital, other hospitals in the Republic of Texas were organized at White Hall, Houston, and Austin, but these communities were of insufficient size to assure the growth and permanence of these institutions. Until the 1870s, when railroads lessened the importance of the ports, commercial and immigrant ships bringing hundreds of settlers from Europe instead gave Galveston and Indianola a role in dictating patterns of growth across the region, including those in medicine. Galveston, rather than San Antonio, emerged as one of the state's first population centers and its first medical center, thereby affirming the idea that the appearance of such centers depends on the rise of cities.

"Galveston," New Handbook of Texas.

Although neither Galveston nor Indianola play a major role in the state's development today, their histories explain why medicine gained a foothold in South Texas before it succeeded in either Houston, Austin, Dallas, or El Paso. Necessity called Galveston's attention to medical issues. Although spared much of the disruption of the Texas Revolution, the port city's Gulf Coast location made it a thriving environment for disease. Throngs of immigrants who arrived during the antebellum period came with or soon suffered from poor health, including bouts of pneumonia, diarrhea, malaria, and smallpox. Records show that yellow fever, cholera and dengue fever epidemics struck repeatedly from the 1830s until the early twentieth century, and that as late as 1920 Galveston's inhabitants even endured an outbreak of the bubonic plague. If, in a clever analogy made up by historians, Stephen F. Austin, who established the first Anglo colony in Texas, resembles Moses leading his people into the promised land, Galveston, in a medical parallel to the story of Exodus, resembles Egypt as the place from which immigrant physicians fanned out across the region as did the chosen people toward the promised land.

Wygant, 236-7;
Ferris and Hoppe, 202;
Nixon, Medical Story of Early Texas, 385-6

Galveston's initial efforts to support the medical profession failed. Faced with suffering, residents of the fragile community put out a call for help, asking city officials to draw up plans for a Galveston hospital and other public health efforts to care for sick residents, newly-arrived immigrants, and the poor. In response the town constructed its first community hospital after Texas incorporated in 1839 but was still a Republic, and supported the effort by placing a tax on passengers arriving at the port. Every immigrant was compelled to contribute one dollar to the maintenance of the hospital, and later the commander of every vessel arriving at the port was similarly taxed. For a small community with few resources to succeed in establishing a permanent medical institution was unlikely, and one observer described the result as "*a shell of misery, and a great coffin of the unburied dead*". "*Located a mile and a half from any human habitation,*" the "*long and ordinary weather-boarded and shingled house looked out on a landscape of wild sea swamp.*" Given the town's frequent bouts with disease, health officials soon realized that better health facilities would be needed.

Wygant, 236-7;
Ferris and Hoppe, 202;
Nixon, Medical Story of Early Texas, 385-6.

Another glimpse of medical conditions along the Gulf Coast can be obtained from the writings of an individual who called herself Mrs. Houstoun. Scholars estimate that all of Texas was perhaps twenty years behind other parts of the country from the start. In her report, the author described the experience of a Galveston deck hand who had been struck with a large iron hook while loading a ship and received a severe eye injury. A Galveston doctor treated the injury in the absence of the ship's doctor, who was ashore and did not approve of the treatment, and the seaman lost his eye. In 1844 Mrs. Houstoun commented that "*I confess I should not much like to trust a serious case in the hands of the Texan doctors. Some of them may be clever and well-educated, but the medicine in general I believe to be bad.*"

Mrs. Houstoun,
Texas and the Gulf of Mexico, or Yachting in the New World, 1844, cited in Red, Mrs. S.C., Medicine Man in Texas, 87

Despite its inauspicious beginnings, however, Galveston had certain advantages that helped medicine take hold there. First, it remained predominantly Anglo when Texas became a state and continued its role as a staging ground for immigrants arriving from Europe and elsewhere. Those responsible for creating the local medical establishment were, like its first settlers, chiefly people from the eastern and southern United States who retained ties with those places while towns such as San Antonio retained their Hispanic (Mexican and Spanish) flavor. Those who managed to create successful Galveston practices tended to be Anglo, educated, interested in maintaining a stable community of medical practitioners, and determined to establish their own medical standards until state standards could be formulated. As the first to arrive and stake a territory, moreover, they were in a position to influence all who came after. Although Sam Houston approved an act in 1837 that formed a Board of Medical Censors for

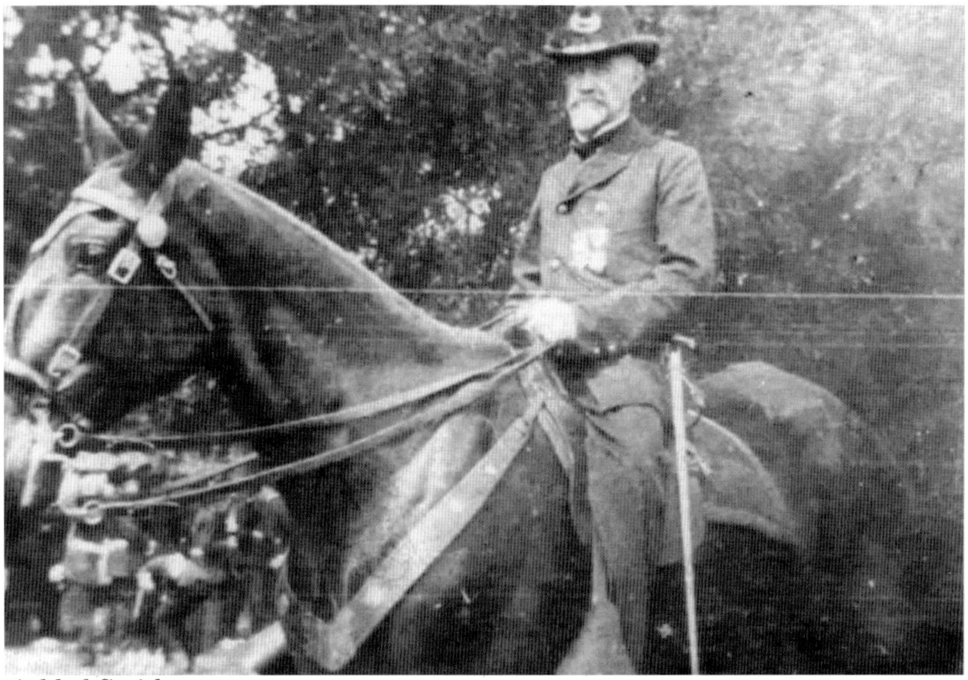

Ashbel Smith

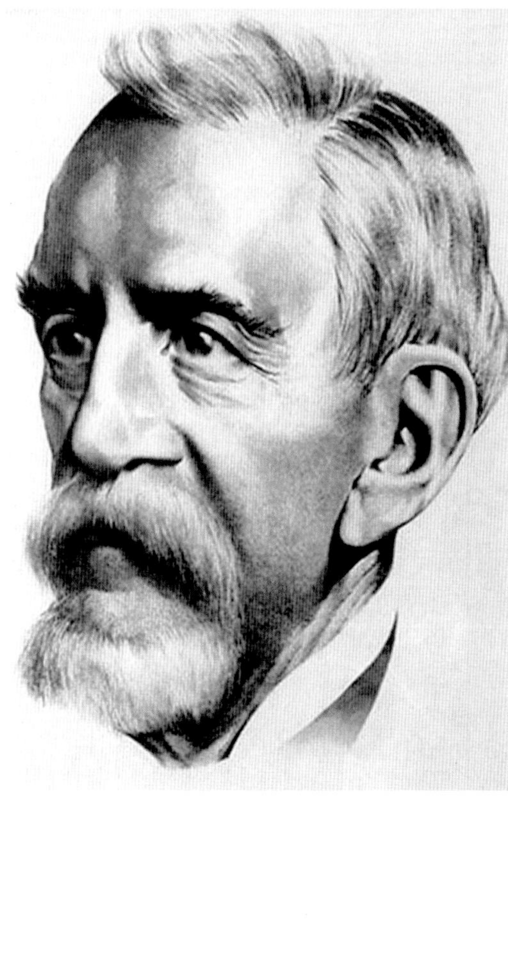

Ashbel Smith

the Republic of Texas with responsibility for granting licenses to practice medicine, that legislation was repealed in 1848. In response, Galveston doctors in 1848 took charge of medical matters by chartering a medical school and creating a local medical society. Mortality at the hospital ranged from 5.8 to 7.7%. By 1851 Samuel Hurlbut contracted with Galveston's aldermen as physician for the City Hospital, earning $1,000 a year and treating between 250 and 500 patients. The Galveston Medical Journal that appeared continuously from the end of the Civil War in 1866 to1871--the first of its kind in Texas--confirmed the importance of the community to the state's medical affairs. At the same time, Galveston attracted the largest number of physicians anywhere in the region.

"Galveston," New Handbook of Texas;
Ferris and Hoppe, 142

Galveston medical practice was relatively sophisticated from the beginning because the physicians who settled there brought with them the benefits of training in medical centers where standards and practices were more up to date. One of Galveston's most successful early physicians, Dr. Ashbel Smith, was an outstanding surgeon who had graduated in 1824 from Yale University, studied medicine in Paris, and treated European epidemics and cholera cases in several eastern American cities before coming to Texas. Arriving during the Texas Revolution of 1836, Smith joined the military when he was appointed Surgeon General of the Army of the Republic of Texas by his close friend, Sam Houston. Later he aided Zachary Taylor in the Mexican War, served as minister to England and France, became a Texas legislator, and worked as Secretary of State under his fellow physician, President Anson Jones. Given his heroism and help in getting the new state on its feet, Smith was a natural choice to lead the Galveston medical profession. When a group of visionary physicians founded the Texas Medical Association in 1853 to obtain support for medicine from the state government, it was Smith who chaired the committee that drafted the constitution and bylaws and eventually served as President of the new association. Later, he was chosen to become President of the Board of Regents of the University of Texas that was proposed in 1839 and opened for classes in 1883.

"Ashbel Smith," New Handbook of Texas.

At the height of his career, Ashbel Smith may have been the most distinguished physician in Texas. His later years are of particular interest to ophthalmologists because of a report he made on a case of malignancy of the eye to the American Journal of the Medical Sciences. While working at the Baylands Orphans Home on the west side of Galveston Bay near Morgan's Point in the area that became the Goose Creek Oil Field, Dr. Smith treated the nine-year old orphan child of a farmer killed in the Civil War. By the age of eleven, Anna Allen suffered from a type of severe eye disease that was never clearly identified, and worked at making candles. Dr. Smith treated her for several months and then took her across the bay to his expansive home at "Evergreen," where he could provide more constant care. There she improved and stayed on as a member of his family. Unfortunately, Dr. Smith never fulfilled his desire to adopt the little girl, although he came to consider her as his daughter and willed to her at his death an estate whose value was greatly increased by the discovery of oil at the site. Smith's general treatment of diseases of the eye, noted in Mrs. S.C. Red's The Medicine Man in Texas, and his own report to the American Journal of the Medical Sciences constitute evidence that early eye care in Galveston was probably equivalent to some of the best offered in the United States at the time.

Silverthorne, 183-4;
Nixon, Medical Story, 330;
Ferris and Hoppe, 118;
"Bayland Orphan's Home," New Handbook of Texas.

## DOCTORS IN THE HINTERLAND

Although the idea of professional overcrowding in the nineteenth century may seem difficult to imagine, many physicians came to Texas to avoid the stiff competition they faced from colleagues elsewhere as much as to acquire free or inexpensive land as did other settlers. Perceptions that medical opportunity in the East was rapidly lessening and that greater possibilities awaited in the newly-opened West motivated skilled physicians to seek new opportunity on the frontier. The story of a steamboat that exploded on a Connecticut River in 1832, drowning a New Hampshire physician, sums up conditions in the Northeast that sent many ambitious young doctors westward. According to the story, "a nearby doctor urged his son to move to fill the vacancy at once, but the young physician arrived too late since three other physicians had already preceded him." Similarly, the Boston Medical and Surgical Journal suggested a level of congestion in 1839 by noting that Cincinnati already had 100 doctors in a population of 50,000, or one for every 500 persons. In other words, by the time Texas won its independence, overcrowding among doctors in the eastern United States was considerable. As a result, Galveston attracted a population of well-trained physicians who were able to foster the growth of early hospitals, professional associations, and journals, and to shape medical practice across other parts of the region as well. Little did they know, however, that competition would follow them to the Southwest.

Ferris and Hoppe, 135; Wygant, 235; Rosen, 31

The fact that the only Anglo town in Texas in 1840 with a population of 1,500 had twenty-five physicians not only suggests that a relatively high standard of medical practice existed in Galveston, but documents the fact that the concentration of doctors was already high and profession competition growing. The fact that the City of Galveston used fees and taxes to support thirteen physicians as city, port, or hospital doctors and that others supplemented their medical practices as druggists, customs collectors, hotel keepers, dentists, and businessmen or by doing contract work further reinforces the idea that Galveston physicians found local competition fierce. At the same time, city officials leased contracts to administer local hospital facilities out in an annual competitive bid process.

Wygant, 238-240

The small circle of Anglo doctors who first set up successful practices staked claims to the territory and pushed those who came after them out along the frontier. By 1860, the number of Galveston doctors reached 100, a density high enough to act as a regulatory device on medical practice as the reputation of more highly-skilled competitors spread and the less-skilled were forced to move to places "*offering greater opportunities*." As a result, many immigrant physicians who arrived at Galveston quickly moved on to nearby towns.

Stiff competition for a place in Galveston tended to make those who succeeded into prominent citizens like Dr. Ashbel Smith. The credentials of physicians who practiced at Galveston between 1839 and 1860 confirms this idea by documenting that fifty-seven percent of those who practiced for five years had some form of college education, five were trained in the Northeast, and a number in Germany. According to the Galveston Tribune in 1896, there were "*more eminent men in the medical profession here than in any other town in the state*" and "*orthodox medicine had become institutionalized in Galveston.*"

Wygant, 238-40, 259; Singleton, Albert O., 2;
Galveston Tribune, May 10, 1896;
Nixon, Medical Story of Early Texas, 414-421.

While Galveston became the first medical center in South Texas, a large number of those who arrived at the port remained for only a few months before they experienced a feeling of overcrowding. According to Galveston scholar Larry Wygant, as many as fifty-five percent of those who arrived before 1860 left the city in under a year. The number of potential patients for each physician steadily increased during the antebellum era, but remained far lower than the ratio in other urban areas. In this sense, San Antonio and other towns benefited from the oversupply of doctors that crowded into the flourishing community on the Gulf, and medical conditions at Galveston for a time dictated medical standards across the entire region. Galveston continued in its role until Houston superceded it and later came to be known as the "*Ellis Island of the West*" when thousands of immigrants, including physicians, made their way inland from the port city to populate states in the Midwest as well as Texas.

Wygant, 237-8, 246 249-53;
Matagorda County Historical Committee et al., v. 1, 154-5

Because of its medical resources and professional excellence, Galveston's influence reached across the South Texas region. Successful medical reputations allowed Galveston doctors to extend their practices beyond the community, the beginning of a tradition that continues down to the present. In a few years, county physician Dr. Joseph E. Burk reported that the "*hospitals of Galveston are well patronized by people from the interior*," suggesting that nineteenth-century patients in the Texas hinterland regularly came to medical centers in urban areas and doctors in the hinterland referred their patients to urban specialists. In retrospect, the concentration of doctors at Galveston appears to have produced a winnowing process that accelerated the pace at which outstanding physicians both established themselves in the city and carried standards of medical care into the hinterland.

Wygant, 183

While Galveston offered the best medical care in the state, however, the need for doctors beyond the Gulf Coastal Plain remained high. Many who came through Galveston's port of entry worked itinerantly or alone in small communities where they were the only doctor for miles around. In these places, medical care before they came had been either poor or non-existent. In nearby Matagorda County, for example, Arda Talbot Allen wrote in her book Miss Ella of the Deep South of Texas that "*there were only three doctors for the whole county; so more often and not the patient was dead before the doctor could even see him.*" Typical medical charges were $15 for consultations, $5 for day visits, $2 for bleeding, and $5 for cupping, often with costs of transportation included. So poor was the population, however, that immigrant physicians often found it necessary to move from town to town in order to establish a sufficiently lucrative practice.

Matagorda County Historical Committee et al., v. 1, 156

Typical of hinterland doctors who could afford to treat the poor by owning farms or performing a combination of other activities were Drs. John W. Brown and Henry Loundes Rugeley of Matagorda County and Dr. E.H. Smith of Victoria, who listed themselves as both doctors and planters, or small farmers. Smith, who had been born in San Augustine in 1831 and grown up in Gonzales County, practiced medicine in Mexico before opening a plantation on the west side of the Guadalupe River in 1858. Rugeley maintained what was described as a "*good-sized plantation.*" In many cases, doctors "*did well if they collected a third of their fees.*" According to one local physician, the average annual income from a rural medical practice was forty dollars. Eye care was basic at best, and doctors continued to rely on emetics and practices of heroic medicine that left patients better off without a physician's care. Much work was needed, in other words, to establish a suitable climate for specialization.

Wygant, 305;
Matagorda County Historical Committee et al., v. 1, 156

Throughout the antebellum period, most South Texas physicians also lacked the institutional and professional support that would enable them to compete successfully with doctors in distant cities. Competition in the period included "*regular and irregular physicians, quacks, physicians in other cities, and self-medication*." While the Lone Star State remained in colonial dependency on the Northeast for manufactured goods, many Texans chose when the need arose to go east to doctors with well-established reputations, leaving local physicians struggling to survive. Many Texans had grown up near urban hospitals that offered the beginnings of specialized medicine before coming to the frontier. Despite the considerable distances involved, these individuals simply went north when illness or disease struck until the Civil War ended the practice. Galveston newspapers regularly advertised facilities in New Orleans such as Dr. Beard's Eye Infirmary that were within a distance reachable by ship or even by horseback and stagecoach, and additional competition came from doctors in cities who diagnosed and prescribed by mail. Among wealthy Galvestonians who went east to find the best available eye care, Sarah Williams, the wife of wealthy Galveston businessman Samuel May Williams, saw a surgeon in Lexington, Kentucky, about her cataracts in 1842 and 1844, and in 1854 went to Boston for a successful cataract operation. The editor of the Galveston News, Willard Richardson, went to Dr. Beard's New Orleans Eye Infirmary as late as 1858. In answer to these problems, the arrival of immigrant physicians from important medical centers in Europe supplied new energy to help the medical profession establish its autonomy.

Wygant, 245-46

## GERMAN IMMIGRANT DOCTORS AT SAN ANTONIO

As one scholar of Texas medicine has noted, "*European surgeons who immigrated to Texas naturally had had the best training*." Given the inadequate medical care in the early years of Texas statehood, the importance of the arrival of waves of German immigrants, including outstanding doctors trained in European medical techniques, cannot be underestimated. According to Texas medical historian P.I. Nixon, "*the most important development, historically, economically, and culturally*" in the period of the Texas Republic was "*the immigration of German colonists*," an ethnic group closely associated with the advance of specialized medicine. German immigration was carefully planned and succeeded in bringing a substantial population into the region.

Singleton, Albert O., 2;
Nixon, Medical Story of Early Texas, 414-421;
"Germans in Texas," New Handbook of Texas.

In 1823 the Baron Felipe Enrique Neri de Bastrop had been appointed commissioner of colonization for an Anglo settlement with authority to issue land titles and helped to secure passage of the act that established a port at Galveston. The man for whom the town of Bastrop, Texas, is named, a former Prussian soldier of fortune under Frederick the Great and the king of Spain, helped Moses Austin to obtain his land grant from the Mexican government and Stephen F. Austin to settle the first Anglo colony. By encouraging settlement in South Texas, the Baron also encouraged the arrival of new medical leaders in the region.

"Bastrop, Baron Felipe Enrique Neri de," New Handbook of Texas

The first Germans to reach the region arrived in the final years of Mexican sovereignty and settled along the Gulf Coast, but larger groups that came between 1844 and 1847 established German settlements in the counties of Comal, Gillespie and Llano, Guadalupe, Kerr, Kendall, Calhoun, Victoria, DeWitt, Lavaca, Colorado, Austin, Washington, Fayette, and Bastrop. Latecomers also settled in Galveston, Houston, Austin and San Antonio. Funneled to the outer edge of the frontier where they served as a buffer to protect East Texas settlements against the Native-American population, middle and upper class Germans succeeded in part because of their skills in dealing with the tribes. Not only did they set up treaties that enabled them to establish and maintain their communities but, by being tolerant of their neighbors and clustering together in towns built according to patterns of settlement developed in the ancient walled cities of Europe, were apparently perceived as somewhat less of a threat to the natives than independent Anglo farmers and planters. Hardly pausing to unpack their trunks, tenacious German newcomers opened shops and built manufacturing enterprises, constructed substantial, elegant homes, and infected their communities with enthusiasm for culture and education. Though some German physicians were able to establish successful Galveston practices, the majority moved to areas surrounding San Antonio, making the port city's loss the Alamo City's ultimate gain.

Nixon, Medical Story of Early Texas, 414-421

If immigration and shipping made Galveston an early medical center, immigration brought the first trained physicians to San Antonio when the old Spanish town became the beneficiary of a plan to bring German immigrants to Texas under sponsorship of a group of German nobles called the Adelsverein. The immigrants who came established permanent settlements and farms at Fredricksburg, New Braunfels, and other new German communities to the north and also settled in considerable numbers in San Antonio, where their influx conveyed powerful European medical knowledge to the community and stimulated development of the town's medical infrastructure. Accompanying the immigrants, three German physicians who arrived at Galveston in particular represented a powerful and potent gift to the new nation. Dr. Ferdinand Ludwig von Herff began practicing medicine in 1856 at New Braunfels, but enjoyed a distinguished medical career that lasted for fifty-years in San Antonio, while Drs. Heinrich Fischer and Charles Weising established successful practices at Victoria.

Nixon, Medical Story of Early Texas, 414-421;
"Herff, Ferdinand Ludwig von, New Handbook of Texas

## DR. FERDINAND LUDWIG VON HERFF

In Dr. Ferdinand Ludwig von Herff, frontier medicine and Texas ophthalmology found a true pioneer. When he arrived in Texas, Herff came with a medical background that included two years at the University of Bonn and a medical degree from the University of Berlin that he received in 1843. He had also studied surgery under the senior Albrecht von Graefe, father of the famed oculist, who helped him to become proficient in cataract surgery. Herff decided to come to Texas after four years service as a soldier in the Hessian Army, in which he fought at least twenty duels with cavalry "*schlagers*" (a saber and a pistol), when he became discouraged with political conditions resulting from a severe economic crisis that caused many Germans to suffer. In 1847 he decided to emigrate, and came to Texas as the leading member of a German society of forty members known as Die Vierziger, organized at Darmstadt by John O. Meusebach, Prince Carl of Solms-Braunfels, and Hermann Spies, who hoped to establish a socialistic community. Herff was one of two physicians in the group of mostly young professionals who landed at Galveston, took a boat to

Indianola to purchase supplies, and then set out for a site north of San Antonio near the clear waters of the Llano River in the rolling hills of west central Texas. Unfortunately, the utopian community they named Bettina failed a year later, and the community joined a growing list of Texas ghost towns where efforts at permanent settlement did not take root. Faced with a need to assimilate to the culture around him, the young German doctor dropped the "von" from his name, confronted the challenges of practicing medicine in San Antonio, and set out to make important contributions to frontier medicine.

Nixon, Century of Medicine in San Antonio, 160;
Ferris and Hoppe, 16-20;
Blode, 1-20.

Along with introducing medical practices that substantially improved the level of medical care in the region, Dr. Herff made an important contribution to ophthalmology when he performed the first operation in Texas for cataract removal. Far from the centers of Europe, the Native Americans Herff saw as patients were so pleased with his treatments that they came to view him as a "*medicine man*" of great stature. One of these was a Comanche brave whose eyes were clouded with advanced bilateral cataracts that physicians of the day believed were caused when the constant flowing of ocular fluid was aggravated by emotions or bodily states and produced an effect like that of a waterfall or cataract, hence the term. Herff and the Comanche brave entered medical history when the doctor, equipped with the "*latest set of ophthalmological instruments of the time*" and knowledge gained from performing cataract surgery in Europe, successfully removed both cataracts from the young man's eyes. Herff later shared the following memories of that notable event with his biographer and grandson, Ferdinand Peter Herff, M.D.

Atkinson, External Diseases, 13;
Herff and Barber, eds., 14;
Ferris and Hoppe, 16-20;
Tomlinson Lone Star Book of Texas Records, 145.

*I knew I was taking a risk, but I was also sure that without surgery this unfortunate Indian would be doomed to permanent blindness, a condition which probably would be blamed on me because of my inaction. Since it occurred in pre-Listerian days, I did not miss the assistance of this technique. In those times we had not yet discovered the use of local anesthesia, but in my medical kit I had brought a eye operations in Darmstadt. Due to the primitive knowledge at that time, the question of infection did not worry me. However, always as a matter of personal cleanliness I was in the habit of meticulously scrubbing my hands before making any medical or surgical contact with a patient. Also, since the conjunctiva is kept clean from dust and other irritating particles by the free flow of tears, it occurred to me that any operative procedure on the eyes should be preceded by copious washings with water. I selected some from a cistern because this was uncontaminated by lime, sulphur, iron, or any other excoriating minerals. As the use of my 160-power microscope showed that the stored rainwater was infested with numerous small moving bodies which I called animalcules, I decided to clear the substance by boiling it. I then felt free to wash out the conjunctival sac with this purified water.*

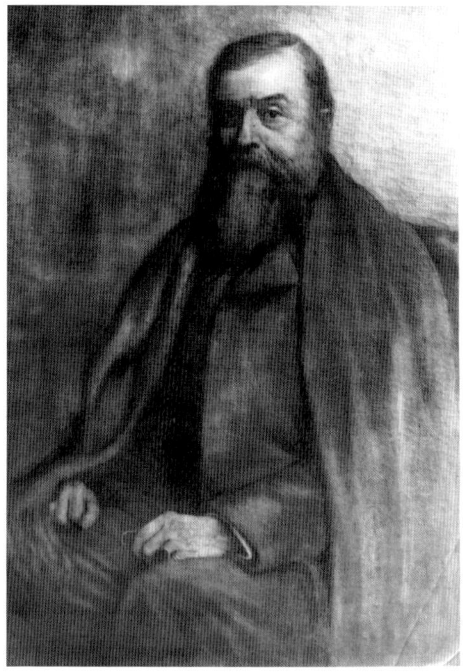

Ferdinand Ludwig von Herff

*Proverbially, one of the outstanding essentials in a cataract extraction is adequate light. In those primitive days the only forms of artificial illumination were candlelight and kerosene lamps whose rays were intensified by magnifying lenses. But the quandry lay in the fact that the only type of anesthesia available was ether by inhalation. The flammable nature of ether definitely contraindicated its use anywhere near a naked flame, so the only solution was to perform the surgery out of doors, aided by the sunlight. I decided to do the work out on a gravel floored patio adjoining the bunkhouse. Requisites were a clear, entirely cloud-free, dustless, windless, insectless day. Surrounding the operating group stood a dozen 40-ers with palm leaf fans to keep the flies away. The patient was put to sleep by my associate physician while the subject's head was steadied by Julie Herf, (the woman who served as the group's cook and housekeeper, no relation to Dr. Herff) and I was ready to go to work.*

Herff's grandson later reported the success of his grandfather's milestone operation had been rewarded in an appreciative, albeit unorthodox, fashion. The recovered patient, who had noticed that Dr. Herff was unmarried, returned about three months later to present his healer with a "*squaw*," a young captive Mexican girl who remained with the German immigrants and later married the colony leader, Hermann Spies.

Herff, 14-15;
"Ferdinand Ludwig von Herff," New Handbook of Texas

Herff returned to Darmstadt to marry Mathilde Klingelhofer, but Texas had captured his imagination and his heart. By late 1849 he opened a new practice in the small German settlement at New Braunfels, and the young couple of aristocratic heritage took up lodgings in a modest three-room adobe house. As Herff's work became known, his reputation in the successful treatment of eye problems spread and he began to draw patients from as far away as Austin and San Antonio. His reputation improved further when he was consulted about a case in which an eye injury resulted in sympathetic ophthalmia. At approximately the same time that the New York Ophthalmic Hospital opened to serve the indigent poor in 1852, Dr. Herff treated a farmhand whose right eye had been pierced by the tine of a pitchfork, resulting in ophthalmitis. Although he had received extensive treatment in San Antonio without showing improvement, the patient was as reluctant to give up the eye as were his physicians to sacrifice it, especially because the traumatized eyeball, although sightless and extremely painful, did not show further signs of infection. Much discouraged but still hopeful, the young man returned to New Braunfels where he soon developed pains and increasing dimness in the healthy eye. At this point he was persuaded to consult Dr. Herff, who told him after careful examination that he was suffering from sympathetic ophthalmia. Bluntly, the doctor warned him that only immediate removal of the injured member would save the good eye. The patient readily agreed to surgery, the success of which became obvious in the restoration of perfect vision to the healthy eye.

Herff, 31-32

As word of his reputation spread, medical leaders at Galveston invited Dr. Herff to move his practice to the prestigious medical community, but he declined, possibly due to his awareness of the intense competition there. Instead, in 1850 the doctor moved his practice and his family to San Antonio, a community with a population of between 3,000 and 3,500 people. Little did he know that only a decade later in 1860, the population would double in size. For a number of reasons, it was a practical step for Dr. Herff to move to San Antonio. According to Heusinger family accounts, Dr. Julius Heusinger opened an apothecary and drug store on Commerce Street on May 1, 1850, that was the first business of its kind in the community. A few months later, he sold the store to German immigrant, Dr. August Nette, a practitioner and druggist who, like Dr. Herff, had moved to San Antonio from New Braunfels. It was reported that Dr. Herff patronized his fellow countryman's drug store because Dr. Nette was the only druggist who could read his handwriting.

Herff, 45;
Nixon, Century of Medicine, 176, 179, 184;
Heusinger, 9

Herff's influence soon reached well beyond San Antonio. When physicians formed the Texas Medical Association in 1853, Dr. Herff was a charter member. He also helped to create The Bexar County Medical Society in the same year to offer the first major professional support to San Antonio practitioners. This institution was the first county medical society formed under the Texas Medical Association. In his subsequent practice, "*cataract extractions and eyeball excisions for arrowhead and rifle-ball wounds and sympathetic ophthalmia*" continued to be an important part of Herff's work. He succeeded in surgically curing a number of cases of strabismus, was credited with having performed the first lithotomy for removal of gallstones in Texas, served as San Antonio City Physician in 1855, and continued the military career he began in Europe by serving as a contract surgeon in the U.S. Army. He may have also played a role in helping the frontier city to endure through peaceful coexistence with the Native-American population, since his former Indian clientele continued to consult him even after he established his practice in San Antonio. By this time he had become fluent in the languages of both the Apaches and Comanches, and this helped in gaining their trust and acceptance. Not long after coming to the city, Herff performed one of his successful bilateral cataract extractions on a young Apache woman who expressed her thanks by presenting him with the gift of a small beaded buckskin pouch containing a necklace made of twenty-peso gold coins. In 1886 he met his grateful patient once again when he accepted an unexpected and puzzling invitation to visit the recently captured Apache chief, Geronimo. The infamous chief had been held in the

Menger Hotel for a time and was now confined at San Antonio's army depot at Fort Sam Houston. While the two men conversed in Apache, they were joined by an Indian woman from Geronimo's band, the same woman whose sight had been restored over thirty-six years earlier.

"Herff," New Handbook of Texas; Ferris and Hoppe, 188

Though there is little to suggest that Dr. Herff maintained communication with physicians in Germany who were developing the idea of specialization, he nonetheless must be credited for helping to lay the groundwork for the idea of specialized medicine in Texas. San Antonio's distinctly German culture created an environment in which the idea of European medical training along with specific European medical advances could be integrated more rapidly than might otherwise have been possible, an important contribution since German science had just given birth to the major breakthrough that created a separate science of ophthalmology. While individual San Antonians were no doubt grateful for his service, Herff's most lasting contribution to South Texas medicine lay in transplanting European attitudes toward medicine to the frontier. In his later years working at the Santa Rosa Hospital to improve the quality of care in the city, Herff introduced medical practices to its staff that established permanent standards that could be passed down through the institution to others.

"Herff," New Handbook of Texas; Herff, The Doctors Herff.

## THE CIVIL WAR

Subsequent South Texas medical history may have been different had not the Civil War altered the course of its development. Americans, who were known in Europe for inventions ranging from Yankee apple parers to hosts of gadgets for which they sought patents announced in the new journal Scientific American, had already begun to redesign and modify the European ophthalmoscope when the war broke out. As German medicine progressed, however, United States physicians became entangled in a civil conflict that obscured the great discovery for nearly a decade while the nation turned its medical attention to support for military efforts and the necessities of war.

The Civil War shook the new nation, enlisted Dr. Herff to serve as brigade surgeon in the Confederate militia, and changed Texas forever. Many stalwart citizens who had once called Virginia, Georgia, or other southern states "*home*" passionately contended for the Confederacy, but many of San Antonio's newly-arrived Germans and much of its Mexican population fervently opposed slavery and just as feverishly resisted forsaking the Union. As in other towns, debate burned hotly as people struggled with their loyalties. Even after Texas seceded from the United States to join the Confederacy--San Antonio voted to secede by a mere 113 votes--the dispute continued and the town was plagued with a climate of suspicion and mistrust that seemed to rend her spirit. San Antonians were alternately harassed by irrational southern patriots, Unionists celebrating northern victories, or placards calling on Unionists to rebel, and in 1862 a Confederate riot on Christmas Eve wrecked the chili stands in the downtown plazas.

Shashid, 594-5; Richardson, 200-224

At the beginning of the Civil War, the U.S. Army Medical Department. had less than 100 doctors and other individuals capable of treating the sickness and injury suffered by the Union troops. Creation of the U.S. Sanitary Commission and the work of George Templeton Strong improved conditions in the North, and field hospital reorganization and ambulance service produced greater effectiveness at Antietam (1862) and the Battle of Gettysburg (1863). Meanwhile, the South established hospitals along the routes of major railroads and relied on the aid of local residents who flocked to temporary hospitals to care for the sick and wounded. In most places, medicine suffered along with other community services in those chaotic years. The infant Texas Medical Association suspended meetings after its first convention, and was unable to gather again until 1869.

"Civil War," New Handbook of Texas;
Nixon, Century of Medicine

The war's worst blow came in the hundreds of soldiers who marched down San Antonio's streets on their way to fight in far-off battlefields, never to return. With them went some of the few physicians in the state, including San Antonio 's Dr. A.M. Dignowity, who left his practice at the outbreak of the war and went north, and others who served the Confederacy. Dr. Ashbel Smith of Galveston had served in the Mexican War and now joined the Civil War cause by organizing the Bayland Guards, participating at the siege of Vicksburg, and later taking charge of the defenses at Galveston. Dr. Reuss of Cuero treated both Confederates and Yankees.

Nixon, Century of Medicine, 170, 207, 214-5; Richardson, 200-224

Before the war began, San Antonio had managed achieved two further indicators of medical progress. Dr. George Cupples had been elected president of the Texas Medical Association at its first membership meeting in San Antonio in 1853 and in 1854 was chosen to be San Antonio's first City Physician, an office in which he was succeeded a year later by Dr. Ferdinand Herff. During the Civil War, Cupples was first surgeon for the 7th Texas Regiment of mounted volunteers in the Confederate Army and medical director of the eastern military district of Texas, continuing in charge until he was ordered to join Sibley's Brigade in Louisiana. In 1864, he was senior chief-surgeon and medical director of the Trans-Mississippi department for all cavalry in the service of the Confederate government until the close of the Red River campaign.

"Dr. George Cupples," Encyclopedia of the New West.

(After the Civil War, Cupples took the advice of Dr. Ashbel Smith and settled in San Antonio with his second wife, the granddaughter of "*Ready-Money*" David Provost of New Jersey, a man who ran the first stage lines to Mexico and was an associate of Cornelius Vanderbilt. Cupples later introduced the use of anesthetics to Texas, initially ether and then chloroform, and was the first doctor to perform a number of operations, including amputations at the hip and knee joints and on cancer of the tongue. Two decades after serving as President of the Texas Medical Association, he served a second term).

The rumbling storm that erupted in 1860 benefited American medicine indirectly by giving doctors the equivalent of research experience as they coped with record numbers of war casualties. In spite of hardships, the War Between the States had positive influences in its power to focus the nation's attention on the importance of medicine, to raise the demand for doctors of all kinds, and especially to heighten awareness of the need for trained physicians.

Edwin Klebs, a German observer who later practiced medicine in the United States, claimed in 1868 that, "*the greatest and most admirable success has been attained by the North Americans in military medical work. The history of the War of the Secession has to show a display of medical and scientific activities that leaves anything that even since has been achieved, way in the background.*" Among other achievements in ophthalmology in that year, Hermann Knapp opened the Ophthalmic and Aural Institute in New York. In this sense, the great civil conflict contributed to forces that would hasten the transfer of specialized medicine from the major cities of Europe to the frontier.

Bonner, 10-11

Most of the injured suffered without the ether anesthesia that John Collins Warren had introduced in 1846, but the horrors of war taught surgeons to ligate arteries and deal with complications of bullet wounds. Better hospitals and some of the nation's first specialized medical institutions were both byproducts of the war. Based on his war experience, William H. Welch made Johns Hopkins a research center, and encouraged General George M. Sternberg to establish the Army Medical School that promoted scientific work by Army medical officers. Cornelius Rea Agnew (1830-88), who had served in the Army, established the New York Eye and Ear Infirmary and improved the structure of military hospitals. In Texas, farmers turned to manufacturing and centers of population expanded. While Galveston established a Charity Hospital that operated after the Civil War, the appearance of medical specialists in South Texas awaited the presence of other cultural factors and influences the military could not provide but that would shortly bring necessary change.

Bonner, 11, 206-227; Duffy, 229; Red, 56

# CHAPTER 5

# THE COSMOPOLITAN FRONTIER: PROFESSIONAL DEVELOPMENT AND THE INFLUENCE OF EUROPE, 1865-1916

*Suppose that crippled eyes were transformed into crippled legs. What a heart-rending parade we would witness on a busy street! Nearly every other person would go limping by.*

Dr. Matthew Luckiesh, "*Seeing and Human Welfare,*" in Aldous Huxley, The Art of Seeing, New York, Harper and Brothers, 1942, 18.

As South Texans rebuilt their farms and established new enterprises in the years of Reconstruction, eye, ear, nose and throat specialists established successful practices that paved the way for the acceptance of the first true ophthalmologists. Although little fighting had occurred on Texas soil during the Civil War, many men did not return from the battlefield and numerous families still faced challenging conditions. During the conflict, the frontier fell back two hundred miles to a line that left Austin and the center of Texas government at the mercy of marauding Native-Americans. The war hobbled both economic and medical development, leaving the region with neither enough manufacturing to overcome its dependence on the northern manufacturing states nor sufficient transportation lines to reach distant markets. So limited was the medical infrastructure in the difficult years of Reconstruction that the possibility specialized medicine might take root in the rough soil of South Texas seemed remote, indeed.

Richardson, 202-224.

Under alternately harsh and supportive Reconstruction administrations, the state of Texas faced political and social problems that weakened it for decades. In medicine, the limited communication that occurred between the North and South in the early phases of Reconstruction—resulting from the desire of some in the government to punish the former Confederacy—translated as resistance to the cultural transfer of specialization. P.I. Nixon had commented on medicine in Texas prior to 1836 that "*Where there is no political or economic progress, medicine must necessarily falter. If medicine in Texas. . . made no advance, the reason is readily found in the uncertain condition of local affairs.*" Local conditions after the Civil War, in many cases, were worse than those a decade earlier. People in the hinterlands who had been too poor to avail themselves of medical services earlier found their situation unaltered. Ophthalmology as yet carried little influence as a formal specialty beyond the eastern seaboard. In 1864 the American Ophthalmological Society was organized to "consult upon the best mode of promoting the interests of ophthalmology in this country," but its influence remained distant and inaccessible. Until the turn of the century, moreover, a more serious problem for medicine prevailed. Many physicians who ventured into Texas could be described as pioneers or, at worst, quacks.

Richardson, 224-245;
Nixon, Century of Medicine, 40;
Chance, 165-7;
Bonner, German Universities, 37;
Albert and Scheie, History of Ophthalmology at the University of Pennsylvania, 111.

## QUACKS AND NOSTRUM DEALERS

No place more clearly demonstrates the importance of professional development in medicine than does nineteenth-century South Texas, and nowhere did specialization play a more important role in advancing the medical profession. The experience of the Civil War left the region without legal standards to govern medical treatment and with little access to medical education. A few physicians spent the war years at home, but chaotic conditions that lasted throughout the Reconstruction years gave charlatans of all kinds freedom to prey on the ignorant and left the state a fertile ground for the growing menace of medical quackery. Little opportunity to improve conditions existed until physicians began to seek training abroad and to organize and institutionalize their profession. The first San Antonio City Directory published for 1877 and 1878 captures something of the flavor of the community with its listing of 13 physicians, 5 public schools, the Santa Rosa Hospital, a Government Hospital at Houston and St. Mary's, and 62 saloons.

San Antonio City Directory, 1877-78.

Frontier towns such as San Antonio created havens for sellers of snake oil and patent medicines and allowed the worst in medical practice to proliferate. As its new role as a shipping point for cattle and farm products emerged, the old Spanish town acquired a bawdy reputation that created a stimulating atmosphere for quack doctors. The tendency for moral behavior to deteriorate as people recover from war has long been recognized, and San Antonians were no different. As prosperity returned, life around the plazas was high carnival, attracting gamblers, drifters, and saloon girls. The open-air, kerosene-lit stands of the Chili Queens on Military Plaza, cockfights, and the swirling ruffled skirts of fandango dancers became common sights. Cowpokes returning from cattle drives frequented the town's vaudeville houses and variety theaters or rode their mounts up to brass-railed bars at rowdy saloons such as the Gray Mule, the Hole-In-The-Wall, and the Revolving Light. Men short on cash traded sets of antlers for a cold mug of beer at the Buckhorn Saloon or kept the brew flowing for an entire weekend with a sack of rattlesnake rattles. Evenings often ended with a flare of gunfire as quick tempers and strong whiskey combined to escalate the slightest offense into a serious and sometimes fatal altercation. The famed evangelist Dixie Williams later denounced what many perceived as *"the wickedest city in the Union, not excluding Washington City."*

Panfield, 3;
Fehrenbach, 3;
San Antonio Express, March 10, 1886.

Numbers of quack doctors who had already established themselves in the region before the Civil War began now flourished. As early as 1837, the Houston Telegraph announced the presence of "*pseudo-doctors more dangerous than the hostile Indians and not considerably less numerous.*" The San Antonio Daily Herald for June 25, 1858 contained advertisements for quackery alongside mention of quality physicians such as Dr. Ferdinand Herff. In this issue, A.F. Kercheval announced the sale of a medical preparation described as "*Dr. Hoofland's Celebrated German Bitters Prepared by Dr. C.M. Jackson, Philadelphia, Pa.*," a preparation promulgated with "*utmost confidence*" for the effectual cure of everything from the "*Deficiency of Perspiration, Diseases of the Kidneys, Liver and Stomach, and Constant Imaginings of Evil to Dimness of Vision and Dots or Webs before the Sight.*" Another outlandish purveyor of "*medicine without doctors*" placed advertisements in local newspapers promising effective cures and treatment without actually needing to see the patient. During Reconstruction, few physicians had enough power to counteract these individuals and quackery thrived.

Grimes, 534;
San Antonio Daily Herald, June 25, 1858;
Jones, 33,
Galveston News, January 17, 1871;
Houston Telegraph, June 24, 1837.

Given the vacuum of professional standards and institutions offering medical training, quack doctors operated in South Texas until after the turn of the century and medical specialty fields failed to take root. Dr. J.A. Jones, who had received his education at "*the best medical colleges in America and Europe*," was described in the Austin newspapers as "*the most skillful operator on the eye and ear in this country*" and claimed to have operated successfully on "*deformed eyes.*" His fee for medicine to treat sore eyes was $30. A colorful individual named J.D. Forest, who received a charter from the Texas Legislature in 1889 to operate a San Antonio enterprise known as the New York Medical College, was a classic later example. Forest taught ophthalmology despite the fact he could not spell the term; his wife taught female diseases; his brother, surgery; and his six-year-old son, pediatrics. In order to put a stop to his enterprise, the Texas Medical Association collected fifty dollars from each of its members to enroll an African American porter in Forest's college. The Association succeeded in closing Forest down when the porter received a diploma in seventeen days, signed by a faculty member who had taken the accelerated course and finished in twelve. In 1871 the Galveston News reported that "*Texas is about as full of quacks as McKinney's Bayou is full of ducks*," and as late as 1900 Texans celebrated a Victoria physician with a large country practice who could "*work miracles with gin and peach-tree-leaf poultices.*" A serious consequence of these practices, unfortunately, was increased hostility toward specialists. Even within the medical establishment there were problems. Dr. Salm of Austin, who listed himself as an oculist and aurist, was expelled from the Texas Medical Association in 1886 for gross plagiarism. Quacks and nostrum dealers competed with legitimate physicians in a contest they occasionally won by showing equal success in curing patients. For years, common opinion in Texas echoed Dr. W.J. Mayo's humorous remark that specialization meant "*more and more knowledge about less and less.*" As late as 1922, H.L. Hilgartner wrote:

*Specialization in the practice of medicine is necessary, but it must be guarded against its two besetting dangers—excessive narrowness and the tendency to fall away from the foundations upon which it should ever stand in structural unity.*

Medical historian George Rosen quotes an American doctor who later noted that "*The word 'specialist' is most unfortunate, for it is only a few years ago that it was solely applied to charlatans and empirics in medicine*," despite the fact that official recognition of specialization had been made in 1869 when the American Medical Association resolved "*that this Association recognizes specialties as proper and legitimate fields of practice.*"

Rosen, 58, 68-9;
Coleman, 52-53;
Burrow, "Economic and Political Policies of the Texas Medical Profession in the Progressive Era," 57-8;
Galveston News, January 17, 1871;
Jones, 33;
Wygant, 252;
Nixon, Century of Medicine, 111-112;
Nixon, History of the Texas Medical Association, 127, 318;
Nixon, Medical Story, 400-410;
Hill, Herbert, "Cooperation Between the Internist and Ophthalmo Oto-Laryngologist," Southwest Texas Medicine, November, 1934, 14.

In spite of these difficult circumstances, opposing forces began to gather strength by the time Reconstruction ended. In 1873 the Texas Legislature passed new laws regulating medical practice. Acceptance of the ophthalmoscope by physicians dealing with eye problems had further implications. "*Specialization in any kind of cultural activity*" is "*a socially conditioned phenomenon,*" as Rosen pointed out. Enthusiasm for the successful use of the instrument increased support for other advances in medical technology, and the scientific interest it represented created a force against quackery and a platform on which to build a tradition of ophthalmic research. At the 1877 meeting of the Texas Medical Association in Galveston, Dr. T.D. Manning's paper, "*A Report on Ophthalmology and Otology,*" indicated that diseases of the eye and ear were "*being segregated*" into their respective specialties. At the 1889 meeting in San Antonio at which Dr. Ferdinand Herff welcomed the membership, a prize was awarded for a paper on "*The Ophthalmoscope in General Practice.*" Ultimately, heroic efforts to rid the state of unlicensed impostors caused attitudes toward specialized medicine to slowly begin to change. One of the first activities undertaken by San Antonio's Bexar County Medical Society was to inaugurate "*a war against these hotbeds of pollution,*" and enlist reputable physicians, including eye specialists, to the cause. The fight against the reign of fraudulent practitioners ended after the turn of the century and was only the first of many steps, but in time the effort succeeded. An equally important if unintended consequence of the fight against quackery was a heightened awareness of the need for greater professionalism. By 1875 the <u>New York Medical Record</u> could report that "*the practice of a specialty*" was now "*considered the sine qua non of success,*" a development soon to be repeated as far away as South Texas.

In the same paper, Dr. Manning indicated that yellow oxide of mercury ointment was being praised for use in eye infections. Faith in Education, 120;
Rosen, 3, 63;
Nixon, History of the Texas Medical Association, 74, 151.

Where no formal standard existed for either medical education or practice, a particular hostility toward specialization came from the profession itself. General practitioners frequently saw both qualified specialists and the throng of quacks doctors as unwelcome competition. Specialists threatened a generalist's sphere of expertise and charlatans, their public reputations. In this climate, one doctor explained, "*professional sentiments were opposed to specialism, and apathy toward ophthalmology was always present.*" Dr. T.H. Nott, a general practitioner, summed up the attitude of many frontier physicians at the 1883 Texas Medical Association Meeting by explaining that he was "*an isolated member of this honorable body, there being no other member in less than seventy-five or one hundred miles of me, and no medical organization nearer than that, while I am without railroad or telegraphic communication with the rest of the state or world.*" Dr. Nott claimed that a specialist was a man who "*sits back on his dignity and grows rich and famous, while we struggle for a living and a small reputation and drum for him.*" As a solution, Nott suggested inserting "*a clause in the article regulating the practice of medicine, which shall forbid any person to practice a specialty in this State who has not done a general practice for at least ten years.*"

Hubbell, 138;
Nixon, History of the Texas Medical Association, 106.

Lack of access to professional training compounded the problem. As Rosen points out, the ophthalmoscope helped ophthalmic medicine to separate itself from general surgery by introducing the use of a new technology. In time, introduction of the technology established the idea that basic training in the specialty was needed to properly utilize it. In the absence of medical schools, however, most doctors lacked authority to formulate training requirements or delineate differences between the practices of specialists and generalists. Few medical schools existed outside the Northeast and Midwest, and many schools required only a two-year course of three to six months each year for graduation until the Flexner Report of 1910 called for improvements. Doctors worked "*for varied periods to learn what was known as to become specialists,*" constrained by preceptorships that limited their learning to assisting a local physician who frequently had little training himself. Specialists in a new field also had their limitations. Treatment for trachoma meant rubbing the lids with a stick of copper sulfate or a swab of boroglycerin. In 1885, a Texas doctor using a four to eight per cent solution of cocaine for eye, nose, and throat surgery was unaware of both the hazard to life and the danger of habit formation. "*Fee splitting*" only made matters worse. In this illegal activity, general practitioners referred patients to specialists who charged high fees for treatment and then split the fee with the man making the referral, thereby increasing the business for both. As a result, some years transpired before the competition between general practitioners and specialists abated. In the meantime, specialists felt considerable pressure to convince the public that their services were both valuable and respectable. The solution to medical quackery lay in institutions capable of overseeing medical training. Fortunately, a powerful force was about to appear on the horizon that would shake the grip of those who preyed on the public and make the necessary institutions a reality.

*Efforts to end quackery, necessary to establish scientific standards for medicine, unfortunately discredited both the midwife and the curandera, although these folk healers continued to practice until the late twentieth century.*

Hubbell, 64, 138;
Vail, 15;
Goar, "Ophthalmology," 82;
Cary, 298-301;
Lesky, 434;
Nixon, History of the Texas Medical Association, 121;
Sykes, 120

## OCULISTS, AURISTS, AND INSTITUTIONAL DEVELOPMENT AT GALVESTON

Although few specialists or permanent medical institutions established a foothold before the end of the century and family doctors commonly treated everything including eye problems, "oculists and aurists" who limited their practices to the eye, ear, nose and throat practiced successfully in South Texas before trained EENT specialists arrived. Dr. M. Josephthall of Waco, who practiced ophthalmology exclusively beginning in 1873, was the first Texas physician on record to advertise the specialty. In South Texas, where hogs, sheep, and goats wandered uninhibited in the city streets until as late as 1875, the Turpin brothers practiced general medicine and Dr. P. Butler Turpin appears to have established himself as a specialist at Corpus Christi around 1874, but initially the pair advertised themselves as "*Turpin & Turpin, Physicians and Surgeons*" in the Corpus Christi Gazette. With a third brother, Phillip, they also operated a perfumerie that sold oils, paints and pharmaceuticals. At the end of that year, P. Butler identified himself in the Gazette as a specialist "*giving special atten-*

*tion to diseases of the eye and all chronic diseases.*" On February 11, 1876 (the year in which the Nueces County Medical Association was founded), however, Turpin notified his patients that he was leaving and recommended a Dr. Hamilton, who had taken over his office, as his replacement. From 1880 to 1909, Turpin practiced on a part-time basis in Laredo and Corpus Christi. In the latter town, Dr Arthur Spohn was forced to use the home of Carlota Verain Rossi and her half sister, Concha Rodriquez, to treat patients from ranches in the county until he established the first hospital in 1905 in the early years of a new century.

The first Spohn hospital was shortlived and succumbed to the hurricane of 1919. U.S. General Hospital No. 15 opened in the Corpus Christi Beach Hotel in 1918; a new Spohn Hospital opened in 1919, and two other hospitals were completed by 1929.

Goar, 82-84;
Corpus Christi Gazette, January 5, 1876;
Ferris and Hoppe, 216;
Nueces County Historical Society, 134-6;
Nueces County Medical Society Auxiliary records.

Reconstruction produced few permanent medical institutions outside Galveston, but here the presence of a successful hospital led to the creation of a medical school that, despite initial failure, eventually thrived. At the start of the Civil War in 1860, local doctors at the urging of Dr. Ashbel Smith had chartered the Galveston Medical College, but were forced to abandon it because of the conflict. In 1873, a mere forty years after the first Anglo settlers arrived in the region, they revived the school, renamed it the Texas Medical College, and began to train medical students, starting with a faculty of eight. This school emphasized "*diseases of the eye, ear, throat, and skin—plus surgical and clinical teaching and lectures*" in the third year of training. Due to the hazards of Reconstruction, however, this effort also failed. Thirty years after the first attempt and after the John Sealy Hospital opened in 1889, Galveston doctors in 1890 succeeded on a third attempt in organizing the University of Texas Medical Department. Opened a year later as the University of Texas Medical Branch, this institution became an enduring success. The British Medical Journal for June 17, 1891 captured the auspicious beginnings of the fledgling institution:

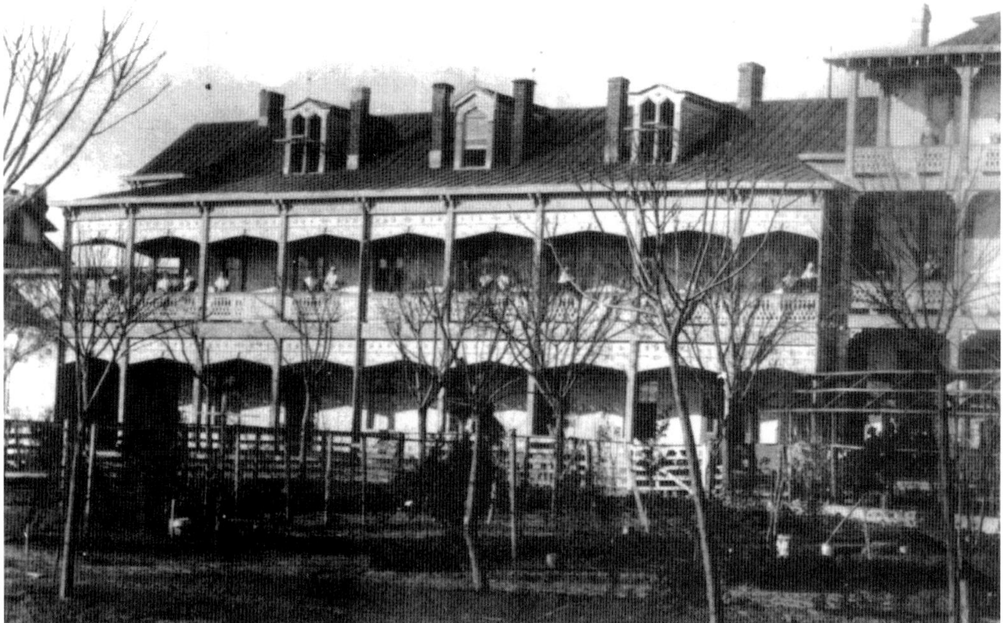

1878- First permanent structure on the present site of the Santa Rosa Medical Center. It was partially destroyed by fire and razed to make way for a larger building in 1884, which lasted until 1966.

*If there are any 'comparatively young men' who would not mind exchanging the barren pavements of London for what Johnson would have called 'the potentiality of growing (well) beyond the dreams of avarice' in the Great West, they might think it worthwhile to apply.*

Brown, 50;
Ferris and Hoppe, 215.

From the start, ophthalmology was a key component of the training offered at the new medical school. Among the faculty of the reorganized college in 1889 was Dr. George P. Hall, a lecturer in diseases of the eye, ear, nose, and throat. Disreputable doctors practiced in Galveston as well, but the community continued to be a lonely island of hope in a stream of medical deficiency. Although the John Sealy Hospital adjacent to the Medical College recorded only eight eye, ear, nose and throat cases among its 2,892 patients as late as 1894, Galveston's reputation swiftly reached distant parts of the state. Records show that "*patients from a large floating foreign population and from different parts of the state*" arrived regularly at what they understood to be "*the nearest point where hospital relief can be procured.*"

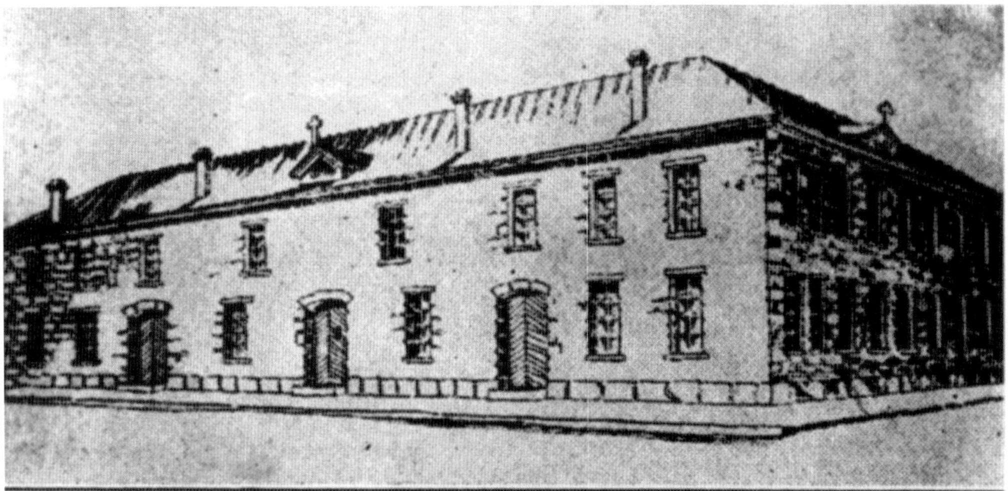

1869- First Santa Rosa Hospital on Military Plaza in San Antonio, which would later become the largest Catholic hospital system in the United States.

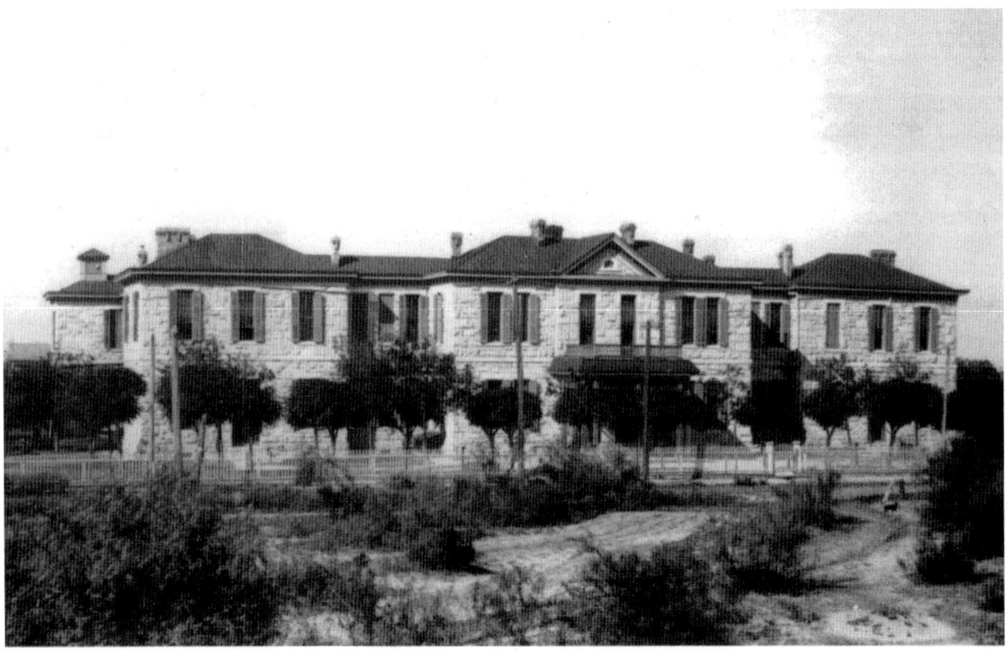

1969. Old City Hospital in San Antonio

In 1860 there were only 7,307 people in Galveston, and only 421,629 in all of Texas.
Faculty and Staff, University of Texas Medical Branch, 17, 20, 83.

In one sense, the University of Texas Medical Branch at Galveston can be understood as simply part of a broad nationwide movement to improve medical education and create general hospitals. This interpretation, however, overlooks considerable differences between conditions in Reconstruction Texas and places where other new institutions began. Institutional development in South Texas, given the level of general development in the region, was both early and significant. Although the new medical school offered neither eye, ear, nose, and throat nor ophthalmology residency training, Galveston Medical Branch faculty employed models of the eye and ear in their teaching almost from the start. American medical education suffered from a lack of patient contact and opportunity for dissection, but contact with Europe soon resulted in the addition of these important educational components. By 1890, when the institution became The University of Texas Medical Branch, Dr. R.C. Hodges lectured regularly on diseases of the eye, ear, nose and throat and, henceforth, specialists were a permanent part of the faculty. Records show that the teaching of ophthalmology was first separated from otolaryngology in 1900 when Dr. John B. Haden and Dr. Henry C. Haden, two brothers, taught there. Outside of Galveston, however, Reconstruction produced few permanent medical institutions in the region.

Faculty and Staff, University of Texas Medical Branch, 8, 17, 20, 35, 83;
Brown, Dayton, 49-53;
Wygant, 30;
Ferris and Hoppe, 217

## INSTITUTIONAL DEVELOPMENT AT SAN ANTONIO DURING RECONSTRUCTION

Without the professional strength of Galveston, San Antonio gained a new medical institution only when lack of proper sanitation made the town vulnerable to epidemics. Concerned citizens and city leaders faced insufficient resources to establish a hospital to care for the stricken when cholera claimed hundreds of lives in 1866, and appealed instead to Galveston's Catholic Bishop Dubuis. Their pleas went unanswered, however, until three years later when another wave of the epidemic threatened and church officials responded. On December 3, 1869, three Sisters of Charity of the Incarnate Word opened San Antonio's first non-military hospital for civilians, an eight-bed infirmary housed in a two-story frame building on Military Plaza at the corner of Commerce and Cameron Streets. The "*City Hospital*" or "*Charity Hospital*" that was the forerunner of today's Santa Rosa Hospital provided eight patients admitted on opening day with quality nursing care, clean rooms, and abundant fresh air and soap, all for fifty cents a day. Fortunately for the new charity hospital, the German doctor, Ferdinand Herff, improved the practice of medicine there by setting medical standards and introducing European medical practices that established a new tradition for local medicine. At the same time, Herff was instrumental in organizing another professional institution, the West Texas Medical Association, which increased communication between doctors across the region. Within a few years the infirmary moved to larger quarters on Zavala and North Concho Streets, and in 1874 the first Santa Rosa Hospital was built on the corner of Santa Rosa and Houston Streets in part of the old San Fernando Cemetery. The cornerstone for a more adequate County and City Hospital would not be laid until July 9, 1888. Today, over 120 years later, the Santa Rosa Medical Center is the largest Catholic hospital system in the United States.

San Antonio Light, October 7, 1974;
Fehrenbach, 4;
Huesinger;
Ferris and Hoppe, 202.

Morrison and Fourmy's General Directory of the City of San Antonio for 1877-78 and 1883-84 shows that, in only six years, the number of "*physicians and surgeons*" in the city doubled from thirteen to twenty-eight while the general population grew from 8,235 in 1860 to over 20,000 in 1880. By 1890, fifty doctors were listed, and in 1900 the number of names exceeded ninety-five. Under "*Oculists and Aurists*," the 1883 Directory listed the names of T.J. Tyner at 268 W. Commerce and N.S. Burnham at 272 Commerce, with a note to "*See advt*" elsewhere in the volume. The advertisement noted that Burnham was a "*Late Surgeon in Charge of Kansas City Eye and Ear Infirmary*" who gave "*Special Attention to the Treatment of Catarrh, affecting the Eye, Ear, Throat and Lungs*." Although nothing is known of his formal education or the scope of his practice, the 1885 directory reveals that Dr. Burnham had become the *"proprietor of the San Antonio Eye and Ear Infirmary, over 13 E. Houston, cor. St. Marys, beds, Vance Hotel"* with a residence at the same address. By 1890 he resided at the *"San Antonio Eye, Ear and Throat Infirmary"* on the northwest corner of E. Houston and St. Mary's, and was also surgeon there. Tyner's San Antonio office notices appear until 1885, but later he apparently had a prominent practice in Austin and was active in matters of medical ethics for the Texas Medical Association. Another institution known as the San Antonio EENT Hospital, established in 1910 as a private 10-bed facility with Dr. Charles H. Edwards as physician-in-charge, was located where the M&S Tower later stood. Beginning in 1901, another EENT Hospital, with Dr. James Hall Bell in charge, was located in the Wright Building at the corner of Houston and Navarro streets. Other names appearing under the heading for *"Oculist and Aurists"* in the 1880s include Charles Deady, Henry Olin and Jerod Wilson, although it is unclear whether any of these were qualified physicians. Medical establishments of the period were frequently the equivalent of a storefront, consisting simply of a room where the doctor conducted his business. Without professional journals or meetings and limited opportunity to consult with others in their field, every general practitioner became a researcher in the effort to learn from experience and search for better solutions. Recognition of the need for greater medical understanding also formed the stimulus for many to seek further education.

Dr. Burnham was included in the City Directory until 1890, but no longer under the listing for "Physicians and Surgeons."

San Antonio City Directory, 1887, 1889-1890, 1897-98, 1905;
Dr. Dan Russell, Jr., interview;
AMA Directory, 1914.

## GERMAN IMMIGRANT PHYSICIANS AND MEDICAL EDUCATION ABROAD

Given the considerable forces at work against professional development in South Texas, specialization might have taken years to develop had not European influence reached the United States at the beginning of the Civil War. At that time, Dr. Elkanah Williams established the pattern for a generation by becoming the first American to specialize in EENT, doing so by studying in Europe. As early as 1816, two graduates of the New York College of Physicians and Surgeons had studied the "*nature and treatment of eye diseases*" at the London Eye Infirmary founded by John Saunders, but Williams' ambition to become a specialist came from studying with Samuel D. Gross, the famous Louisville surgeon who also did eye surgery. On graduating from the University of Louisville Medical School in 1850, only a year before Helmholtz invented the ophthalmoscope, Williams set out for Europe. There he studied in Prague and Berlin, and eventually decided to specialize after a meeting with Albrecht von Graefe. As a result, it was Dr. Williams, rather than one of his European colleagues, who introduced the ophthalmoscope to London's Moorfields Hospital in 1854 and then brought ophthalmology's key diagnostic tool back to the United States. Instead of remaining on the East Coast, moreover, Williams moved to Cincinnati, then still close to the frontier, where he founded an eye clinic "*according to the European plan.*" Elected in 1860 to a professorship at Cincinnati's Miami Medical College a school (which was founded only in 1852), the "*first pioneer surgeon west of the Alleghenies*" made ophthalmology the first specialty recognized by any medical college in the United States).

Vail, 11-17;
Bonner, 89;
Rosen, 33;
Hubbell, 144

Williams's success produced such enthusiasm in the United States for the idea of specialization that hosts of other medical students soon followed his lead. Chief among the offerings sought by American medical students was ophthalmology. Of all the clinical specialties, ophthalmology was the first and most profoundly affected by the advances made in German universities. According to Bonner, "*it was ophthalmology which drew the first significant numbers of Americans to German universities, well before the general exodus after 1870.*" Virtually all prominent American eye specialists in the second half of the nineteenth century studied in a German-speaking country while the idea was in vogue and, in many of America's great cities, the "*pioneers in ophthalmology were German-born or trained.*" Hermann Knapp, considered America's leading nineteenth-century ophthalmologist, served as Graefe's assistant, set up both his own clinic and a professorship at Heidelberg, and went on to train many outstanding

American specialists who practiced across the country.

Bonner, 88-92;
Nixon, Century of Medicine, 261;
Vail, Derrick, 13.

German doctors established a model for specialization in medicine everywhere, and those they trained in turn "*fought hard for the inclusion of ophthalmology in the curriculum of the medical schools and its establishment as a specialty in medical practice.*" The German influence in ophthalmology further extended beyond the invention of the ophthalmoscope to the setting of new medical standards. "*It was the example of European specialization in eye diseases that convinced Americans abroad to inaugurate ophthalmology as a separate branch of medicine in this country.*" Both Drs. Elkanah and Henry Williams worked to include the subject in northern medical school curricula, while Dr. Christian Fenner pursued a similar objective as a leader in the South.

Elkanah Williams, perhaps the first eye specialist in the Midwest, criticized the medical profession for neglecting eye disease and leaving the field open to quacks in 1857.

Rosen, 57-59;
Vail, 13;
Bonner, 88-92.

Although physicians from the Northeast were the first to seek overseas training, a handful also went abroad from the South and former Confederate states and their proportion gradually increased. In time, a European medical education replaced the conventional preceptorship with a well rounded, scientifically based education that gave medical students permission to work directly with patients. Contact with European science not only introduced medical practices that would have taken a good deal longer to evolve locally, but constituted a major force for eradicating the flourishing medical quackery that put specialists at hazard. In little more than a decade, doctors with European training transformed frontier medicine, established successful eye, ear, nose, and throat practices across the region, and paved the way for ophthalmologists as the new century began.

Not all the factors needed for professional specialization to flourish were yet in place, however. Faced with a lack of medical facilities and a contentious medical climate, the period from the 1890s to the 1920s came to be known as the Golden Age of EENT rather than the Golden Age of Ophthalmology. At the 1969 meeting of the American Academy of Ophthalmology and Otolaryngology, the membership later acknowledged that "*The combined specialty came to be a natural one*" and that "*this was strictly an American phenomenon.*" Access to European medical education dramatically accelerated the growth of knowledge in the field of ophthalmology in the U.S., and in Texas as well. Although one hundred and fifty American medical schools opened between 1834 and 1892, however, much of American medical education was a matter of business rather than professional training, especially in areas where quackery prevailed. Until American physicians caught up with their overseas counterparts, many hospitals offered such poor conditions that patients were safer at home. A total of only six books made up the shelf of the well-informed eye doctor in 1850. Ignorance of the field abounded, including unproven ideas like that of an American physician named Loring, who on examining the eyes of New York school children was among the first to believe that "*modern education" had the "power to change the shape of the human eye.*" Depending on the doctor, treatment could be entirely unreliable. Those who obtained a credential to practice medicine frequently possessed limited knowledge and less experience. The American system of post-graduate or residency training did not develop for another generation, but roots of the idea can be traced back to the nineteenth century when young doctors began their studies at American medical schools and then went abroad for post-graduate training in specialty medical fields in Germany and Austria. According to scholars, "*between 1870 and 1914 a large proportion of the most talented and ambitious of American medical men studied abroad in German universities.*"

In 1908, there were seven medical schools in Texas, four of which were in Dallas.

Vail, 14; Cary, 298-301; Bonner, vii, 3-6;
Chance, 186;
Faculty and Staff, Galveston Medical Branch, 97

South Texas received an additional boost from German immigrants who continued to arrive and settle in San Antonio and nearby German communities. According to Rosen, "*of all the clinical specialties ophthalmology was the first and most profoundly affected by advances in the German universities.*" Not only were many physicians influenced by overseas training but German immigrant physicians, who brought with them the benefit of training, "*added to the luster of American ophthalmology.*" Julius Hirschberg believed "*immigrant specialists from Germany had made the greatest contribution to*

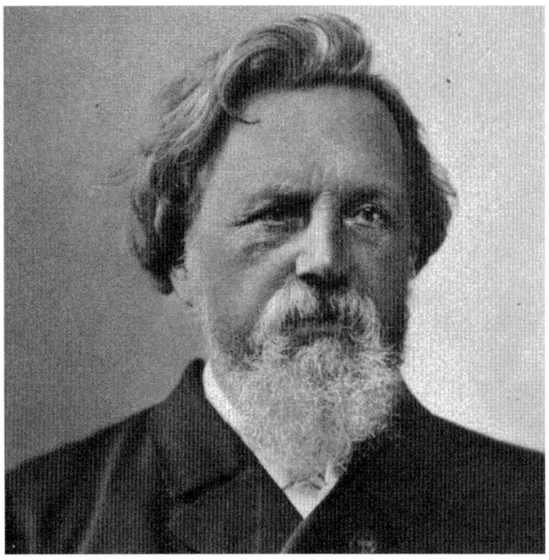

Frans Cornelis Donders (1818-1889)

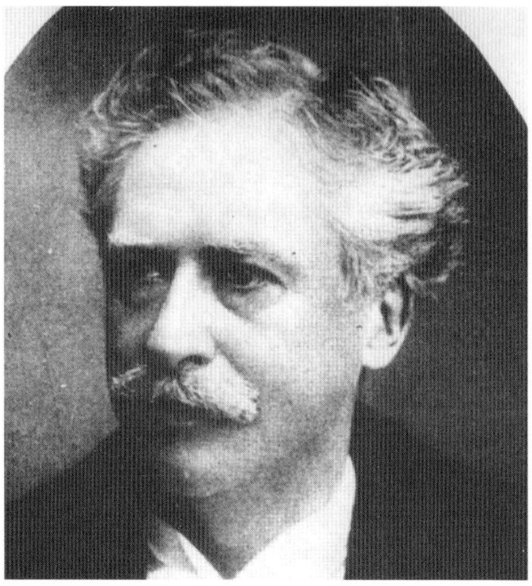

Hermann Snellen (1834-1908)

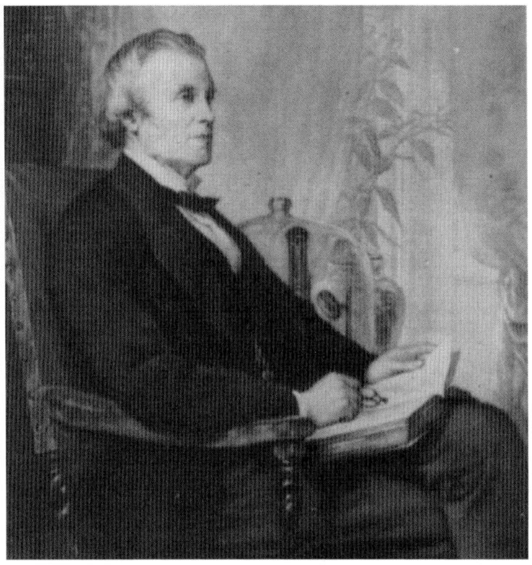

Sir William Bowman (1816-1892)

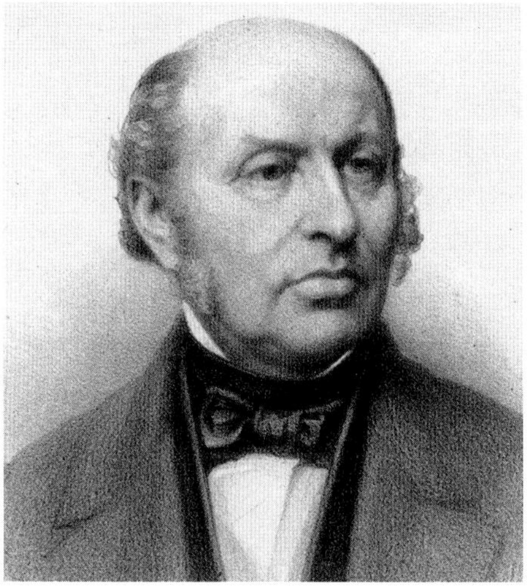

Jules Sichel (1802-1868)

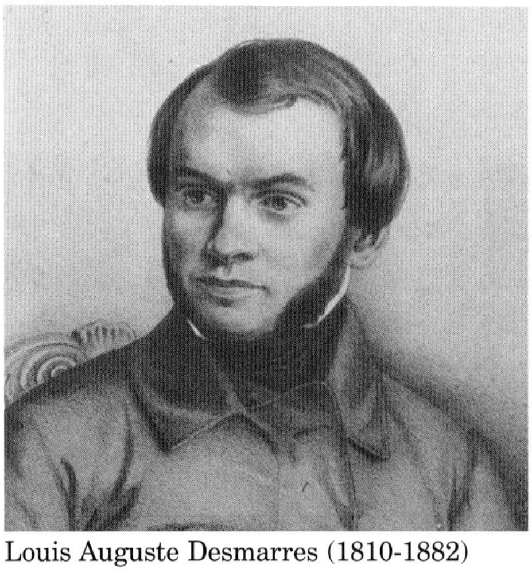

Louis Auguste Desmarres (1810-1882)

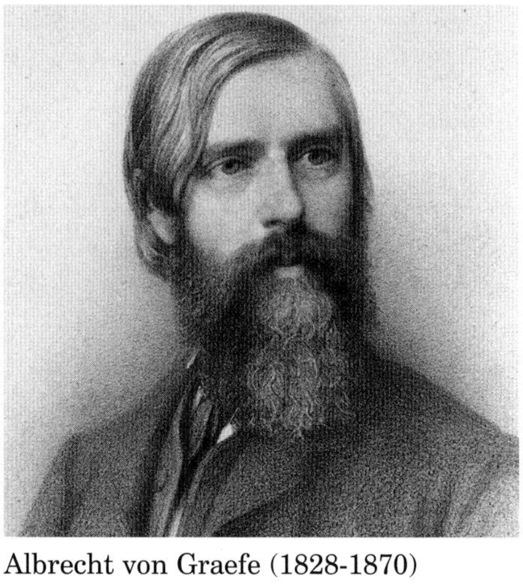

Albrecht von Graefe (1828-1870)

*American ophthalmology*." And in South Texas especially, European medicine became a tangible presence because of the region's large German population. A significant population of Germans and of German physicians helped to accomplish the transfer of European medical knowledge to the frontier that otherwise would have taken years to complete. German doctors such as Dr. Ferdinand Herff not only introduced a more scientific approach to medicine, but also maintained an appreciation for the rigors of European medical training and important links to European medical schools and hospitals. Dr. Charles Weising, who came from Germany before the Civil War in 1856, or Dr. Heinrich Fischer, who was born in 1817 and practiced for twenty years in Victoria County, represent this first generation of German immigrants. At a time when many people lacked familiarity with specialists or found consulting one unacceptable, German physicians heightened public consciousness about standards of medical care available overseas and laid the groundwork for those who went overseas for training.

Bonner, 37, 90-92

Awareness of German culture encouraged native Texans to follow in the footsteps of immigrant doctors trained in Europe. "*Many of the early Americans to study medicine in Germany were the sons of German emigrants*." An 1867 edition of the <u>Lehrbuch der Anatomie des Menschen</u>, the famous anatomy text by Joseph Hyrtl, housed at the Bexar County Medical Library in San Antonio, contains a letter written by Hyrtl to a medical student named Rudolf Menger at Leipzig. Menger was the son of German immigrant, Joseph Menger, the founder of San Antonio's Menger Hotel located adjacent to the Alamo. Born five years after his parents arrived in Texas from Germany, Menger went to study at Vienna and graduated in 1874. The letter suggests the kind of experience those who went abroad might have had:

*Most honored Sir,*

*I have presented your case to our Dean Dr. Prof. Braun and received word from him that there is no obstacle to your admission as "ordinary listener" of medicine in our university.*

*When you have heard all the prescribed scientific subjects, partly in*

*Leipsiz and partly here in Vienna, there is no objection to your graduation here after passing strict examinations. You have then only to present a Revers that you as a foreigner will not practice in Austria. (It is understood that you can receive a dispensation). What your admission to the medical examination requires re certificates for collegiate subjects heard: Anatomy, Physiology, Mineralogy, Zoology, Botany, Chemistry, General Pathology, Pharmacology, Clinical Medicine, Ophthalmology, Obstetrics, Pathological Anatomy, Veterinary Arts, and Forensic Medicine. One studies here five years in order to hear all the subjects. You will meet here many of your countrymen. This is all that can be told to you by*

*Your devoted*
*J. Hyrtl*

"Notes and Queries," Southwestern Historical Quarterly, XI (1956) no. 1, n.p.

South Texas doctors found the antidote for quackery when they began to seek specialty training abroad. Improvements at San Antonio's Santa Rosa Hospital alone would not likely have produced the level of medicine South Texans enjoyed by the late nineteenth century had not medical students, less than fifty years after the Texas Revolution, soon joined other American physicians on their way to distant capitals to avail themselves of the best medical training offered anywhere in the world. Undaunted by their circumstances and the difficulties of transportation, these individuals completed their medical education in Germany, Vienna, Paris, or London and returned to the region with sufficient skills and experience to turn the once primitive and violent frontier into a place with a decidedly cosmopolitan flavor. Their impact not only contributed to the diversity and sophistication of places like San Antonio, but, coupled with the well-trained doctors from outside the state who also established practices in the region, succeeded in heightening doctors' prestige in their communities and improving public attitudes toward specialization.

In the second half of the nineteenth century, Vienna overtook Paris and London as the most popular destination for aspiring American physicians. Frank E. Brawley said "*For the idea work, Vienna certainly is the place to go*." American industrialists had traveled abroad to learn about technological processes, machinery, and craft knowledge from Europe's Industrial Revolution. Now, in a parallel "*medical revolution*" , medical students took a similar route to gain the knowledge and experience necessary to specialize.

At the turn of the century, Vienna was the medical center of the world. America owes its pre-eminence in the medical sciences of our own time, in no small part, to the thousands of medical students who went to Vienna at a time when the standards of American medicine were scandalously low.

Janik and Toulmin, 35

Centralized facilities at a cluster of Viennese clinics known as the Allgemeine Krankenhaus or General Hospital provided unique access to anatomical material and private courses. Working in the hospital's wards, clinics and dispensaries, medical students could concentrate on their specialty and consult with other specialists. In the process, they learned both the science and practice of medicine, "*acquired the spirit of research and expansion of knowledge*," and learned more about emerging fields of specialization. Most of these individuals adopted the paradigms and practices of their teachers, and subsequently influenced the direction of medical practice and accelerated the pace of change when they returned to the United States.

Bonner, 5, 70

Statistics on the high number of doctors who completed their medical education abroad capture the extent of Viennese and German influence on Texas medicine, showing that a majority of Americans studied in Europe between the years of 1850 and 1890, and a total of 10-15,000 individuals studied at over twenty-eight universities in Germany, Austria-Hungary, or Switzerland between 1870 and 1914. Of the latter group, two thirds went to Vienna and twenty percent to Berlin.

Bonner, 23-7; Hun, 3-7

Theory and factual knowledge circulated freely in an open exchange between countries when American physicians studied with

Donders and Snellen in Holland, Bowman in London, Sichel and Desmarres in Paris, von Graefe in Berlin, and Arlt and Jaeger at Vienna. Helmholtz, for much of this period, was at Heidelberg. Some Americans went for a full degree, but the majority completed postgraduate training programs in a specialty that ranged from a six-week private course to two or three years of intensive research in a German laboratory. Between 1877 and 1881 a total of 765 North Americans attended Ernst Fuchs' courses, influencing the professor so strongly that by 1879 he had begun to offer courses at Vienna in English. By 1912 the Blue Book of the American Medical Association of Vienna used by American students as a guidebook to the city listed thirty-eight courses being offered in ophthalmology, of which twenty-five were taught in English. Such courses generally introduced the use of the ophthalmoscope, allowed the student to witness eye operations, and provided study of eye diseases and anomalies of refraction. Young ophthalmologists looked forward to meeting and working with the most outstanding doctors of their time, and were not only conversant about science, but travelers aware of a wider world by the time they returned to their hometowns.

Bonner, 23ff., 36, 75, 80-1; Hun, 36; Lesky, 445

European medical training had other influences on the medical profession in the United States as well, giving rise to professional societies and journals. Specialists had learned medicine in the laboratory and hospital settings, "and this brought a growing interest in the segregation of men interested in the eye, ear, nose and throat. Fewer of these specialists were interested in the general practitioner as an audience. Instead, they became interested in their own knowledge and the interchange with fellow practitioners in the same field." Ultimately, this impulse led to the development of both the first professional societies for specialists and a growing interest in research. In the North, two German physicians who studied with Albrecht von Graefe—Hermann Althoff of New York and Ferdinand Karl Hotz in Chicago—along with Hermann Knapp in New York trained many others when they returned from Europe. A German immigrant physician who had studied with von Graefe and Sichel published the country's first ophthalmological journal, the American Journal of Ophthalmology. A German doctor who had taught at Heidelberg started the Archives of Ophthalmology, first published in 1869. In South Texas Dr. Sofie Herzog, the daughter of a well-known Austrian surgeon who came to the United States from Vienna in 1886 just after finishing "*the best medical training that Europe offered at the time*," also demonstrated the power of European influence. After practicing briefly in New York, Dr. Herzog moved to Brazoria, Texas, and, remarkably for the time, established a successful practice as a female physician, performing so many operations to remove bullets that she proudly displayed the extracted missiles strung onto a necklace. Herzog also served as a surgeon for the Gulf Coast Lines, riding on boxcars, handcars and locomotives in an effort to reach her patients and enjoyed a private life in which she bore fifteen children.

Dr. Josephine Kingsley, San Antonio's first female physician, arrived in 1878. In general, both immigrants and American doctors who trained overseas, helped to heighten the awareness of general practitioners and the public regarding the practices of European medicine and, within a generation, to make European medicine a tangible presence in Texas, manifested by the arrival of trained specialists. Another outstanding immigrant ophthalmologist in the region was Houston's Dr. Ray Karchmer Daily from Lithuania, one of the first women to graduate from the Galveston Medical Branch. Dailey went on to complete her training in Vienna.

Bonner, 23ff.; Scheie, 24; Hun; Red, 83-4, 106; Cary, E.H., 300.

## GERMAN INFLUENCE AT CUERO

The contribution of German immigrant physicians and German medicine to South Texas was particularly significant in the town of Cuero in the Rio Grande Valley where, along with Galveston and San Antonio, a South Texas medical center developed in the last half of the late nineteenth century. Here, a large immigrant population helped the frontier to overcome provincial attitudes and quackery and established new potential for growth in medicine. Because of its German population, Cuero, rather than older communities like San Antonio, became an early center for medicine in the region.

"Cuero," "Indianola," New Handbook of Texas

Cuero's history begins with that of Indianola, the coastal town founded in 1844 that for a time rivaled Galveston as a major port and the destination of a large number of German immigrants. Known originally as Powderhorn or Karlshaven, Indianola became a center for regional trade because of its location at a natural deep water port. Morgan Line steamships carrying European immigrants arrived regularly from New Orleans and as far away as New York City before Galveston gained fame as the "*Ellis Island of the West*" or Houston became the state's chief railroad terminus or managed to dig a channel to the Gulf. (Historically, the two major Gulf Coast cities—Houston and Indianola on the west shore of Matagorda Bay and Galveston—dominated the state before the effects of urbanization reached Texas. In its hey-day, Indianola supplied thirty-four inland military forts, including those in West Texas, maintained several plants that slaughtered cattle for the hide and tallow business, and shipped live cattle to Cuba and the Northeast as early as 1849).

"Indianola," New Handbook of Texas.

Ships from Europe brought 4,000 Germans to Indianola in 1846, but between 1,000 and 2,000 swiftly succumbed to epidemic disease despite the fact that several physicians accompanied the party, including Dr. Wilhelm Keidel, who had attended the University of Goettingen and who served in the Mexican War soon after he arrived, and Dr. Hermann Nagel, who had studied at Halle, Wurzburg and Berlin. Before the Indianola City Council established a $3-a-day hospital and provided a city physician in 1855, disease in the community induced many of these immigrants to move inland to New Braunfels, although epidemics pursued them there as well, making an improvised hospital on the banks of the Comal ineffective against the onslaught of the disease. The remaining population eventually moved to Cuero.

Nixon, Medical Story of Early Texas, 389, 414-25;
"Indianola," New Handbook of Texas

In 1872 Gustav Schleicher, a German engineer, created Indianola's legacy when he surveyed the Cuero townsite (a word that meant "hides' in Spanish) near Cuero Creek roughly half way between the coast and Austin in central DeWitt County. To replace Indianola's dependence on water transportation, he also laid out a route for a new branch of the Gulf, Western Texas and Pacific Railroad from Indianola to San Antonio through the community. When a series of powerful hurricanes between 1875 and 1886 destroyed Indianola, Cuero, protected by its inland location, profited from the port city's demise. With Indianola in ruins, families gathered their belongings and took the railroad seventy miles inland to rebuild, creating a highly-sophisticated community at the new location almost overnight. Indianola homes were dismantled and their boards numbered and packed on the railroad to be reassembled in Cuero, where much of their original construction can still be seen today. The San Antonio and Aransas Pass

Railroad linked Cuero to Houston after the 1886 hurricane, acknowledging a population that had nearly doubled to 2500 people, while at Indianola destruction of the railroad wharves and the effects of a fire demolished the town so completely that scarcely a trace remains today.

Pridgen, Dr. James, interview, April 23, 1997;
Pridgen, 5;
"Gustav Schleicher," New Handbook of Texas.

Of those who made the trek to Cuero, a significant portion was German and also highly educated. According to James E. Pridgen, M.D.: *"The majority of the German intelligentsia from Indianola settled in Cuero during the 1870's, along with similar people from the Green DeWitt Colony. Interest in literature, music and other cultural accomplishments was at a high level."* Pridgen also notes that, although the town had a population of less than 5,000, it sent the second highest number of students from any city in Texas to the University of Texas in 1883, an indication of both its educational interest and level of culture. A community that might have otherwise taken years to develop soon flourished such that by 1873 the town had a bank, a school, drug and hardware stores, a weekly paper, and a school called the Guadalupe Academy. Cuero soon rivaled San Antonio and the northern German towns as a seat of growing cultural sophistication. While other places remained preoccupied with the issues of Reconstruction, the relatively new town of Cuero—rather than an older community like San Antonio—became the state's newest medical center. Thanks to the efforts of a German doctor, Dr. Joseph Reuss, Cuero developed several excellent medical institutions and soon enjoyed the practices of two outstanding eye, ear, nose, and throat specialists.

Nixon, Medical Story, 400-25; Pridgen, 5-10;
Texas State Journal of Medicine, 26 (June 1930), 67-69; 35 (June, 1939), 151-2;
DeWitt County Historical Commission, 67.

Members of the Reuss family who moved to Cuero brought with them traditions of German medicine that established a powerful new cultural force in South Texas. Joe Henry, the elder Reuss had been to Vienna, Paris, and Heidelberg, and became part of a distinguished group of physicians that included the Drs. Mayo and Lahey. During the Civil War he treated both Confederates and Yankees and, when the conflict ended, transferred his drugstore from Indianola to Cuero in 1872 and his medical practice in 1892. (Today the enterprise, founded in 1845 at Indianola, remains the oldest drugstore in continuous operation by the same family in Texas). Joe's son, Joseph, attended Cuero's German English School and then availed himself of the best training in the region as part of the first class to enter the University of Texas, the year it opened in 1883. Before 1891, when he returned to Cuero to enter his father's practice, he had completed a degree at the Medical College of Physicians and Surgeons at Columbia University and postgraduate surgical training at the New York Polyclinic. For postgraduate work he spent a year at the teaching hospitals of Berlin and the Allgemeine Krankenhaus in Vienna.

Pridgen, 4; Pridgen, James E. interview.

Reuss then took an important step. Transferring what he had learned in the country's most advanced medical institutions directly to South Texas the year he returned, he established the Salome I Hospital in the upper story of the town's Catholic school in 1892. When facilities there became inadequate, ladies of the community raised funds to build a new hospital, the Salome II, in 1894. Reuss went on to organize four hospitals in all, and for fifty years Cuero served as the primary medical referral center "*from the Gulf Coast to San Antonio*." Before the turn of the century, Cuero was one of the best places in South Texas to find quality medical care.

Pridgen, 2-5;
Pridgen, James E., interview

Evidence suggests that the Salome Hospital, which according to Paul Starr's theory constituted the kind of medical institution necessary to support specialists, did in fact attract them. When Reuss left Cuero in 1904 to set up a surgical practice in Dallas and organize the Marsalis Sanitarium there, he left the hospital under the direction of two eye, ear, nose and throat specialists. Though neither was German, their success relied on both the nature of the community and Reuss' achievement. The first, Frederick Kirkham (1859-1910), from Norfolk, England, had received his medical credentials in 1882 from the University of Cambridge, completed another degree at the University of Edinburgh, and served as town surgeon at the Royal

Ophthalmic Hospital in London before making the decision that brought him to Cuero in 1900 to open a practice in EENT. His choice suggests that the South Texas community had a reputation as the type of place where a doctor might do well. He later practiced at Brownsville on the Gulf, and died there on September 19, 1910, at the age of fifty-one.

Texas Medical Association membership records

The other EENT specialist, Dr. John W. Burns (1866-1939), was descended from the first Anglo-American child born in DeWitt County named Columbus Burns, who had been a stock farmer and government freight agent. The village of Burns Station through which the Gulf, Western Texas and Pacific Railroad passed to reach Cuero took its name from the Burns family. Born here in a log cabin in 1866, Burns took his medical degree in 1891 at Vanderbilt in Nashville, Tennessee, and did postgraduate work in New York in 1892, 1894 and 1897 to specialize in diseases of the eye, ear, nose and throat. Early in his practice when Cuero was a city of roughly 5,000 people, Burns drove a horse and buggy or rode horseback to reach his patients. He nonetheless went off nearly every year for further study, traveling to Vienna and other European cities in 1899, 1902 and 1908 and returning to the frontier Southwest with the ability to practice state-of-the-art medicine. It is likely that Burns returned to his native city rather than going to Houston or Galveston where competition was strong in part because of Salome Hospital and the sophistication of the town's German and European culture. There he developed a circuit practice to Yorktown and worked along the stagecoach line from Victoria to San Antonio.

Texas State Journal of Medicine, 26(June 1930), 67-9;
Burns, John W., 68-70;
Pridgen, Dr. James, interview.

Given the limited nature of medical facilities in Texas, it is difficult to believe that at one time the small town of Cuero had two fully accredited medical facilities so early in its history. Dr. Burns built the Burns Hospital in Cuero named for his father, in 1911 and with his two sons, both of whom were doctors, also built up the collection of books that later formed the backbone of the core collection at San Antonio's University of Texas Health Science Center and Medical School. Transfer of the Burns collection over a century later, therefore, represents a direct link between the beginnings of specialized medicine in South Texas and its most recent institutional developments.

University of Texas Health Science Center News Release,
May 14, 1970 on dedication of the Burns Memorial Library Collection;
Texas State Journal of Medicine (June 1939), 151.

## HEALTH SEEKERS AND PROFESSIONAL DEVELOPMENT IN SAN ANTONIO

Before the century's end, Cuero blossomed and San Antonio experienced a peaceful period that allowed physicians to establish new roles in the community. Despite the distance to essential markets, poor railroad rates, and a lack of surface water and mineral resources that limited local industry to cement-making and brewing, the Alamo City never welcomed innovation with greater speed or vitality than in the last thirty years of the nineteenth century. In 1877 a throng of citizens carrying flags, Chinese lanterns, and hundreds of flaming torches had celebrated the arrival of the first railroad to serve San Antonio with regular passenger trains. Doors had opened to robust new hotels, banks, retail stores and office buildings, and Colonel Belknap's mule-drawn streetcars carried residents for a nickel to San Pedro Springs Park, where local newspapers advertised "*Dancing, Swinging, Rowing*." By the mid-1880s, water flowed through a new distribution system and electric incandescent lamps had replaced the gaslights that had defined an era. The area in front of the Alamo commonly referred to as a "mudhole" had been transformed into a park, and Julius Joske and his sons had vacated their modest Austin Street adobe building and relocated their dry goods store on Alamo Plaza next to the Menger Hotel. By 1900 the Alamo City had become a major distribution center, a mercantile and financial center for the military and the cattle industry, and the state's largest community. Infected by the sweep of recent progress, the Evening Light newspaper vividly described the "*new*" San Antonio as follows:

*"It is such a boom, such a rush, such good natured busy prosperity that our people do not realize its magnitude. This Commerce Street rush*

*has overflowed into Houston Street, and from a quiet residential place it too has become a busy street with hotels and bazaars of all kinds.... A city of 30,000 people doing the business of a city of 100,000".*

Huesinger, 6;
Everett, 134-5;
King, 321;
Panfield, 2-3.

San Antonio's medical resources further increased when the federal government, accepting the responsibility to close the frontier, sent cavalry troops to protect outlying settlements from the last Native-American encroachments. Realizing the value of military support, San Antonio city fathers in 1875 offered to donate land to the U.S. Army to build soldiers' quarters and stables. The government responded by reestablishing a military headquarters in the city and, to back up the federal troops assigned to the region, made plans to replace the original log cabin dispensary. The first real post hospital was built in 1885 and, by the century's end, San Antonio's military facility had become the Army's prime administrative headquarters in the Southwest. By 1907, the year when the post was renamed Fort Sam Houston in honor of the first President of the Republic of Texas, an eighty-five-bed hospital had been constructed, and by 1912 Fort Sam Houston was the largest Army post in the United States. Creation of the Southern Department of the Army in 1913 led to further improvements at area military installations. In World War I, the base would occupy a total of 17,274 acres.

"Pocket Guide to Historic Fort Sam Houston," San Antonio, Fort Sam Houston Museum, 1994, 19; McBride; Huesinger, 40.

By 1900, the San Antonio City Directory listed the Bexar County Hospital at the Poor Farm near Rock Quarry Road, the San Antonio City Hospital, the Santa Rosa Infirmary, a South Pacific Company Hospital, and an Insane Asylum one mile south of the city. An earlier institution, the Graves and Cross Infirmary for women established in 1888, had disappeared. Rates at the Santa Rosa were seventy-five cents to one dollar for the General Wards, and between $1.50 and $3 for a private room. Now, as San Antonio expanded, the area that included Bexar County, Boerne, Austin, Fredericksburg, and

Uvalde became a popular destination for invalids, commonly referred to as the "Sanitarium of the West." A newspaper article in 1873 boasted that "there is not State of greater healthfulness than Texas, while many portions of the State, as Austin and San Antonio and hilly regions farther north and west, are the resort of consumptives who almost invariably recover and live many years." The "Sunset" line of the Houston and Texas Central Railway carried an annual flock of the sick and infirm to Sulphur Springs, Luling Springs, and Sutherland Springs. M.K. Taylor praised the area in 1888 in a piece called "The Climate of Southwestern Texas and Its Advantages as a Winter Health Resort" for the Transactions of the American Climatological Association, and in 1892 M.D. Littlejohn published an article in the New York Medical Record on "San Antonio and Southwest Texas as a Winter Resort," foreshadowing the coming of the Snowbirds, or "*winter Texans*," who today migrate to the area during the winter months. Among famous people drawn to the region were Max Krueger, the German-born president of the San Antonio Machine and Supply Company; Jay Gould, who went to El Paso in 1892 for his health; and cereal producer and health promoter, C.W. Post, who established a Texas town bearing his name.

San Antonio City Directory, 1189-90, 1899-1900;
Jones, 103-115;
Littlejohn, 235-239;
Coleman, 78

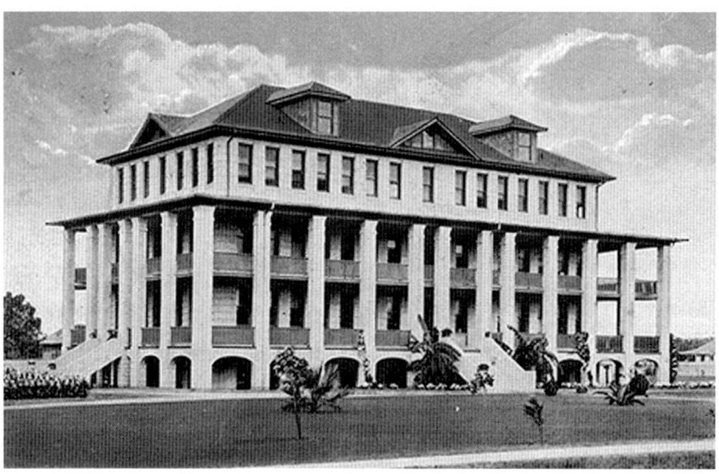

The Burns
Hospital in Cuero

## FREDERIC H. TERRELL BEGINS A TRADITION OF COMMUNITY SERVICE

San Antonio's thriving and increasingly cosmopolitan community permitted local doctors to make significant strides in professional development. In 1881 the Encyclopedia of the New West boasted that, "*the medical profession in San Antonio is ahead of Philadelphia and New York because the surgeons have full control of their cases, the climate and active habits of the people enabling them to undertake what in the North and East would not be ventured on. They have also made new departures in several directions with success.*" Dr. Frederic H. Terrell, a distinguished general practitioner who also offered specialized eye care, further improved the South Texas medical climate by serving as a model for a new, more complex and sophisticated role they might adopt in their communities. Terrell, with his successful career as a San Antonio city leader, represents the beginnings of community involvement by doctors that would in time lend further support to the acceptance of specialists.

Encyclopedia of the New West, 181

Terrell was born in Indiana in 1856, came to San Antonio through Indianola with his family in 1867, and attended the German-English school that later became San Antonio Junior College. At the time, Germans represented a strong influence in San Antonio in addition to the strictly German towns of Fredericksburg and New Braunfels. By the 1880s a German merchant elite at the center of San Antonio society built lavish homes in the King William district and created many new institutions. Men gathered in the Casino Club, exercised at the Turnverein athletic association, and held lavish annual Volksfest parades. In 1881 Scholz' Palm Garden between Alamo Street and Losoya, was the most popular place for the elegant and tasteful, and by 1895 local Germans constructed Beethoven Hall and brought a level of musical culture to the city unrivalled in the Southwest.

Fehrenbach, 4, 6; Light Years, 3-8.

Anglos organized the San Antonio Club in retaliation against the Germans, opened the Grand Opera House at Alamo Plaza, and introduced a game called polo played by riders mounted on mustangs. The enduring Catholic presence introduced by the imperial Spanish and the town's Anglo, German and Hispanic populations would never be fully absorbed

By this time, several of San Antonio's most distinguished physicians were German specialists. Eye, Ear, Nose and Throat specialist Dr. Abraham Sachs had been born in Austria in 1872 and came to the United States with his parents as a small boy, but returned to Europe for his medical training in Odessa. Sachs practiced at Cincinnati, Chicago and New York for a time, but for reasons that are not clear, he then came to San Antonio where he opened an office in the Conroy Building and became an active member of the German community. In addition to the Harmony Club, Beethoven Männerchor, Hermann Sons and other organizations, Sachs' interests extended to medical research, and his work on "*aural vertigo*" foreshadowed that of researchers after World War I on medical aspects of flight.

Coleman, Bexar County Medical Society Records

Dr. Berthold E. Hadra, an outstanding surgeon educated at the Universities of Breslau and Berlin, served in the German Army before coming to San Antonio in 1870; Dr. Julius Braunnagel, a native of Alsace-Lorraine who arrived in 1870, "*developed a large following among the German people whose language he spoke as well as his native French*." Dr. George Moechel, an immigrant with a degree from Germany's University of Tuebingen, arrived in the 1890s, established an office on Alamo Plaza where he worked as an "*oculist*," and became a prominent member of San Antonio's Beethoven Mannerchor.

Bexar County Medical Society membership records;
San Antonio City Directory

Terrell's introduction to medicine, however, took a different route, starting at the military barracks located where the Gunter Hotel stands today. As a young boy, Terrell accompanied his father on his rounds as paymaster for the troops in a vehicle that also served as an ambulance. His inspiration came from Dr. Dallas Bacle, an Army surgeon from Philadelphia who had been stationed on the San Antonio frontier. Terrell later served as acting assistant surgeon for the United States Army, but first graduated from De Pauw University in Indiana and in 1881 received a medical degree from Harvard University before he returned to San Antonio to practice medicine.

Although Terrell did not receive a credential in ophthalmology at Harvard, the human eye had already become one of his major interests. According to the San Antonio City Directory, by 1890 he shared his practice with Dr. John Victor Spring, a graduate of the Philadelphia College of Medicine and Surgery who described himself as an oculist and aurist, the equivalent of an ophthalmologist before qualifications for the specialty had been formally established. Henceforth, the two advertised as "*Spring and Terrell, Oculists and Aurists*," indicating that Terrell also considered himself capable of treating eye problems.

BCMS Membership Files; San Antonio City Directory.

Established at the center of the community, Terrell and Spring also became active in advancing the medical profession through organized institutions. As early as 1887 Spring was appointed to a committee with Drs. Hilgartner of Austin and Hodges of Galveston to formulate plans for a state ophthalmological and otological society, and in 1907 he was nominated for the Legislative Committee that pursued professional improvements in medicine at the state level. In addition, the young specialist gave a number of papers at the Bexar County Medical Society, including one entitled "*Neuroses of the Eye Due to Stricture in the Male Urethra.*" In 1889, Spring practiced on West Commerce Street, and by 1914 he had moved to the Moore Building, indicating that he had established a separate and successful practice as a specialist after the turn of the century.

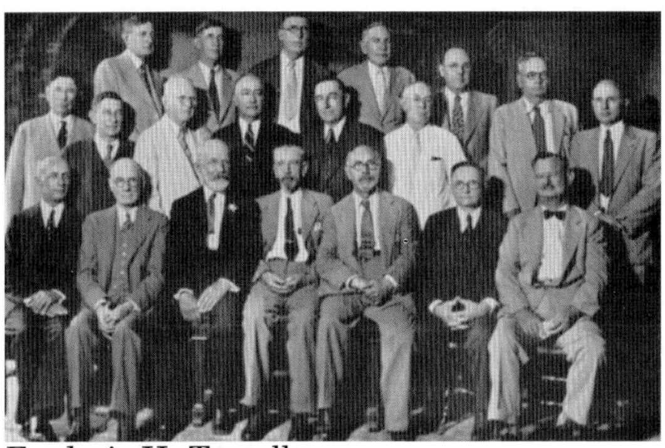

Frederic H. Terrell
(seated, third from the left)

Bexar County Medical Society records

Dr. Terrell, meanwhile, gained a distinguished reputation and become a San Antonio civic leader. The Terrell family home originally occupied the downtown site on which the St. Anthony-Wyndham Hotel now stands, but by the late 1920s the physician began to promote the area to the northeast as a residential addition. Terrell's efforts gained recognition in 1936 when the area known as Terrell Hills was incorporated into the community. Terrell went on to serve as San Antonio Mayor and Alderman, president of the school board, and director of the local Carnegie Library, and to represent the region as a delegate to the National Republican Convention in St. Louis. In business he served as a Director for the San Antonio Public Service Company and Alamo Dressed Beef Company and participated actively in local banking. His local social prominence led to memberships in both the San Antonio Country Club and Casino Club. In sum, these activities established a new paradigm for others to follow that removed the association of physicians with quackery and placed them solidly amid others most interested in and dedicated to improving the community's welfare. Terrell's personal success in the community also increased public awareness and support for medicine, and for specialization in particular.

## OCULISTS, AURISTS AND OTHER SPECIALISTS

By the end of the century, physicians who advertised themselves as oculists, aurists, and eye, ear, nose, and throat (EENT) specialists were well accepted in San Antonio and others had established successful practices across the region. Individual specialists still represented differing backgrounds and a wide range of expertise, but many had European training and together their numbers and experience amounted to a formidable medical community. Koch's discovery of cocaine in 1884 led to painless eye operations, and the rapid development of many new procedures. Texas medical journals reveal that by 1898 numbers of specialists had done enough research to report their findings publicly, as shown by articles on "*chronic granular conjunctivitia or trachoma*" and the "*transplantation of the rabbit cornea.*"

Transactions of the Texas Medical Association, 30:286-898;
Daniel's Texas Medical Journal, 3(9): 367-69;
E.H. Cary, 298.

Among others listed as "*oculists and aurists*" whose San Antonio careers reflect a high level of expertise was San Antonio specialist, Dr. George W. Johnson, who hailed from a family of physicians from Virginia. Born in Hickory Plains, Arkansas, Johnson had attended Vanderbilt and completed his premedical studies at Holbrook

College in Lebanon, Ohio, later Oberlin College, before graduating from Eclectic Medical College in 1883. Johnson did postgraduate work to specialize in eye, ear, nose and throat at the New York Polyclinic before he set up his Bexar County eye, ear, nose and throat practice, but in 1891 he was still listed in the city directory as an oculist and aurist. In this way, Johnson presented himself in terms familiar to the local community while offering that community a higher quality of medical care. As late as 1905, San Antonio specialists calling themselves oculists, aurists or experts in diseases of the eye, ear nose and throat included Dr. N S. Burnham, Charles Deady, Henry Olin, T.J. Tyner, Jerod Wilson, James Hall Bell, Eugene Clark, John V. Spring, George W. Johnson, Frederick Terrell, William Netter, and George Moechel.

San Antonio City Directory, 1905; BCMS Member Files.

North of San Antonio, one of the last specialists to be referred to as an "*oculist*" was an outstanding Austin specialist trained in Europe. The son of immigrants Ludwig and Kunigunda (Dietz), Hilgartner, Dr. Henry Hilgartner, had been born at Baltimore in 1868, completed his medical degree at the University of Maryland in 1889, and done post-graduate study at Baltimore, New York, and in Vienna before moving to Austin in 1891. Two years later he was appointed oculist for the Texas School for the Blind, beginning a lifelong interest in problems of the blind. Referring to the Swiss model for infant eye care, Hilgartner proposed that legislation be passed to protect babies from ophthalmic neonatorum. In 1895 an Eye, Ear and Throat Charity Hospital incorporated in Austin and operated at Brazos and then Colorado Streets. In 1896 Dr. Hilgartner founded the Texas Eye, Ear Nose and Throat Hospital, later known as the Texas Sanitarium, where he served as a surgeon and chief of operations from 1896 to 1912. From 1932 until his death he also served as oculist for the Texas School for Colored Deaf and Dumb. A "*regular and valuable contributor to ophthalmic medical literature*," Hilgartner spoke on a range of topics, including "*Thiersch's Skin Grafts for Pterygium*" at the Texas O&O Society, and is credited as the first Texas physician to use x-ray in the treatment of retinoblastoma.

Coleman, 78;
Ferris and Hoppe, 207;
"A Glimpse into the Past," 100-03;
"Hilgartner, Henry Louis," New Handbook of Texas.

In the early years of the twentieth century, doctors began to advertise using the term "specialist" or at least to refer to themselves as practitioners of EENT, including native South Texans and others who had enjoyed the benefits of European training. Dr. Henry Redmond, who practiced at Corpus Christi, was the son of Henry Redmond and Refugio Cuellar Diaz Stakes Redmond. The future eye, ear, nose, and throat specialist was educated by a private tutor at San Ignacio and later attended Hidalgo Academy at San Patricio and schools at Corpus Christi. Redmond was part of one of the first classes at Texas A&M College, attended Vanderbilt University, and received his medical degree from the University of Pennsylvania in 1886. After a year's practice at Galveston, he went to Europe for three years to study the eye, ear, nose, and throat in Berlin, Vienna and Paris. Part of this experience included serving as first assistant to Professor Hirschberg at the Von Graefe Eye Clinic in Berlin for two years, and later as first assistant to the surgeon to Her Majesty, Queen Victoria, at the Royal Ophthalmic Hospital in London. In 1893 Redmond returned to Corpus Christi, where he became an influential medical leader. In practice continuously until 1933, he also studied yellow fever in Cuba, worked during vacations at Chautauqua, New York and at Monterrey, Saltillo, and San Luis Potosi, Mexico, and became a charter member of the Nueces County Medical Society.

BCMS Member Files

Dr. James Slaughter Steele, born in 1871 at Fayetteville, Arkansas, also received his medical training in Europe. A graduate of the Coronal Institute in San Marcos, Texas, Steele received his medical degree from Vanderbilt in 1892 and completed his training by studying diseases of the eye, ear, nose, and throat at Chicago. Steele then extended specialized medicine into Mexico, establishing an eye, ear, nose and throat practice that lasted for fifteen years in Monterrey, Mexico, and serving as consulting oculist for the Mexican National Railways. He then returned to Texas, where he worked for two years at Dripping Springs. In 1911, however, Steele was off again, this time to Vienna for postgraduate study. Among his most notable professors was Ernst Fuchs. When Steele opened his San Antonio eye, ear, nose and throat practice in the Gibbs Building in 1912, he was a cosmopolitan and highly-trained physician.

BCMS Member Files

Native EENT specialist Dr. Frank Douglas Boyd practiced for a time at San Antonio before doing postgraduate work in New York, Vienna, Berlin and London. He later wound up in Fort Worth, where he became the senior member at Boyd and Boyne Hospital. Dr. Oscar Hunt Judkins, a native Texan who graduated from the Galveston Medical Branch in 1907, did his postgraduate work at Tulane and the University of Vienna and by the 1920s was associated with San Antonio's Eye, Ear, Nose and Throat Hospital.

Judkins later became a principal stockholder in the Fredericksburg and Llano Railroad. At the start of World War II, however, he applied to the War Production Board and the Interstate Commerce Commission and sold the line for scrap.

BCMS Member Files.

Dr. Frank H. Rosebrough was not a native Texan, but was among those who carried the benefits of specialization to the region by practicing in Texas. He was born in St. Louis, Missouri, in 1878 and graduated from St. Louis University in 1904. Rosebrough then turned to ophthalmology and studied at Vienna and other European centers. From 1914 to 1922 he practiced at Brownwood before coming to San Antonio, where he joined the staffs of the Nix and Physicians and Surgeons Hospitals. His interest in microscopic laboratory research on disease conditions of the eye reflected the influence of his European education, and by 1940 Rosebrough was one of five strict ophthalmologists at San Antonio. Rush Medical College graduate Dr. Albert R. Beal worked in Illinois and Iowa and spent time as a surgeon with the U.S. Public Health Service before coming to Texas, where he served as an examiner for several insurance companies. Dr. Beal eventually limited his North Presa Street practice to the eye and may have preceded Dr. John Burleson, most frequently thought to be the community's first ophthalmologist, as San Antonio's first true ophthalmologist.

BCMS Member Files.

## THE END OF THE CENTURY: THE SPANISH-AMERICAN WAR AND THE FLEXNER REPORT

The Spanish-American War was among the last major events to affect South Texas in the nineteenth century. Dr. Leonard Wood organized and assembled three cavalry regiments at San Antonio, and many Texas physicians responded in the tradition of their predecessors and joined the fight. Among those who participated in the conflict was a career military man named Dr. Frederic H. Thorne, who would subsequently become an ophthalmologist and play an important role in the region's history. Another was Dr. Clarence Lucien McClellan, a specialist in diseases of the eye, ear, nose and throat, who came to Texas from Mississippi and was a member of the first class of the University of Dallas Medical Department that became Baylor University College of Medicine. McClellan received his medical degree from the Physicians and Surgeons College at St. Louis in 1905, and then spent three years in Mexico. He subsequently practiced at Rockport, Aransas Pass, Groom, Odessa, and DeLeon, and then went to New Mexico, but eventually found his way back to Texas.

Nixon, Medicine in San Antonio, 312

The custom of going to Europe for medical training persisted until World War I. In 1912, only four medical schools survived in all of Texas: Baylor University College of Medicine in Dallas, Southern Methodist University Medical Department in Dallas; Medical Department of Texas Christian University, and the University of Texas Medical Department in Galveston. For South Texans, only Galveston provided ready access to medical training. A Carnegie Foundation survey in 1910 that resulted in publication of The Flexner Report on Medical Education produced an outpouring of interest in standardizing and improving medical training and practice nationwide. Dr. Abraham Flexner's visit to Galveston in 1909 resulted in praise for the University of Texas Medical Branch facility. Henceforth, medical development in South Texas would be perceived as part of a growing national system. World War I would sever links with Europe that German settlers and frontier doctors had forged, ending America's nearly forty-year dependence on European medical training, but the new century would give birth to a powerful American medical system where new types of training in specialized medicine could develop.

Faculty and Staff of the University of Texas Medical Branch, 101;
Lesky, 445-6;
Fuchs, Ernst Autobiography;
Bonner, Th. N., 1912;
Carnegie Commission on Higher Education, 25.

By 1903 the founding of the American Medical Association of Vienna to aid American physicians studying there established a last link with Vienna and European science. This organization survived the first World War and enjoyed a golden era thereafter, when international postgraduate courses were organized that formed the basis for the present Academy of Postgraduate Medical Education. The arrival of immigrants also continued for some years, bringing ophthalmologists Drs. Fred Frueholtz and Paul Suehs, both of who were born in Germany, to South Texas. By World War I, however, new traditions had begun to emerge. Creation of the Western Ophthalmological and Otolaryngological Society in 1896 at Kansas City, a key step in the development of specialized medicine in the western states, had little effect in Texas but would ultimately effect the profession everywhere in the United States. Started in part "*to spite the snooty Eastern Seaboard American Ophthalmology Society*" thought to be composed of aristocrats who looked down on the "*peasants' of the midwest*," the new organization strengthened the foothold of specialized medicine at first primarily in states to the north. By 1902, however, the WOOL Society, as it was known, renamed itself the American Academy of Ophthalmology and Otolaryngology. Creation of the American Board of Ophthalmology in 1916, the first organization in the field to be created, rested on the cumulative accomplishments that preceded it. Its requirement of seven years of graduate training was a clear reflection of the significant advances in the field. It would take another twenty years before specialists in the Southwest unified their profession and established a similar institution at the regional level, but a foundation had been laid.

Vail, 11

# CHAPTER 6

## THE FIRST GENERATION OF SPECIALISTS: 1890-1914

*The success of specialism has turned the heads of half the rising generation of medical men. It seems with them to be an accepted fact, that not to be a specialist of some sort is to be nothing.*

"Specialism as a Practice," New York Medical Record, 1875

*This Association recognizes specialties in proper and legitimate fields of practice.*

American Medical Association, 1869

*And there were only three doctors for the whole county; so more often than not the patient was dead before the doctor could even see him.*

Arda Talbot Allen, Miss Ella of the Deep South of Texas

San Antonio ophthalmologists today follow traditions and paradigms established by the "*first generation*" of specialists to practice in the region, a cohort of contemporaries who received their training at approximately the same time and who arrived in South Texas around the turn of the century. The purpose of this chapter is to give the reader a sense of the adventures, vicissitudes, and rich professional life experienced by early ophthalmologists. Before World War I, only a handful of physicians outside the Eastern Seaboard and along the recently closed Texas frontier devoted their practices exclusively to ophthalmology, yet within a generation ophthalmologists or their contemporaries in eye, ear, nose and throat were established their specialties in both major Texas cities and the rural hinterland. With growing prosperity in the region came new medical innovations, a new faith in medical science, and rapid progress in specialized medicine.

A detailed account of three representative men—three early South Texas specialists—not only clarifies the scope and substance of this achievement but captures the flavor of medical life at a time remarkably different from our own. Taken together, the stories of Drs. John Burleson, Donald Atkinson, and Edwin Meredith Sykes provide a wealth of detail about how professional advances transformed old-fashioned oculists and aurists into full-fledged ophthalmologists and otolaryngologists. In particular, their stories demonstrate the importance of professional organizations, permanent medical institutions, and medical standards in supporting specialization; the beginnings of a tradition of research; and the lasting contributions that made physicians leaders in their local communities. Dr. John H. Burleson's life demonstrates that ophthalmologists played a leading role in building a healthy environment for statewide medical development and emphasizes Cuero's early role in the state's medical history (one that has generally been overlooked). Dr. Donald T. Atkinson's career demonstrates how a "horse and buggy doctor" achieved the cultural transfer of the latest American and European medicine to the frontier and started a tradition of ophthalmic research there. Finally, the experience of Dr. Edwin Meredith Sykes captures an element common to the stories of all three as a prominent citizen who helped San Antonio become a cosmopolitan city and a major medical center.

# DR. JOHN H. BURLESON AND PROFESSIONAL DEVELOPMENT

San Antonio's Dr. John H. Burleson came from a line of "*preachers, Indian fighters and statesmen.*" The first Burleson family representative in America, Burleson's paternal grandfather, was an Irish immigrant who had arrived in Maryland in 1723, toured the Southwest in 1824 with a group of explorers and hunters from Tennessee, and obtained Spanish land grants from Moses Austin to bring his family into the region. Four of the original Burleson brothers who came to Texas received grants of 400 acres each on the Colorado River between Smithville and LaGrange, and Jacob Burleson, a relative, had been killed at the Battle of Brushy Creek near Round Rock. Dr. Burleson was proud of the fact that his parents were native Texans and that his roots went back to the time when the Texas colonies first sought their independence from Mexico. He himself had been born in November 1867, in a log cabin at Bastrop near the Colorado River in the dark days of Reconstruction when the state still suffered from the ravages of the Civil War. Members of his family fought for the Confederacy, and a Texas county would eventually be named for the pioneering Burleson clan.

Dr. John M. Smith interview;
Dr. John Burleson obituary;
Bexar County Medical Society Records

Why John Burleson decided to pursue a career in medicine is uncertain, but was no small accomplishment given the difficulties of his early life. His parents had died while he was still a child, and poverty forced him to take his first job as a newspaper boy in Austin when that town was still located on the edge of the Texas frontier. His fortunes improved, however, when General Edward Burleson, a distinguished relative and former Lieutenant Governor of the Texas Republic, adopted him. As a result, Burleson was able to attend the University of Texas in 1886 and 1887, and from there went on to receive his medical degree in 1890 from Missouri Medical College, one of the earliest institutions to offer medical training in the American West. As a newly-minted physician, Burleson spent the next five years as a general practitioner and country doctor at Huntsville in Walker County in Southeast Texas, one of the region's most highly populated areas at the time.

It may be noted that in 1889, as the Texas State Medical Association received its second charter, the Texas Legislature called for the establishment of a medical department at the University of Texas—one of its first major efforts to support medical education in the state. Later the Missouri Medical College at St. Louis became the University of Missouri that merged with Washington University.

Dr. John M. Smith interview;
Bexar County Medical Society Records;
Ferris and Hoppe 188

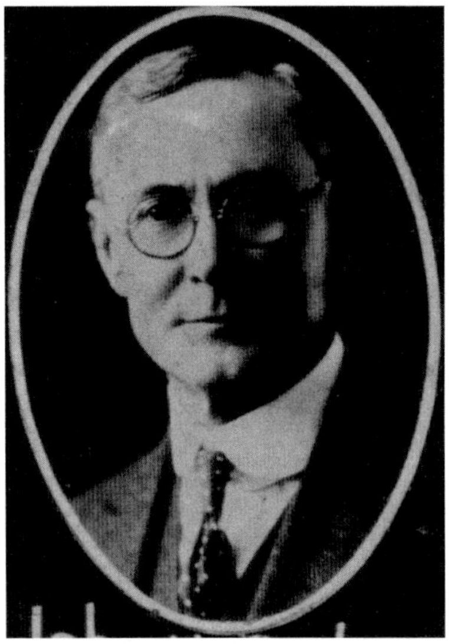

Dr. John H. Burleson

Records show that poor health limited Burleson's ability to undertake the strenuous tasks of such branches of medical practice as surgery, and may have been a factor in his decision to specialize in eye, ear, nose and throat. For post-graduate training, he studied diseases of the eye, ear, nose and throat at the Ochsner Clinic in New Orleans and spent another year in New York before returning to Texas in 1897. This time he did not go to Huntsville, but instead followed members of his family up the Colorado River to establish his first eye, ear, nose and throat practice at Lampasas in the Texas hinterland. Discovering that he missed the pace and professional climate of urban life, however, he soon moved on to the emerging medical center at Cuero where the substantial German immigrant population of Indianola had gone after that community's demise in a hurricane.

Dr. John M. Smith interview;
Dr. John Burleson obituary

Before Victoria replaced it, Cuero served as a major railroad crossroads and cotton center for much of South Texas. Despite a population of less than 6,000 residents, the town also was already recognized as a medical center. Due to the powerful influence of the Reuss family and its economic role, Cuero retained its importance until economic change and World War II defense contracts helped Houston overshadow every other community in the region. Before the turn of the century, however, San Antonio's "first surgeon" caught the train

Medical License of
John H. Burleson, M.D.,
to practice medicine in Texas,
dated 1908.
Dr. Burleson was one of the
early San Antonio
ophthalmologists. mentor, and
later partner of
Dr. Marion W. McCurdy
Courtesy of The Gordon Library,
Department of Ophthalmology, UTHSCSA

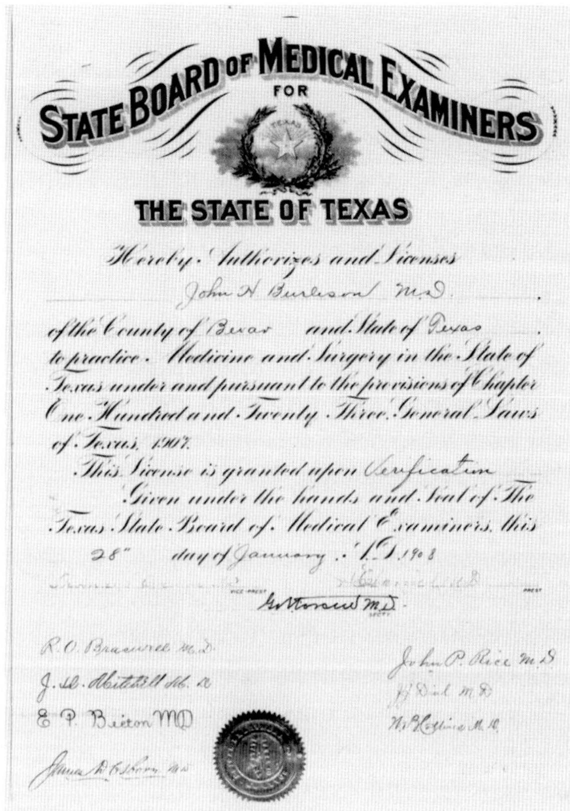

STATE BOARD OF MEDICAL EXAMINERS
FOR
THE STATE OF TEXAS

Hereby Authorizes and Licenses
John H Burleson M.D.
of the County of Bexar and State of Texas
to practice Medicine and Surgery in the State of
Texas under and pursuant to the provisions of Chapter
One Hundred and Twenty Three General Laws
of Texas, 1907.
This License is granted upon Verification
Given under the hands and Seal of The
Texas State Board of Medical Examiners, this
28" day of January A.D. 1908

to operate there and doctors across the region referred patients to Cuero's Salome Hospital. As a result, Cuero no doubt afforded more opportunity for a young doctor than Lampasas. Burleson settled there some time between 1897 and 1899 at approximately the same time as Dr. Frederick William Kirkham. It is probable that both Drs. Burns and Kirkham served as Burleson's mentors, introducing him to new ideas and sensitizing him to medical issues of the time.

The railroad that went from Houston to Waco and Flatonia was likely the San Antonio and Aransas Pass.

Dr. John M. Smith interview;
Bexar County Medical Society Records;
"Cuero," New Handbook of Texas

To support himself as he built up his Cuero practice, Dr. Burleson performed "contract work" for the railroads that passed through the community—a common means for many doctors at the time to supplement their local practices. Contract practices offered full medical service for men working for the railroads, and usually their families as well, at minimal cost. This old-fashioned way of providing medical service resembled a "*circuit practice*" since it required the doctor to travel by train or stage coach line on a regular route; in this case, between Victoria and San Antonio. Cuero's strategic location at the terminus of the railroad that stretched from Indianola to the inland trade territory west and south of the Colorado River made it easier for Burleson to expand his practice and develop a network of patients and colleagues that reached deep into the hinterland. Witness to his early reputation is the story of a horse race at which a man was struck in the eye after trying to dissuade another man from cursing in front of ladies. Dr. Burleson, described as "known locally as a top specialist," was sent for and came by special train to Victoria to attend the injured man. By the time physicians bidding for contracts became a threat to the goals of the Texas Medical Association, he had risen to become a spokesman for organized medicine, working for a Medical Practice Act to regulate the profession. At a meeting of the Railway Surgery Section of the Texas State Medical Association some years later, Burleson recalled working with injured railroad workers as a learning experience. "*This phase of ophthalmic practice has been particularly brought to my notice on account of my connection with railroad work, and the great number of accidents I am called upon to treat.*" Railroad doctors typically removed cinders from workers' eyes with toothpicks wrapped in cotton and sharpened a match or used the point of a pocket knife to remove foreign bodies, but the job nonetheless provided valuable experience and prepared Burleson for his next step.

Drs. Scott and White, who later founded a major hospital in Temple, Texas, did contract work for the Santa Fe Railroad that extended their practices from Amarillo to Galveston.

Mrs. Bell Louise Stevenson interview;
Dr. John Smith interview, April 5, 1996;
Dunlop, 160-1;
Burrow, James G., 59;
Burleson, John, "First Aid to Injured Eyes;"
Dr. Marion W. McCurdy interview

Although by 1905 Cuero had the capacity to support medical specialists, Burleson was sufficiently established to strike out for a place where he could develop a more lucrative practice. He may have moved to San Antonio in part to avoid the ongoing competition between Drs. Reuss and Burns, which may have limited his ability to more fully realize his own ambitions, but there were other reasons as well. When he set up his Moore Building office, San Antonio was no thriving or dynamic metropolis, but had begun to show signs of more substantial development. Although conditions around 1895 were such that two Germans set up a trout line on the San Antonio River in downtown San Antonio and caught sixteen pounds of fish in two hours, a more cultivated atmosphere had begun to develop alongside less savory elements of the community. In 1897, two local ladies of some prominence, Miss M.B. Fenwick and Miss Sara Hartman, published a Directory of Societies and Ladies Address List that served "*as an index to San Antonio's progress in all those things that tend towards the development of culture and refinement in any community.*" Church on Sunday morning might take place in a hall over a Saturday night saloon, but Catholic and Protestant religious services were regularly conducted in at least four languages—Spanish, English, German and Polish. For inhabitants with finer sensibilities, not all of the evening amusements were of the raucous sort still to be found in the plazas. More stable denizens now sought social clubs and more sophisticated entertainments. The Casino Association's dazzling Mardi Gras Carnival, one reporter declared, "*compared favorably with those of other more populous cities on this continent,*" and the French Social Club and the Turner Association or Turn-Verein staged similar fetes. Expansion of the Guenther Mills in 1900 and a new Swift meatpacking plant built in 1903 improved the business climate.

In Cuero, the Reuss-Burns conflict continued until 1911 when Burns honored his father by founding the Burns Hospital, a modern institution that came to be known for its early use of therapeutic and diagnostic techniques, including electrocardiography and radium therapy. Reuss returned from Dallas briefly to head the medical department of the San Antonio and Aransas Pass Railroad before leaving again to study at Berlin's teaching hospital and Vienna's Allgemeine Krankenhaus. Missing his intended passage on the maiden voyage of the Titanic on April 20, 1912, he returned to Cuero convinced of the need to build an even larger hospital and subsequently erected the Reuss Memorial Hospital to honor his father. In retrospect, the act looks suspiciously like a case of one-upsmanship, but one that nonetheless made the tiny town of Cuero into a first-rate medical center. The elder Dr. Reuss published articles on his work in Philadelphia on cholera between1845 and 1875, learned surgical techniques in Germany, and was acquainted with both Lahey and the Mayos.

Fehrenbach, 3; McCurdy interview; San Antonio City Directory.

More important for the young physician, San Antonio possessed the basic medical infrastructure needed to support professional specialists, including the Bexar County Medical Society and several permanent medical institutions. When Burleson arrived, the county medical society was decades old and had been reorganized in 1903 according to the guidelines of the American Medical Association. A year after Burleson arrived it was actively engaged with the *Ladies Home*

*Journal* and *Colliers Weekly* in a crusade against patent medicine. According to one local ophthalmologist, the Bexar County Medical Society served as an "*arbiter of the profession*" that steadied competition and established communication among practitioners. The new Physicians and Surgeons Hospital downtown, just completed in 1903, gave medicine a more visible presence in the community. By 1908, when Dr. Ferdinand Herff performed his last operation at the Santa Rosa Hospital, that facility had newly-expanded operations. Herff died in 1912, but by then a legacy of excellence had been established. Each of these achievements formed part of the foundation on which a successful ophthalmology practice might be established.

Bexar County Medical Society Minutes, February 1906;
Dr. Dan Russell interview;
American Medical Association Directory, 1909;
Burrow, James G., "Economic and Political Policies of the Texas Medical Profession in the Progressive Era"

Burleson eventually limited his practice to ophthalmology when younger colleagues with more recent training in the specialty joined him. "*Dr. John*," as he came to be known, was the first San Antonio ophthalmologist, however, to own a tenometer to check for the pressure of glaucoma and was credited with modifying the technique for cataract surgery devised by Lieutenant Colonel Smith of India. The Bexar County Medical Society Journal documents his clinical research work with patients from both the Anglo and Hispanic communities in reports on "*The Granulation of the Conjunctiva*" and "*Some Observations Concerning the Etiology of Glaucoma*." As a founder of San Antonio's first Eye, Ear, Nose and Throat Hospital, he also was instrumental in creating the city's first specialized hospital facility, opened in 1931 on Main Avenue behind the present Baptist Hospital.

Dr. John Smith interview;
Bexar County Medical Society Journal 1905, 1910-14;
San Antonio O&O Society Minutes, March 3, 1931;
Bexar County Medical Society Records.

Burleson also looked beyond his specialty to the profession as a whole. Experience had taught him the value of organized medicine, and he clearly understood the need for standards to regulate medical practice. Despite regional achievements, Texas medicine at the start of his San Antonio career was likely to be relatively primitive and unsophisticated. Important attitudes necessary for the public to accept specialized medicine had not yet taken hold. The lack of standardization led to one Texan's recollection that his grandmother generally called in not one, but several, doctors to improve the odds that an ailing family member might receive effective treatment. Dr. E.H. Cary, Dean of the University of Dallas that became Baylor University, remembered that in Texas as late as 1901, "*countless persons who had become blind with glaucoma had been told they had cataracts that could be removed when they became blind.*" Many people in rural outposts retained the provincial belief that little could be done to combat illness or put their faith in native doctors and curanderas who offered only comfort and patience. One of the more noticeably unfortunate cases of the period was referred to simply as "*Strabismus Bill.*"

Cary, E.H., 299;
Ferris and Hoppe, 214;
Nixon, Century of Medicine, 84.

Dr. Burleson also understood the common philosophy held by frontier physicians, as indicated by his comment that "*Most of us practice medicine as individuals; we reach our conclusions as the result of personal experience.*" But it was this condition, in a sense, that he wished to improve by uniting physicians around a shared standard. As Rosen pointed out, a specialty could be said to exist "*only when there are bonds between practitioners, which take shape within an association based upon like interests and common problems.*"

John Burleson, First Aid to Injured Eyes;
Rosen, 36

Almost as soon as he arrived in San Antonio, Burleson developed a presence and made important contacts in the community. Records show that he and Captain T.E. Moore were injured in a baseball game between San Antonio doctors and lawyers in 1905, and that he had become a Mason and a member of St. Luke's Episcopal Church by year's end. As a charter member of the Order of the Alamo he established links with prominent citizens who staged the city's annual Fiesta celebration, and later he owned a controlling interest in the professional baseball team, the San Antonio Missions. Once established as a community leader, the doctor described by P.I. Nixon as a man who "*ran things*" was now in a position to serve as a leader and spokesman for the medical profession as a whole.

*The team ultimately proved to be a bad investment when the Ball Park burned. According to an associate, Burleson later suffered heavy losses in the Depression when the City Central Bank failed, but by then his practice was less important and he often treated old friends for free.*

Nixon, Century of Medicine, 202;
Dr. John M. Smith interview;
Bexar County Medical Society Records;
McCurdy, Anne Ayers Lide, 147

Faced by the need to regulate aspects of the medical profession over which no control existed, Burleson became an institution builder and leader in professional organization. Throughout his distinguished sixty-year career, he acted as a spokesman on current issues, bound physicians together by raising their awareness, and along the way gained social sanction for specialized medicine from the community at large. Initially, he took on one of the most urgent problems of the day by confronting the quackery that dominated frontier society. Some idea of the conditions he faced can be garnered from the work of San Antonio EENT specialist Charles David Dixon, who documented South Texas medical swindlers in his book The Menace: An Exposition of Quackery Nostrum Exploitation and Reminiscences of a Country Doctor, published in 1914. In particular, Dixon mentioned two "*eye specialist humbugs*" named Craig and Neuman, who claimed to be doctors of optometry with the ability to "*correct every defect of vision, such as cross eyes, headache, sleeplessness and astigmatism.*"

Dixon, 32;
Dr. Joseph DeGasperi interview;
Cary, 298-301;
BCMS Minutes;
TMA Records.

Dixon, a San Marcos native, had attended Tulane and Jefferson Medical College in Philadelphia and practiced briefly at Junction, Texas, before coming to San Antonio. He later did postgraduate work at Chicago's Eye, Ear, Nose and Throat College and the New York Polyclinic before limiting his general practice to eye, ear, nose and throat. Apparently a well-respected member of the community, Dixon was on the staff of the Santa Rosa Hospital and later joined the staff of San Antonio's R.B. Green Hospital when it opened in 1915. He also served as president of the Bexar County Medical Society, offered professional services at the Mexican Christian Institute, the Home of Neighborly Service, and San Antonio Salvation Army Home at San Antonio, and served in the Medical Corps of the U.S. Army in World War I).

Offering "*a concise history of the work of ridding the county of quacks and nostrum exploiters*," Dixon's book demonstrated that standards were needed to end Texas' tolerance for quackery, expose false claims, and protect the public. According to his findings, most quacks obtained their education in a "*fourth class medical college or some summer or night school.*" Unable to compete with better-trained physicians, Dixon's typical villain resorted to advertising to get business. One notorious consumption cure known as "*Mexicantuberculogetwell*" and the "*great goat lymph treatment*", he learned, had been made from substances found in the "*back yard and woodpile.*" Dixon regularly sent people disguised as patients to incompetent practitioners and then filed charges against them for practicing medicine without a license, fraudulent use of the mails, or even vagrancy. Most individuals either fled the state, paid a fine, or spent time in jail. One man alone, however, could not put an end to the threat of quackery. A more lasting solution depended on the backing of medical professionals, working together under the leadership of someone capable of organizing their efforts.

Dixon, 15-30

In 1873 the thirteenth Texas Legislature had passed an act that provided for some regulation by permitting Texas counties to register doctors coming into the state, established Boards of Medical Examiners, and required medical degrees, or "*certificates of qualification*" from all physicians practicing in the state. Stronger laws were clearly needed, however. In the course of his career, Burleson confronted A.B. McCanna, an "*electro therapeutist*" who claimed to have an electric battery made in France that could cure all the diseases of mankind. Dr. N.A. Haizlip provided "*painless and quick*" medical solutions at the Gunter Building, and the obscure, but intriguing, Dr. Tom L. Miller offered simply "*something new in medicine.*" Both of these individuals eventually were run out of town, but Dr. Phenomenal managed to maintain his practice until 1910. A more notable case was that of a seventy-five-year-old German lady who had her eye removed and mailed to Dr. W. O. Coffee of Des Moines for repair and return, one of a number of quacks who advertised the ability to diagnose by mail or cure without operation. Dr. J. Harvey Moore claimed he could cure cataract by the "*absorbent method*" and straighten crossed eyes without surgery. "*The skilled practitioner was a rarity along the frontier,*" according to one historian, who also said:

"*It was difficult to distinguish between practitioners. A diploma was easily obtained, and often none was needed. There were few standardizing medical boards and certifying agencies, no real authority, and no real science of medicine*".

No specialist could practice successfully surrounded by charlatans, and hosts of patent medicine salesmen only further confused the pub-

lic with false promises and misinformation about science.
The new Texas Constitution of 1875 provided for the Legislature to pass laws establishing minimum qualifications for medical practitioners. A year later, the Legislature repealed the 1873 law and enacted a new one that remained in effect until 1901.

Nixon, Century of Medicine, 212;
Dixon, 26;
Jones, 27-28;
Ferris and Hoppe, 191

For two years after he arrived in San Antonio, Burleson led the effort that produced the Medical Practice Act of 1907, motivated by a desire to create a standard for medical practice based on attainment rather than length of study. Working with members of the Bexar County Medical Society and representatives of the Texas Medical Association, he organized an effort to approach the Texas Legislature on behalf of the cause. It would be one of his most important contributions to the profession. In an article on the conflicting interests of optometrists and ophthalmologists, Burleson stressed, "*that the eye, ear, nose and throat men of the country must establish a standard or suffer the consequences*." To overcome resistance, medical leaders needed to convince the Texas Legislature that physicians' demands were made in the interest of improved public health and disease prevention, rather than selfish protection. In time, the Texas medical profession adopted "*the subtle strategy of association, assimilation, and absorption*," resulting in the legislature's adoption of one examining board for all physicians.
(The Medical Practice Act of 1901, described as "ineffective and subject to abuse," was supplanted by the 1907 act.

Ross, A.A., 72;
Burleson, "Standardization of Ophthalmology and the Ethical Attitude of Its Members," 52;
"Health and Medicine," New Handbook of Texas;
Burrow, 56-7;
Nixon, Century of Medicine in San Antonio, 145;
Bexar County Medical Society Records.

The effort also enlisted practitioners and medical societies at the national level. Representatives of the American Medical Association traveled across the state to publicize the need for better public health regulations while Burleson and the others went to Austin to plead the case. As part of the delegation, the young doctor attended three successive legislative sessions before winning support for the legislation that assured the growth of the profession and no longer required young medical school graduates to compete with fraudulent doctors for patients. The resulting "*Act to Define and Regulate the Practice of Medicine*," later recognized as one of the best laws of its kind in the United States, remained in force until 1981. This fundamental legislation provided for a single Board of Medical Examiners and required applicants for medical licenses to be graduates of "*a reputable medical college*." Not only did the law allow the state to prosecute offending quacks, but it gave the profession some control over licensing, income, and the contract practice of railroad and East Texas lumber companies that sought to organize and exploit the medical profession.

Dr. John M. Smith interview;
BCMS Records;
"Health and Medicine," New Handbook of Texas

Passage of the Medical Practice Act was only the first of Burleson's efforts on behalf of the medical profession in South Texas. In 1910 he took another important step to strengthen the profession by introducing the idea of a statewide organization for ophthalmologists and otolaryngologists. A year later he initiated statewide discussion of the subject in an article on "*The Necessity for Ophthalmic Organization in Texas*" in the Texas State Medical Journal. In 1907 eye, ear, nose and throat specialists already had established the Harris County Oculists and Aurists Association at Houston, but no specialist organization existed across the rest of South Texas. It would take nineteen ears for Burleson's dream to be realized, but credit for the creation of the Texas Society of Ophthalmology and Otolaryngology that became an advocate for the profession at the state level goes to this outstanding San Antonio pioneer.

Texas State Medical Journal, 1911;
Moursund, Walter H., 442

Burleson spent the rest of his career in medical politics handling economic and policy problems facing the profession, working as a spokesman for medical ethics, and struggling to set standards for specialists. In addition to his other achievements, he served as sixty-ninth president of the Texas Medical Association and President of the Bexar County Medical Society. He also helped thirty-one county medical societies receive their charters. During the Progressive Era, he worked with Texas Medical Association legal counsel and lobbyist Philip Overton and others to obtain a new medical practice act, board of health, pure food and drug act, and anatomical laws for Texas and from 1931 to 1934 served as Councilor of the Fifth District of the State Medical Association and as chairman of its board in the latter year. "*Some years ago, when I was chairman of this section of the State Medical Association*," Burleson said, "*I advocated the formation of an ophthalmologic society and the establishment of a standard.*" A nineteenth-century observer might have described his work as the forging of a chain or the setting of stones in a perfect necklace, but modern metaphors of systems and networks better explain the group of linked institutions he helped to develop. Seen from the perspective of nineteenth century medicine, Dr. Burleson's accomplishments were impressive, indeed.

Southwest Texas Medicine for November 1934 notes that Burleson limited his Nix Building practice to the eye, although the date at which he did so is not known.

Dr. John M. Smith interview;
BCMS Minutes;
E.H. Cary, 298-301;
Burleson, "Standardization of Ophthalmology and the Ethical Attitude of Its Members," 52.

## DR. DONALD TAYLOR ATKINSON AND OPHTHALMIC RESEARCH

The second representative in the triumvirate of San Antonio pioneer ophthalmic specialists left his most important legacy in research. Dr. Donald Taylor Atkinson, seven years Dr. Burleson's junior, spent much of his colorful career on the frontier yet made significant medical advances. Atkinson contributed to his profession primarily by carrying his knowledge of the importance of research to Texas; not only was he instrumental in bringing medical practices developed in New England and Europe to South Texas, but his experience clearly demonstrates the manner in which medical knowledge could be successfully transferred from one place to another embodied in a single individual. Atkinson's training managed to draw on everything from the teaching of Ernst Fuchs in Vienna to Darwin's evolutionary theories and the values of a nineteenth-century classical New England education. His most remarkable feature was that he made use of everything he learned.

Donald Atkinson came from humble beginnings. Born the son of a small farmer in the rural town of Little Shemogue, New Brunswick, in 1874, he hauled nets on a lobster boat as a boy and dispensed brandy and tea on the deck of a Prince Edward Island iceboat to keep the passengers warm. Though others with his background might not have aspired to a profession, Atkinson decided to become a doctor at the age of ten or eleven after assisting a local doctor to amputate the mangled arm of a man who caught it in a threshing machine. Atkinson watched the entire operation and helped the doctor by clamping a forceps around the man's artery. For the rest of his life, he kept the forceps the doctor left behind after performing the operation.

Atkinson, Dr. Donald Taylor, Texas Surgeon, 1-15

Atkinson's powers of observation, a characteristic common to all good scientists, first emerged when he was a teenager working two thousand feet underground in a coal mine near the family home. While older men used their strength to extract the coal, boys hitched cars loaded with coal to a cable that pulled them up to the surface. Despite the hard labor, Atkinson observed something of scientific interest around him. Fossil ferns lay embedded in the shale next to the veins of coal. Though ignorant of the evolutionary theories of Charles Darwin then under public discussion, Atkinson examined and drew pictures of his discoveries, employing a habit of scientific illustration that would last a lifetime. He later showed his drawings to the doctor who attended him after the mineshaft collapsed and left him paralyzed for several weeks. Realizing the young man had potential, the doctor encouraged Atkinson to pursue his education. The event marked the first step on the path that eventually led Atkinson to Texas and ophthalmology.

Atkinson, Dr. Donald Taylor, Texas Surgeon, 1-15;
Atkinson obituary

Like many a New England farmer who abandoned the land in the 1890s, Atkinson left rural life behind and soon found his way to Boston, where he lived for a time in his Aunt Lavinia's Scollay Square rooming house. Fascinated with the great ships docked in the port, he next shipped out on a voyage to Barbados, but the life of a sailor did not suit and he soon returned to Boston. A job as coachman for a wealthy family in the fashionable community of Newtonville was another dead end, but he used his spare time to read books at the Newton Public Library. Surprisingly, it was his job as an express company freight handler that led to his first opportunity in medicine. Deliveries to Tufts College in Medford took him past Harvard University where he became acquainted with several professors who encouraged him to attend classes in English, Chemistry, Biology and Latin at a local school. This training paid off in 1894 when, while making deliveries in Belmont, he discovered McLean Hospital—the most humane and advanced institution for the mentally ill operating in the United States at the time. Seeing the hospital as an avenue to his dream of becoming a doctor, Atkinson inquired about an opening and was accepted as a student nurse. Soon he not only found himself tending patients but taking classes at Massachusetts General Hospital. By the time he graduated as a psychiatric nurse in 1899, he also had acquired a Harvard Medical School mentor who allowed him to sit in on classes in anatomy while he remained unable to afford Dartmouth Medical School. Instead, he went to work for a private Brookline mental hospital called Bournewood and continued to read medical books in preparation for the next stage in his medical career.

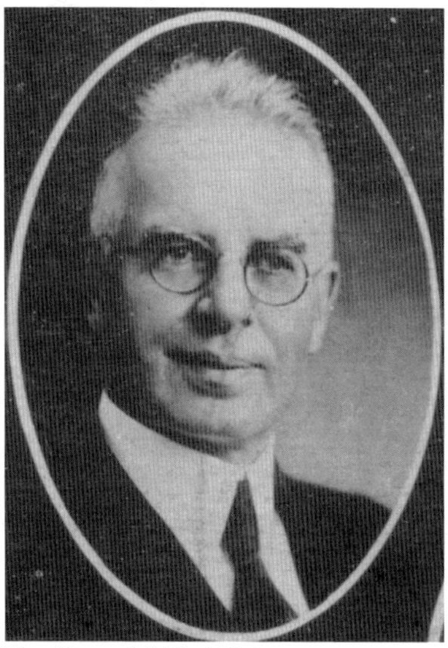
Dr. Donald T. Atkinson

Atkinson, Dr. Donald Taylor, Texas Surgeon, 17-34;
Atkinson obituary

Until this point Atkinson's only connection with the West was a great uncle, John Atkinson, who had been shot by a firing squad in the El Paso Salt War, a political struggle over title to salt deposits at the foot of Guadalupe Peak in West Texas. When his parents separated and his mother and brother moved to California, however, his attention shifted to new possibilities in the West. His next job took him to South Dakota accompanying a new patient, an affluent young antiquarian with an interest in military forts who wanted to investigate military installations there. When Atkinson arrived on the frontier,

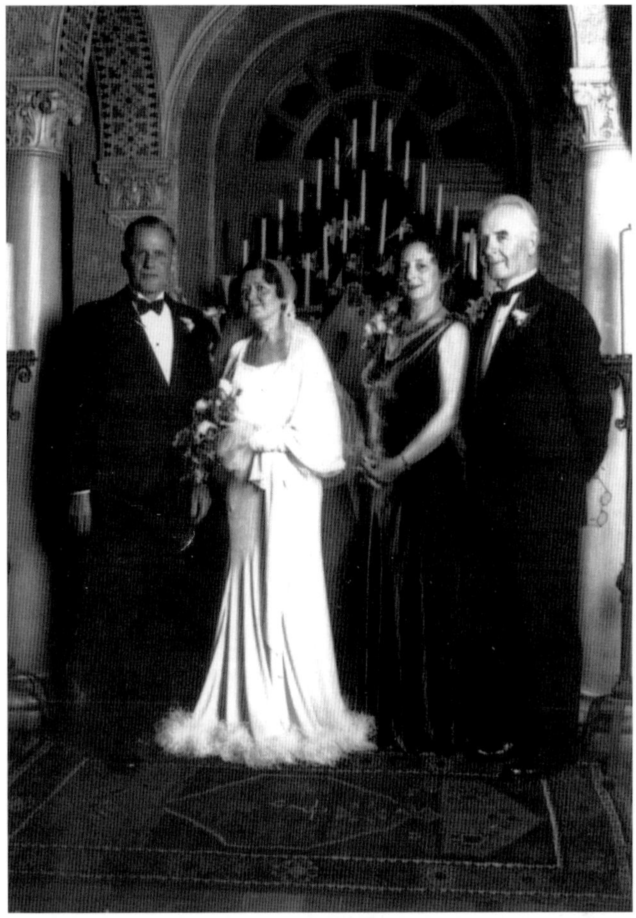

L to R: Mr. and Mrs. Eugene Hall Winkworth, Marion K. McNay and Dr. Donald Atkinson, her third husband, at the McNay home, which later became the McNay Museum of Art.

however, he saw an opportunity to advance his education and left the young man's employ to enroll at a tiny prairie college called Pierre University (Huron College). Here he could pay for classes by cleaning stables and doing chores and widen his education by attending lectures on the Chautauqua circuit. He also could afford to spend a year preparing at Centre College in the Kentucky town where Ephraim McDowell had recently done some of the nations' first major abdominal surgery. Now he was ready for medical school. Entering the University of Louisville, then the Hospital College of Medicine, Atkinson met doctors interested in ophthalmology for the first time and graduated in 1902.

Atkinson, Dr. Donald Taylor, Texas Surgeon, 50-80;
Dr. Joseph DeGasperi interview

Destiny led Atkinson when he tried to open a practice in Louisville, but ran headlong into formidable competition. Others also wished to settle near the medical school, he discovered, and forced later graduates to strike out for new territory. The predicament caused by competition in the period is captured by the following humorous account by the Minnesota doctor, T.H. Shastid:

*"About the only ophthalmologists that I know of now-a-days that quarrel are Dr. David Tilderquist and myself. We, from time to time, take our trusty ophthalmoscopes, and, motoring out to Fairmount Park, Duluth, enter into the strong cages of the "Zoo," and then, locking the iron doors behind us, we, in the midst of wild birds and howling beasts, wage out a fearful ophthalmoscopic duel. Sometimes Dr. Athens accompanies us, and we have a triangular battle"*.

(Shastid, 599)

In medical school Atkinson had met the first Texans he had ever known, and now they urged him to accompany them to Texarkana and take the state medical boards there. He later said, "*there was a time, I can attest, when the Texas spirit drew men like a magnet, because I was one of them.*" Carrying with them a partially dissected cadaver packed in formaldehyde to study, the young graduate and his friends boarded a train and headed for Texas, where he successfully passed the boards in 1903. Atkinson stayed long enough to boil down and divide the bones of the cadaver and buy a horse, and then—a full-fledged doctor at last—rode off to practice medicine on the frontier.

Atkinson, Dr. Donald Taylor, Texas Surgeon, xi, 81-96;
Scheie, 107

More like the Midwesterners who founded Dallas than the immigrants who arrived on the Gulf Coast or came from states in the Old South, Atkinson followed the path of those who entered Texas from the north. At first he did not venture too deep into Texas, but practiced in Bonanza in the blacklands in the northeastern part of the state, a region where poor farmers worked as sharecroppers or raised cotton as tenants after the Civil War. In 1885 this small community boasted a grist mill, cotton gin, Baptist and Presbyterian churches, a hotel, blacksmith, two grocers and a population of 100. Here Atkinson found an ideal place to test and improve his skills, enjoying what he described as "*freedom of the spirit*" and a place where "*the land is wide and hope as wide as the land.*" Given the rough circumstances of the frontier, Atkinson delivered babies, cared for men with gunshot

wounds and snakebites, and watched local residents with hookworm disease eating dirt, wool, and rotten wood with the voracious appetite caused by the disease. The experience also provided the chance to observe a wide variety of other cases, including those of poor people prone to eye problems.
Some time later after a hurricane passed over the area, Bonanza became a ghost town. The post office closed in 1906 and the population in 1940 was only 40.

Atkinson, Dr. Donald Taylor, Texas Surgeon, 81-96;
"Atkinson, Dr. Donald Taylor," New Handbook of Texas.

The event that stimulated Atkinson to begin the research he pursued for the duration of his career occurred when he struck out next for the Oklahoma Indian Territory to work with the Native-American population there. Faced with a host of unknown eye problems among the tribes, he began to categorize and classify diseases, observing cases unique to a population that lived largely out of doors. For much of his life, he suspected that a relationship existed between the appearance of cataracts and the high exposure to ultraviolet light experienced by those living in the Southwest, although he never obtained proof. He also treated a common occurrence among ranchers and farmers that urban physicians never saw called pterygium, an external condition of the eye suffered by those who spent their lives on the dusty plains. In this disease, constant irritation produced by the harsh environment caused the conjunctiva repeatedly to grow over the cornea, requiring surgical removal. Many of Atkinson's patients with little experience of medicine beyond that of the shaman or military doctor no doubt returned to their lives praising the man who had learned to treat the condition successfully.

DeGasperi,
Dr. Joseph Interview;
Atkinson, Dr. Donald Taylor, Texas Surgeon, book flap, 97-112,179

In the same year Dr. Burleson went to San Antonio, Atkinson found himself in the prime of life and wealthy enough at last to afford a horse and buggy. Possibly fearing again the competition he had discovered in Louisville, Atkinson chose not to move to an urban center in 1905, but instead left Oklahoma and headed for the town of Del Rio on the Rio Grande border in deep South Texas. At the time, a considerable influx of population from Mexico into the region was underway. For many years this area had been part of disputed territory known as the Nueces Strip in the No Man's Land area that lay between the

United States and Mexico. Whether Pancho Villa asked him to serve as a military surgeon for his men or he tended Judge Roy Bean may be open to question, but Atkinson did treat Mexican bullfighters gored in the ring and also likely served a clientele made up largely of Mexican-Americans. Frontier doctors treated all comers, despite the fact that different ethnic groups often lived in separate neighborhoods. His accumulated photographs of cases he treated, including many Hispanic individuals, prove that Atkinson saw all members of the community, an experience that increased his knowledge of eye diseases and stimulated his interest in further research.

Nixon, Century of Medicine in San Antonio, 223;
Atkinson, Dr. Donald Taylor, Texas Surgeon, 97-112

Although he had conducted his practice far from any established medical institution, Atkinson now decided to specialize—a remarkable decision given conditions in South Texas and the distance to established medical centers. Clearly, it was not a matter of income. A Texas Medical Association study published in 1906 or 1907 shows that doctors received an average fee for house calls during the day of $2.50, and $5 for night visits. Seventy-nine physicians practiced in Galveston, of whom twenty-seven barely made a living and only fifty-one earned more than their expenses. A South Texas physician earned an average of $4,100 per year, and had expenses of $3,000. According to one source, "*the average income of Texas physicians was only slightly more than the income of mechanics*," a situation only made worse by the popularity of and competition from quacks. "*Over one-half of the physicians of Texas were unable to afford the study and equipment necessary to do the best work.*" Other reasons, therefore, must account for Atkinson's decision, particularly the knowledge of specialists he had acquired in Boston. In any case, Atkinson set out for New York City's Manhattan Eye and Ear Hospital to seek training in diseases of the eye, ear, nose and throat, undeterred by the lack of transportation and other difficulties. His earlier experience no doubt made the trip easier than it would have been for many a Texas native, but the effort was no small feat.

Texas State Journal of Medicine, 3:60-68, June 1907, quoted in Sykes;
Wygant, 25-30, 236-7;
"Dr. Donald Taylor Atkinson," New Handbook of Texas

When he returned to Texas, Atkinson practiced only a short time before a new dissatisfaction with his level of knowledge prompted the young doctor to pursue additional training. Aware that the best training in ophthalmology was to be found in Vienna, Atkinson paid sixty dollars, boarded a Galveston freighter bound for Bremen (Bremerhaven), and soon found himself walking the streets of European cities and taking classes from some of the greatest doctors in the field. In Myth and Magic, Atkinson noted the "*fame of the Vienna School*" which, he explained, was "*not an organized institution but a group of inspiring physicians.*" "*What a massive change it was, and what an adaptation, suddenly coming from rural Texas to the heart of an ancient city, layered with history and culture.*" The Emperor Franz Joseph still resided in the Hofburg when Atkinson went to Mass in "*the chapel overlooking the Schweizerhof where the famous Vienna Boys' Choir sang.*" Before going home to the frontier, Atkinson received his postgraduate degree from the University of Vienna, took further training at the Royal London Ophthalmic Hospital, and conducted research in the British Museum.

"About the Author," in Atkinson, Myth and Magic; 135, 320;
Texas Surgeon, 113-1315

Of his European teachers, Atkinson said, "*These learned and generous men drew me up to their superior plane of effort, excited my intellect, and stimulated capacities which would otherwise have remained abortive.*" He later credited his skill in the intricacies of surgery to the highly innovative medical techniques he had observed at the Allgemeines Krankenhaus, the common hospital where all patients who died were subject to autopsy under Austrian law. In recognition of his powerful experience, Atkinson was made a fellow of Geneva's International College of Surgeons and became a lifelong member of the American Medical Association of Vienna that supported medical students who followed in his footsteps.

Atkinson, Dr. Donald Taylor, Texas Surgeon, 113-131,
Atkinson obituary

Atkinson's experience in Europe enabled him to transfer the best of German and other European science—including the latest ophthalmological knowledge and techniques—to South Texas. Unique cases he encountered when he returned now provided a powerful stimulus to his scientific interest. Back in Texas, he resumed his surgical practice in Dallas and the nearby rural town of Hillsboro, was elected to office in several North Texas medical associations, and began to write or edit for a number of medical journals. Among his interests were those reflected in his speeches to the Dallas Medical Society in 1908 on "*Some Observations on Trachoma,*" between 1909 and 1910 on "*Some Results of Nasal Stenosis*" and "*The Technique of the Radial Mastoid Operation*," and in 1911 on "*What the General Practitioner Should Know about the Eye.*" In contrast to Dr. John Burleson's interest in stabilizing the profession, Atkinson was more interested in undertaking scientific research to learn more about specific diseases and developing corresponding new surgical techniques.

According to some scholars, experimental ophthalmology probably had its start in America when Dr. Silas Weir Mitchell, between 1853 and 1860, discovered that an injection of sugar solution into frogs caused cataract formation before death.

Albert and Scheie, History of Ophthalmology at the University of Pennsylvania, 112;
Atkinson file, Daughters of the Republic of Texas archives;
BCMS Records;
Texas State Journal of Medicine, 1908-1912;
Atkinson, Dr. Donald Taylor, Texas Surgeon, 132,148

Atkinson's research, however, was interrupted briefly by the unfortunate case of tuberculosis that brought him to San Antonio. After recuperating at the Kerrville Sanatorium, he moved "*to San Antonio and the sun, there to live in a hotel until my lungs were healed.*" In the process, he fell in love with the city and decided to stay, establishing a practice in 1912 "*for reasons of health and of personal liking.*" When he arrived, the city was a retail and shipping center with 214 factories, a population of 96,614, elegant depots, six national banks, and 198 physicians. Three railroads traversed the area and there were two fine hotels, but few individuals who had accumulated significant wealth. Atkinson's move was motivated instead by the community's medical institutions. As he put it, he "*could delay no longer settling where there were complete hospital facilities.*" He arrived in 1903 just as a group of physicians, businessmen, and other community professionals organized the San Antonio Associated Charities to build the four-story Physicians and Surgeons Hospital. Located at Romana Plaza, a typical Southwestern plaza with a church and a monument to Mexican Independence leader Father Hidalgo, the hospital used horse-drawn ambulances to bring in patients for medical care at rates of $1.50 to $4 a day. Here Atkinson's practice soon attracted patients from "*Dallas to Brownsville and El Paso to Houston,*" and he began to pursue his interests in research.

The P&S Hospital later merged to become the Baptist Memorial Hospital on the plaza's eastern boundary in 1948, and underwent a major expansion in 1960.

"Romana Plaza in Evolution;
"Atkinson, Dr. Donald Taylor, Texas Surgeon, 140-5, 155

No American medical school could afford to pay full-time researchers and few Texas institutions offered sufficient infrastructure to support any type of research, although in 1903 the Galveston Medical Branch acknowledged the need when Dean Allen J. Smith said:
*"The medical school at Galveston, the most southern medical institution in the United States and one closely related to the tropics by trade conditions, is in an exceptional position for the study of tropical and subtropical diseases. . . . Such work should be done as a matter of justification for the existence of the school."*

Until World War II, institutions rather than individuals received the bulk of research funding, and in Texas only a few professors studying the cardiovascular system and metabolic processes at the Galveston Medical Branch received small amounts of money from pharmaceutical companies and the American Medical Association. "*Some work was being done in original investigation, but few records were kept of research underway at the young school, and as yet no graduate had followed a career in medical research.*" Without the benefit of institutional support, therefore, Atkinson worked alone using the knowledge he had gained in Europe to conduct medical research and participate in national and international efforts to advance ophthalmological knowledge.

UTMB at Galveston, 104;
Albert and Scheie, 107;
"University of Texas Medical Branch," New Handbook of Texas

By 1915, when visits to European clinics were in vogue, Atkinson began to adapt techniques he had learned in Vienna for new purposes and to develop new procedures of his own. Until the 1920s and 30s, cataract surgery had been done without the benefit of sutures and surgeons removed cataracts within their capsules through an "*extra*" capsular process. Potential for breaking the capsule was considerable, however, and once broken, the condition was difficult to correct. Intracapsular surgery, which left the capsule in tact, achieved a higher rate of success. Patients in Atkinson's time were forced to spend eight or nine days flat in bed with both of their eyes blindfolded for four days and their heads immobilized between sandbags. On the fourth day, they sat up in bed, but the entire process could take up to two weeks. Atkinson's successors used two, three, and later six or seven sutures that enabled a patient to move about in a few days, rather than weeks. Later generations, using sutures invisible to the naked eye, did a better job with twelve to fifteen sutures under a microscope, conducting the operation on an outpatient basis that required no time in bed at all, and eventually learned to complete the process more effectively by developing a new procedure that eliminated sutures once more.

Nixon, Century of Medicine in San Antonio, 261;
Drs. John Matthews, Jack Lee interviews.

According to a colleague, Atkinson became an expert surgeon who did a great deal of eye surgery and considerable plastic surgery on the eyelids as well. Another associate recalled that the doctor had the skill to take a patient's glasses and neutralize them accurately by selecting correctly from his array of lenses almost as fast as a person using a lensometer. Noted for his work on glaucoma, Atkinson "originated a number of instruments and operative methods in eye surgery," and wrote extensively, often illustrating his works with his own drawings or models that employed his considerable artistic skill. Among other innovations, he is credited with developing the Valude-Atkinson tenotomy for strabismus. In addition to several books published between 1914 and 1916, when he became a U.S. citizen, his more important *Handbook of Eye, Ear Nose and Throat Diseases* came out in 1924 and his *Outline of Eye, Ear, Nose and Throat Surgery* a year later. He then went on to study cancer of the larynx, to perform other innovative operations, and to study tropical diseases including yaws and goundou in the Caribbean. He also consulted regularly with physicians in Mexico and Cuba, and conducted expeditions to Mexico and Haiti to research leprosy and other diseases in remote areas. Pursuing science largely on his own, Atkinson worked without the benefit of institutional support outside the Bexar County Medical Society, which he joined in 1917. During World War I, he served as ophthalmology editor for the Texas Medical News and associate editor for a Chicago eye, ear, nose and throat journal. In recognition of his efforts, he was awarded a medal of merit in 1947 from the University of Florence in Italy for his "original research." By then, he claimed to have done research on five continents and collaborated with a number of educators and surgeons.

Atkinson also published articles on "corneal ulcers," "injuries of the eyeball," "rare lesions of the eyelid," trachoma," and congenital anomalies of the external eye" in Texas Medical Association publications.

Dr. Joseph DeGasperi, Dr. Marion W. McCurdy, and Dr. John Matthews interviews;
"About the Author," in Atkinson, Myth and Magic, 320;
Atkinson file, Daughters of the Republic of Texas archives;
Bexar County Medical Society Minutes, 1917;
"Dr. Donald Taylor Atkinson," New Handbook of Texas.

According to Texas medical historian P. I. Nixon, Atkinson's *External Diseases of the Eye*, first published in 1934, was one of four most important things to come out of San Antonio medicine in the early part of the century. At 674 pages including the author's illustrations and others, the work reveals that by the 1930s Atkinson had formed important international contacts and considered himself to be working on the frontier of ophthalmological science. Using his artistic talent, he illustrated texts with his own drawings and gathered photographs of unusual cases from doctors in Mexico and South America and archives around the world. Atkinson acknowledged Dr. R. Seefelder of the Augen-Klinik der Universitat, Innsbruck, Austria; Dr. A. Green Brinton of the University of Witwatersrand, Johannesburg, South Africa; Dr. Ignacio Barraquer, Facultad de Barcelona, Spain, and Dr. Jose de Jesus Gonzales, Academic Nacional de Medicina, Mexico, along with several physicians from Canada for help in preparing the manuscript. Photos were attributed to local specialists including Drs. Dan Russell, Sr., Ray K. Daily, Dr. Bloyce H. Britton in El Paso, Dr. C.S. Sykes at Galveston, Dr. W.D. Gill, Dr. Owen R. O'Neil at Paris, Texas, and others in Iowa City, Memphis, and Chicago.

Atkinson, Dr. Donald Taylor, External Diseases of the Eye;
Nixon, Century of Medicine, 375

Although its value to the profession is uncertain, Atkinson may have had the frontier physician in mind when he wrote the volume and might have wished to provide a helpful tool for this particular audience. His purpose, according to the "Preface," was to focus on the anterior segment of the eye and to offer information about diagnoses that could be done without the benefit of the ophthalmoscope or other instruments. *The Journal of the American Medical Association*, which listed Atkinson as a consulting ophthalmologist at the Santa Rosa Infirmary and the Nix Hospital in 1934, claimed that the *External Diseases of the Eye* was "*a distinct contribution to the English speaking physician*," but noted that the book's references were incomplete, its methods wholly empirical or out of date, and its texts filled with inadvertent misstatements. The *New England Journal of Medicine* recommended the work for orienting general practitioners, but indicated that recent medical graduates would be disappointed to find little on the bacteriology and histopathology of ocular lesions, suggesting that Atkinson was not familiar with the corneal microscope or slit lamp.

New England Journal of Medicine, 1934;
Journal of the American Medical Association, 1934

No mention in the journal reviews, however, is made of other topics Atkinson discussed at some length such as the fungus diseases of the external eye common in the South and diseases such as yaws and leprosy that may have constituted an important part of his contribution. Atkinson also mentioned such rare practices as tattooing the cornea that could be traced back to ancient cultures. The book's objective may have been to serve as a practical tool for the practicing specialist. Here could be found a catalog of the effects of diseases in advanced stages—tumors left without treatment, adaptations to severe injuries, and similar topics that would have been useful to those in the hinterland. Dr. Archibald Fletcher Clark, Sr. recalled studying Potter's Field cases, but research opportunities were still rare. Although detractors claimed that he sent copies to general practitioners, used his books to advertise his practice, and did not add significantly to the literature, Atkinson's considerable body of work contributed to Texas ophthalmology by acknowledging the importance of research as an activity appropriate to practicing ophthalmologists.

Clark, Archibald Fletcher, n.p.

Atkinson's interest in art—an appreciation of links between ophthalmology and the visual properties of paint—led to his social success as well and, indirectly, to another important gift to the San Antonio community. As a young man, the doctor not only drew the fossil ferns he discovered on the walls of a coal mine, but became an amateur painter. When he met Marion Koogler McNay, the daughter of a wealthy family who had worked briefly at the Chicago Institute of Art before coming to San Antonio, the two shared an interest in both medicine and painting. McNay's father was an Ohio country doctor and Santa Fe Railroad surgeon who bequeathed her a fortune when oil was discovered on the Kansas land he gave her. She arrived in San Antonio after two brief failed marriages in a "state of melancholia," but her discomfort disappeared when the beauty of the place inspired her to take up painting again. In 1926, after meeting the distinguished local surgeon, she married Atkinson in Austin, who promptly enlisted her to make drawings of some of his operations.

Dr. Joseph DeGasperi interview

Back in San Antonio, the couple soon acquired modern French artworks by Modigliani, Derain, Picasso, Toulouse-Lautrec, Dufy, Vlaminck, Van Gogh, and Forain, but set out to build "the finest home in San Antonio." Atkinson bought up the Gonfacio Rodriquez farm on the Austin Highway and proceeded to build a $250,000 estate inspired by Mediterranean and Spanish design, which was completed in 1929. Of the property, a local resident later recalled, "*often I had watched the forty or more peacocks spread their fan-like tails and proudly strut around its miniature gardens and cactus beds or the acre or more of natural park surrounding this mansion. Then I had wished that I might live there.*" The couple also raised Nubian goats and Irish terriers. According to one observer, "*the double iron gateway to the estate was never closed and many strangers who wandered off the highway and into the grounds thinking they were in a public park were hospitably received and frequently invited inside the house.*" Ultimately, the home Atkinson built for Marion McNay indirectly became a lasting legacy to the city. When she died in 1950, years after divorcing him, Marion McNay bequeathed to the city of San Antonio the largest single gift in its history.

Elizabeth Moorman Holm, 141ff.;
"A gift to the "illimitable public," 67;
Atkinson owned 40 acres in Alamo Heights, including the space formerly occupied by the Woodmen of the World Hospital.
Dr. Joseph DeGasperi interview

From horse and buggy doctor, Atkinson now rose to the ranks of San Antonio's wealthiest citizens. Due in part to his community presence, he also found himself in competition with Dr. John Burleson despite the differences in their respective interests and accomplishments. The city's two most outstanding practitioners were opposites. Burleson had arrived in San Antonio in 1905, and no doubt considered Atkinson—who came in 1913—an outsider and an upstart. Where Burleson was socially adept, Atkinson was reticent, a poor public speaker. Where Atkinson's interest lay in broadening the knowledge of the specialty, Burleson focused on stabilizing medical practice of all kinds. These differences likely account for the feud that developed between the two men. Though both were described as "*fine gentlemen,*" a colleague said in later years that, "*Dr. Burleson and Dr. Atkinson got along like two cats in a sack.*" Other doctors in the city divided into camps on opposing sides in the feud. Physicians in the Medical Arts Building tended to be "*Atkinson people*" and those in the Nix Building "*Burleson men.*" Hostilities reached the point that members of the two groups didn't speak while riding on a common elevator, and colleagues compared the two rival doctors to the famous feuding families, the Hatfields and McCoys.

Dr. Jack Lee and Dr. Marion W. McCurdy interview

Dr. Atkinson rounded out his life of world travel and research, and died in 1958. Although many of his colleagues remained unaware of his activities, his contribution to South Texas ophthalmology was to create a tradition of clinical research that laid the foundation for more substantial research to follow. Questioning the nature of eye diseases encountered in his practice, Atkinson was a cataloger and classifier who performed the important function of categorizing and summarizing what he had learned. By providing general practitioners with a useful tool, Atkinson helped ophthalmology and specialized medicine to reach from established medical centers all the way to the frontier.

Atkinson, Dr. Donald Taylor, Texas Surgeon, 167-172;
Atkinson obituary

## DR. EDWIN MEREDITH SYKES WIDENS THE COMMUNITY ROLE FOR OPHTHALMOLOGISTS

Dr. Edwin Meredith Sykes, a native of Texas, who took his Boards in otolaryngology but practiced ophthalmology, created a third tradition for South Texas ophthalmologists by becoming a prominent citizen and contributor to the San Antonio community. While participation in local society may seem to have little to do with the development of ophthalmology, social relations have often had a good deal to do with improving the climate for medicine. If general practitioners had long been respected citizens, specialists who joined the ranks of the local upper class increased public acceptance for their profession by being active members of their communities. Dr. Sykes' career demonstrates the kind of local activities and affiliations that added stature to the profession and helped the first generation of specialists to advance beyond its predecessors.

One of the first true specialists from the region, Edwin Meredith Sykes was born at Galveston on September 12, 1885, and much like Donald Atkinson worked as a boy for a line of English freighters that frequented the port. When the Galveston storm of 1900 destroyed the town, he was serving as an office boy at the local YMCA. He came from a medical family, the son of general practitioner Dr. George Sherbourne Sykes, who had been inspired by a man educated in Heidelberg and at the Sorbonne but never had the opportunity to specialize. In 1880, George Sykes graduated with a degree signed by Ashbel Smith from the precursor of the Galveston Medical Branch, the Texas Medical College. Unable to pursue further training, he took jobs as a pharmacist at the Aschoff Drug Store and steward at the Galveston City Hospital, where he also lived for a time. His brother, Clarence Sykes, pursued medical training in Vienna and Klagenfurt, Austria, and then returned to Galveston to join the faculty at the Galveston Medical Branch. Edwin Sykes followed in his father's footsteps and in 1908 graduated in a Galveston Medical Branch class of twenty-five only a short time after John Burleson succeeded in obtaining passage of the Texas Medical Practice Act that cleared the state of quacks and charlatans.

Charles Ganahl inspired Sykes.
BCMS Records; Sykes, 1-20.

Sykes interned at the Provident Sanitarium in Waco, and then left the state to join the house staff of Chicago's St. Joseph's Hospital. There, after a year and six months of general medicine, he became interested in eye pathology and decided to specialize in the still-combined field of eye, ear, nose and throat. He spent a year working at the Contagious Disease Hospital of the City of Chicago Health Department, and then took a position on the house staff of the distinguished Brooklyn Eye and Ear Hospital that had been in founded in New York in 1868. Although he did not get to Europe to complete his education, Sykes translated Albrecht von Graefe's text on eye pathology during his New York residency in 1912, and so managed to touch base with German expertise in ophthalmology.

BCMS Records;
Sykes, 1-20.

Sykes returned briefly to Galveston in 1914 but, like Burleson before him, went north to set up his first practice. His biographer offers no particular reason for this choice, but presumes the young man may have wished to avoid competition with his father in Galveston's bustling medical marketplace, and likely preferred the more open medical environment to be found in San Antonio. There his early living arrangements reflect the humble nature of his circum-

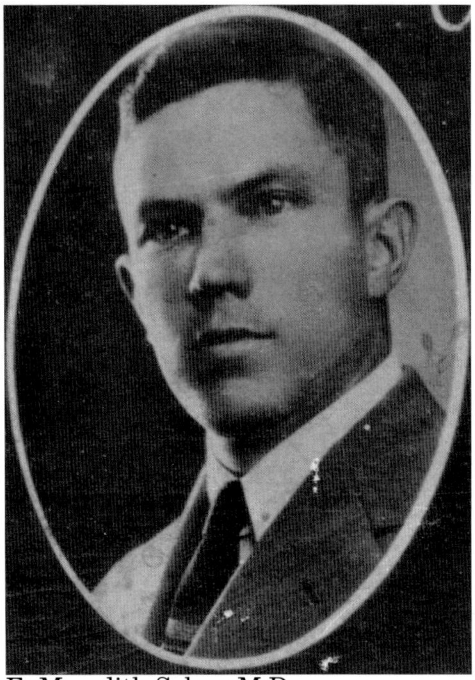
E. Meredith Sykes, M.D.

stances. Although his office at room 421 in the Moore Building was acceptable, he lived at the San Antonio YMCA until 1915 and then moved to a boarding house. In order to buy equipment, Sykes had to ask his father to co-sign the necessary bank loans. A year later, however, he was well established as an oculist and aurist, and had become an attending physician at the City Hospital and an examiner for boys referred from the local Peacock and West Texas Military Academies, for which he received an annual income of $2,000. He also was comfortable dealing with San Antonio's Hispanic population because he had learned to speak Spanish by translating English medical articles into that language and had conversed with educated Mexican patients at Waco during his internship there.

Sykes, 20-35

By the time Sykes arrived, San Antonio had become a bustling urban center. The San Antonio Country Club had opened in 1908, by which time the town had become the wealthiest in the state and a health resort for the cure of throat and lung trouble. The population, reported by federal census as 53,321 in 1900, doubled in a decade as an Anglo majority for the first time outnumbered the Germans, Hispanics and African Americans who controlled the city previously. A new city hall rose next to the farmers' market, the annual Fiesta began, and a gala complete with banks of fresh flowers, gold watch fobs for the gentlemen, hatpins for the ladies, and songs by a "*noted Italian opera star brought from Rome*" celebrated the opening of the city's new Gunter Hotel. Andrew Carnegie donated $50,000 for a new public library, and reporters noted new life in the building trades. Although the San Antonio River remained something of a health menace, electric motor cars replaced mule-drawn streetcars and a Denver investment company and syndicate of local capitalists acquired the land to develop Alamo Heights, an area characterized by beautiful drives and park-like terraces. The familiar chili stands in Alamo Plaza would be gone by 1920, and the hay wagons on Military Plaza as well.

Fehrenbach, 3; San Antonio City Directory, 1903-4

Acceptance for specialists in a community where quacks were a recent memory was not exclusively a matter of skill, and Sykes now took the necessary steps to establish himself socially. In New York, he had not only attended the Metropolitan Opera but had become a local handball, tennis, golf and bowling champion. He also loved to dance. According to a contemporary, Sykes spoke French, Spanish and German and, after study in New York, had a concert-quality voice that could sing opera. Building on referrals from college and family friends, the handsome, blue-eyed young man joined San Antonio's Beethoven Maennerchor, French Club, and Travis Club, and quickly became a social favorite. As he rose in local social circles, Sykes also met and married a young woman who had been a "duchess" in the annual Fiesta event that maintained the social dominance of the community's oldest Anglo families. In a lavish coronation rite equivalent to debutante parties in the Northeast, daughters of San Antonio's finest donned dresses with fifteen to twenty-foot trains costing thousands of dollars to stage a public spectacle equal to those of European royalty. Sykes' wife gave him connections to the Order of the Alamo that hosted the event and an introduction to the city's civic leaders, including John Burleson. After their marriage in 1916, the couple bought a newly-built house near Incarnate Word College in Alamo Heights and spent summers in Boerne at a family home nicknamed Puccoon or at James Park near Comfort, Texas.

Sykes, 120; Dr. Francis Weixel interview

By 1925 Sykes was successfully established, and purchased two-thirds of an acre on Charles Road in the developing suburb of Terrell Hills from Dr. Frederick Terrell. There he constructed a $20,300 house in a prestigious suburb, where new social contacts enabled him to join the San Antonio Country Club and the Conopus Club, noted for its high-spirited enthusiasm and motto "We Do Nothing But We Do It Well." He also joined the Kiwanis Club, El Patronato, and the Alliance Francaise. Later he developed friendships with a group of men he referred to as the "3Ds," or doctors, druggists, and dentists, and joined the Doctor's Round Table which met regularly for Saturday luncheons. Among its members was Dr. P.I. Nixon, the foremost historian of medicine in Texas.

Sykes, 40-60;
BCMS Records

Professionally, membership was necessary to join the staff of any local hospital and Sykes quickly joined the strong local medical organization, the Bexar County Medical Society, soon after he arrived. Society Minutes record the importance of professional organization for specialists and the communication that occurred among practitioners. In 1908, Dr. Russell Caffery spoke on the "Necessity for Early Treatment in Concomitant Strabismus," Dr. B.F. Stout spoke on the "Importance of EENT Work among School Children," and another specialist, Dr. Abraham Sachs, joined the organization. In 1909 Dr. Robert E. Moss made a "Few Remarks on Chronic Glaucoma." A year later, Dr. J.V. Spring spoke on the "Neurosis of the Eye Due to Structure of the Urethra," and Drs. T. B. Askew and T.H. Walthall joined the organization. Dr. S.S. Beakley's 1911 paper on the "Affection of the EENT in Relation to General Surgery and Medicine" discussed a cataract removal done for $35, and between 1912 and 1913, the *Bexar County Medical Society Bulletin* noted papers on "Glioma of the Retina" given by Dr. S.K. Beck, "Some Observations on the Effect of Salvarsan From the Standpoint of the Specialist in Eye and Ear Disease" by Dr. Moss, and a discussion of "Hygiene of the Eye in School" by Dr. R.F. Miller. Sykes delivered a paper on tonsillectomy there early in his career.

BCMS Minutes

As his reputation grew, Sykes expanded his practice to outlying towns and took on other professional and community roles. His World War I Medical Corps experience at Fort Sam Houston's Base Hospital (also covered in the next chapter) was important from a community standpoint since it helped set the precedent for strong local military-civilian relationships. From 1922 to 1946 he published articles in the *Texas State Journal of Medicine* on eye injury, fungal infections, and cancer of the eye, wrote on the surgery for glaucoma for the *EENT Monthly*, and handled a medical liability suit involving a prescription for eye drops, but in 1926 was certified to practice otolaryngology. After working in the Medical Arts Building across from the Alamo and the Nix Building, Sykes was among the first to move from the city center to the suburbs when he established new offices at 428 Baltimore. In the 1950s, he was joined in practice by his sons, one of whom, Edwin M. Sykes, Jr., served in World War II with the Medical Corps at the 48th Field Hospital in Europe.

Sykes, 62-86

If Dr. John Burleson was an institution-builder, Sykes possessed the necessary social skills to mobilize others behind a good idea. In 1921 it was Sykes' charismatic personality that won support for Burleson's effort to create the San Antonio Ophthalmological and Otolaryngological Society. In recognition of his role, Sykes was chosen as first president of the new society. Seen from a later perspective, Sykes is a prototype for Dr. John Matthews, who assumed a similar role in the next generation. Further testimony to Sykes' social skills comes from the fact that he successfully rode out the Depression simply by relinquishing his life insurance policy. He maintained his practice despite many who were unable to pay for his medical services, and could be found in 1933 helping survivors after a hurricane struck Rio Grande communities at Brownsville, Harlingen, Edinburg, Raymondville, and San Benito. In the 1940s, his practice stabilized once more, Sykes helped to found the San Antonio Chamber Music Society, participated in the Turner Club, and celebrated his fiftieth birthday by doing a handstand. The third of the triumvirate of early San Antonio specialists, Sykes added a vital component to Burleson's professional contributions and Atkinson's research achievements that advanced the cause of both ophthalmology and specialized medicine.

Sykes, 86-125

## EYE SPECIALISTS IN SAN ANTONIO AND THE HINTERLAND

Burleson, Atkinson, and Sykes were the most visible of the first San Antonio generation of specialists and the vanguard of a movement that brought a remarkable group of eye, ear, nose and throat specialists to San Antonio and the hinterland along the recently-closed frontier. Those with EENT practices in the Rio Grande Valley and the German communities to the north benefited from professional networks fostered by the Bexar County Medical Society and the Texas Medical Association, and funneled cases requiring greater specialization to ophthalmologists at San Antonio or Houston. A brief account of some of these contemporaries suggests the range of experience represented by the generation.

Dr. James Hall Bell, who may have preceded Dr. John Burleson as San Antonio's first trained ophthalmologist, graduated from Jefferson Medical College at Philadelphia in 1884. After establishing his San Antonio practice around 1897, he served as an ophthalmic surgeon at the Southwestern Hospital Dispensary and wrote a treatise on ophthalmology. Between 1903 and 1904, he directed the Eye, Ear and Nose Hospital in the Wright Building at 501 Navarro on the corner of Houston Street, and later he served as a consultant and "demonstrator of anatomy" at the R. B. Green Hospital. Bell was an early member of the West Texas Medical Association and served as second vice president of the American Medical Association. His interests included ocular manifestations of conditions in the body including nephritis, and the treatment of infectious diseases. Associated with Bell until his retirement in 1920 was Dr. T. B. Askew, an eye, ear, nose and throat specialist born in Iowa who completed his medical degree at St. Louis, first practiced in Iowa, and later served as president of the San Antonio O & O Society.

BCMS Membership Files;
BCMS Minutes, 1905

Among the last among practicing South Texas oculists and aurists was Dr. Wesley A. Rape, born in Nacogdoches County in 1864 and graduated from St. Louis' Missouri Medical College. After establishing his first practice at Ballinger in 1888 and joining the Runnels County Medical Society, he moved to the larger town of Victoria in 1894, where the Valley View Hospital was founded three years later. Recognizing his need for further training, he went to New York City a few years later for specialty training in eye, ear, nose and throat. Back in Victoria, he served as an oculist and aurist for the Southern Pacific Railroad and later specialized in otolaryngology before his death in 1922. Dr. Rape's successor, Dr. William L. Ward, who came to Victoria in 1890, is considered the first eye, ear, nose and throat specialist in that community. Ward graduated from the University of Louisville in 1881 and practiced for ten years at Lone Oak and Abilene before moving to Victoria. Dr. William C. Swain of Galveston replaced Rape as "oculist and aurist" for the Southern Pacific Railroad in 1898, but moved to Cuero in 1901 and later to Dallas. His replacement was the eye, ear, nose and throat specialist Dr. F.L. Sargent, who practiced in the area for roughly twelve years and in 1905 served as secretary of the Calhoun County Medical Society.

Grimes, 533;
BCMS Membership Files

Other new South Texas specialists also came from distant places to settle in large and small communities across the region. Dr. Benjamin Franklin Houston, born in Lewisburg, Tennessee, graduated from the University of Tennessee in 1887 and established his EENT practice at Corsicana, Texas. Dr. Summerfield Taylor, born at Batesville, Virginia, graduated from the Galveston Medical Branch, and practiced at Austin. Dr. Richard Youngblood went to Pleasanton and Dr. Norman Wood to Uvalde. Dr. Thomas Proctor practiced in Sulphur Springs and Dr. William Morgan in Lockhart, Texas. Mississippi natives Dr. Joseph Camp Phillips and Clarence McClellan practiced respectively at Port Arthur and Kerrville. EENT specialist Dr. S. S. Beakley came with his family to Gray Rock and Paris, Texas, from his birthplace near Nashville, Tennessee. Graduated from the University of Nashville Medical Department in 1900, he enjoyed a successful general practice at Seguin, Texas, for nine years before deciding to specialize. After training in New York he completed postgraduate work in eye, ear, nose and throat diseases at New Orleans, set up a San Antonio practice, and in 1909 joined the Bexar County Medical Society. The city directory listed him as an oculist and aurist, but Beakley served as Associate EENT Chief at San Antonio's newly founded R. B. Green Hospital with Dr. R. E. Moss in 1917. Later, for recreation, Dr. Beakley raised registered Jersey cattle on a farm at Robstown.

San Antonio City Directory, 1909;
BCMS Membership Files

Many of those who came were now trained exclusively in the United States. Of practicing South Texas eye specialists in 1900 trained in the Midwest, Dr. William Rhodes attended the University Medical College in Kansas City; Dr. Charles Pinckney, born in Iowa, attended the University of Nebraska; and Dr. Charles Metz the Miami Medical College at Cincinnati in the state where he was born. Nebraska native Dr. Frank D. Walsworth, graduated from the University of Kansas and completed his specialty training in eye, ear, nose and throat at Kansas City before beginning a forty year practice in Harlingen in 1923. Others attended Washington University Medical School at St. Louis, Northwestern, Hahneman Medical

College and Hospital, the University of Pennsylvania, the University of Illinois, Indiana University School of Medicine, the Homeopathic Medical College of Missouri, and Cincinnati College of Medicine and Surgery. Representative of those trained in places farthest from Texas were Dr. A Wessells, who became a specialist in South Africa, and Dr. Charles Boehs, who trained in England. Other young South Texas specialists went to Jefferson Medical College in Philadelphia or Barnes Medical College in Chicago; Dr. James A. Miller, born in Summershade, Kentucky, trained at Rush Medical in Chicago before beginning his career at McAllen. Dr. Arthur Padilla came from Nicaragua, received his medical education at San Salvador University, and completed his specialty training at Philadelphia before opening an EENT practice in Corpus Christi. Dr. Otto Louis Zanek from Industry, Texas, grew up in Brenham, graduated from the Galveston Medical Branch, interned in Oklahoma City, and trained at the Massachusetts Eye and Ear Infirmary. Later Zanek worked in Houston, served as instructor of clinical ophthalmology at Baylor and Galveston's John Sealy Hospital, and in 1939 came to San Antonio to work at the R.B. Green Hospital.

BMCS Membership Files;
Texas Medical Association Membership Files

By 1900 new patterns in South Texas medicine indicate that ophthalmology had nearly reached maturity there as a profession and a science. The generation of specialists who received their degrees in the late nineteenth and early twentieth century rooted ophthalmology firmly in the region and made significant contributions to their communities, while those who moved to rural towns introduced the benefits of innovations made at distant medical centers. Despite the fact that many counties still had few medical facilitates of any kind, a number of hospitals were built, including specialty hospitals, and more would follow. A Throat, Eye and Ear Charity Hospital, first on Brazos Street and then at 1511 Colorado Street, was completed in Austin by 1896 with the support of charity balls and benefits, and a similar institution built in Nueces County around 1906. San Antonio emerged as a thriving medical center and a leader in both eye care facilities and specialists. By the turn of the century, formal training for ophthalmologists within Texas remained limited, but specialists practiced there who had trained in some of the country's finest institutions. Both distinguished and accomplished, the generation including Drs. Burleson, Atkinson, and Sykes represented a force for cultural transmission that would enable the Texas frontier to rapidly catch up with eastern centers of science, and, in many ways, soon surpass them.

Nueces County Historical Society, 135;
Ferris and Hoppe, 207;
Coleman, 78

# CHAPTER 7

# WORLD WAR I AND ITS LEGACY: AVIATION RESEARCH AND ADVANCES IN OPHTHALMIC SPECIALIZATION, 1914-1918 AND AFTER

*The story of ophthalmology is many stories in one, for ophthalmology is many sciences in one.*

Arrington, History of Ophthalmology

The use of airplanes made World War I different from all other wars in history. This development also produced a specialty field within military medicine known as aviation medicine, in which ophthalmology eventually became a specialty field. Ophthalmologists treated injured soldiers just as their predecessors had in earlier wars, but those whose principal duty was to treat pilots not only devised new forms of treatment but took part in some of the nation's first ophthalmological research addressing entirely new visual objectives. Pilot demands put ophthalmology on the cutting edge of medicine and swiftly led to a host of advances with both military and civilian applications. In South Texas, where military aviation began before the war and expanded during it, aviation-related ophthalmological research soon added a new component to both the region's and the nation's medical infrastructure.

Payne, Lt. Col. Brittain F., 488

Medical scholars have long agreed that the battlefield serves as a "*transformative force*" in medicine. Discussing this process, medical historian John Fulton explained that war creates conditions that necessitate research and frequently gives rise to innovations in medical technique. Efforts to treat the wounded frequently allow physicians to conduct research in that they present numerous cases with uncommon injuries. Both civilian physicians and medical officers in the armed services have made major medical advances "*working under the stimulus of wartime exigency*." In essence, the wide range of battle injuries duplicates the conditions in which large numbers of cases first spawned research in the major cities of Europe. The need to create faster, more effective methods to treat large numbers of the injured encourages physicians to improvise in ways they would not otherwise, spurs innovation, and often produces improvements in ways to routinize care. In addition, until the Great War, few systematic efforts had been made to expand visual capacity beyond the introduction of glasses, or, for that matter, to establish goals for discovery in eye science. What Fulton did not anticipate was that World War I aviation, by requiring military personnel to function in a new environment, would lead to the development of an entirely new branch of medicine.

Fulton, John, "Medicine, Warfare, and History," cited in Naythons, Matthew, 8

Before 1914 few civilian or military institutions in South Texas had undertaken ophthalmological research of any kind. During World War I, however, forces converged at San Antonio that focused medical attention on the problems faced by pilots conducting the air war, and this gave rise to the region's first organized research in ophthalmology. At the war's end, military ophthalmologists and aviators came together to address the problem of “blind flying”, a condition in which visual experience plays a key role. While most Texas ophthalmologists who went overseas brought back new medical knowledge when they returned, pilot William Ocker and ophthalmologist Dr. Fredrick H. Thorne contributed something new to the emerging field of aviation research at San Antonio's School of Aviation Research laboratory. Their experiments not only laid the foundation for ophthalmological research in the region, but also established associations between aerospace research and Texas and precedents for NASA's Manned Space Center that only later came to fruition.

## THE NATIONS MOBILIZE TO IMPROVE THE TREATMENT OF INJURED SOLDIERS

World War I began in Europe in 1914, but not until April 6, 1917, did American forces join the conflict. When the war began, however, United States military medical officials, realizing that American troops would inevitably be needed in Europe, organized a Subcommittee of Ophthalmology to consider options for making an effective response when the time came. Their analysis quickly showed that specialists would be essential to any successful effort. Casualties in the Spanish-American War had been few (a total of 284 men out of 235,631 participants), but, nonetheless, the Army Medical Department had come to "*realize the value of general hospitals (such as Tripler and Letterman) for treatment of patients requiring special therapeutic measures under the care of specialists.*" Originally, U.S. medical divisions had been formed with no provision for specialists, but by the end of 1914 specialists in operative surgery, bacteriology, and ophthalmology were approved for both general and stationary hospitals.

Military Medical Manual, 511

To mobilize the large number of specialists that would be required, the War Department turned of necessity to private practice and local hospitals. When the war began these institutions employed the majority of American ophthalmologists capable of conducting the most difficult ophthalmic surgery, and now there was insufficient time for the military to develop personnel of its own. As hospitals mobilized for the theaters of war, the Army Medical Department followed the British example and assembled civilian medical specialists, calling upon "*the panorama of the health sciences*" for epidemiologists, sociologists, and nutritionists from "*hospital centers, independent hospitals, and laboratories*" across the nation. Among the specialties represented, "*ophthalmology was one of the most important, it being among the oldest and most distinct specialties and one that the average physician knew little about.*" A later statement that ophthalmology was "*logically one of the first (specialties) to impress on the Medical Department of the Army the need for its adequate recognition*" suggests that ophthalmology played an important role in the organization of efficient American medical operations abroad.

MacPherson, W.G. et al., v. 1:44; v. 2: 499;
"Ophthalmology in the American Expeditionary Forces," 659;
Dammin, 1456

Initial U.S. Medical Department estimates showed that at least 500 highly trained ophthalmic surgeons would be needed to conduct the ophthalmic work required at home and abroad. To supply the personnel, training camps and base hospitals taught courses to Medical Department officers and enlisted men, and civilian institutions made their facilities available to train others. Between August 12 and December 24, 1918, the Army School of Ophthalmology set up and ran a four-week ophthalmology training course at General Hospital No. 14 at Camp Greenleaf, Georgia, that qualified 93 student officers to practice. Courses on the basics of ophthalmic practice there provided "*review and postgraduate work for experienced ophthalmologists, special training in military ophthalmology, and basic training in ophthalmology for men who were interested in the specialty and who by examination proved that their current knowledge was sufficient to warrant additional training.*" School facilities included a laboratory equipped with trial cases, perimeters, stereoscopes, giant magnets, and tonometers, in which operations were done on pigs' eyes and sheep heads. Students spent an hour on the X-ray localization of foreign bodies in the eye and plastic surgery to permit them to "*approach their duties from the military standpoint and its necessities.*" One-third to almost half the time was devoted to studying cases with the ophthalmoscope to "*demonstrate ophthalmic changes peculiar to ocular and general diseases.*" Such programs ultimately served not only to prepare personnel, but also to heighten awareness of and interest in ophthalmology.

U.S. War Department, Surgeon General's Office. VII: Training, 124-130;
"Ophthalmology in the American Expeditionary Forces," 3, 659, 669ff.;
MacPherson, W.G. et al, v. 1: 44-50;
Military Medical Manual, 346

Between the time when war broke out and the U.S. entered the conflict, U.S. medical officers further benefited from the experience of their European counterparts. As the fighting intensified in Europe, the British medical system faced demands that "*taxed the ingenuity of ophthalmic specialists to the full, both in preserving and restoring the best possible acuity of vision.*" "*Not even in the districts of large steel works in England,*" *one observer wrote,* "*has there been in a given time such a wide experience in penetrating injuries as that which occurred at the chief operating ophthalmic centers in France*." In response, British ophthalmologists organized an effective system to treat soldiers injured at the front. The volume and severity of injuries challenged the system, but military ophthalmic surgeons responded so successfully that care of military personnel quickly outstripped the level of service provided at home. In 1915--still prior to the time American Expeditionary Forces went abroad--a group of U.S. ophthalmic surgeons went to France and England to observe conditions there and determine how an American ophthalmic service might enhance existing operations already in place. So successful was this experience that all American ophthalmologists were sent to the French, English and Italian fronts for two weeks of observation to learn methods of caring for war-related eye wounds then in use at English eye centers. As the war continued, returning doctors reinforced the idea that ophthalmologists and other medical specialists were essential to the war effort.

MacPherson, W.G. et al, v. 1: 44, 49; v. 2: 667

To handle high numbers of casualties, English specialists devised and American ophthalmologists eventually adopted a teamwork approach that saved manpower and moved patients through the system with a high level of efficiency. In this carefully-orchestrated process, men injured at the front were taken first to "eye huts" or casualty clearing stations only twenty by sixty feet in size. Doctors at these stations administered basic treatment or issued ophthalmic labels that identified individuals for transfer to facilities equipped entirely for ophthalmic surgery and care. After more extensive procedures, patients were moved to base ophthalmic centers and convalescent depots. Due to the limitations of the physician's formulary, surgical techniques performed near the battlelines remained relatively primitive. Instead of ether, surgeons used local anesthetics such as novocaine that deadened the eye for over two hours but allowed continued movement. Standard procedure indicated inserting a needle behind the eye and performing most operations in only forty-five minutes. Morphine was used to quiet and relax injured patients. Another decade would pass before retrobubar injections were developed to allow the placement of anesthetics behind the eyeball to immobilize the eye and permit more successful surgeries.

MacPherson, W.G. et al., v. 1: 44-50

In the American Medical Department, the last and largest divisional units in the chain of evacuation were field hospitals located between three and eight miles from the front line and often grouped for convenience to permit ambulance access and easier exchange of patients. Dressing stations sent casualties to these hospitals to receive a higher level of care, and they in turn sent stabilized patients on to evacuation hospitals. Among the main functions performed by doctors at field hospital sites was channeling men with shell-fragments lodged in their eyes to central units where giant electro-magnets removed magnetic foreign bodies that had entered their eyes; later, mobile units took portable magnets to the patient.

MacPherson, W.G. et al, v. 1: 44; v. 2: 499-500;
Military Medical Manual, 350-1

By the time U.S. forces entered combat, a total of 131 Army station hospitals, four general hospitals, and five temporary base hospitals with a total bed capacity of 9,530 had been set up. Initially, 276 ophthalmologists were assigned to "*base, port, post and general hospitals*" abroad. Before General Pershing arrived in Europe in May 1917, six fully equipped base hospitals were there to meet him, ready for operation. Base hospital units sailed to the aid of the British Medical Service whose bases in Boulogne, Rouen, Etaples, Calais and LeHavre included buildings for ophthalmic outpatients carefully designed and equipped for all emergencies. Nuns trained in ophthalmic nursing were assigned to these bases to further improve the level of care they provided. The number of beds at each center varied, but at Boulogne and Rouen there were between 120 and 170. Hospitals, Overseas Hospitals, and Head Surgery fell under the Division of Sanitation, and officials established a new and independent division for the Air Service. By June 1917, the Medical Department of the American Expeditionary Forces comprised 5,198 officers, 2,539 nurses, and 30,574 enlisted men, and these numbers increased substantially before the war ended.

Military Medical Manual, 341-347;
"Ophthalmology in the American Expeditionary Forces," 659-728;
MacPherson, W.G. et al., v. 2: 505

In addition to the medical officers sent overseas to Great Britain, France, and Italy, American medical schools and university hospitals organized base hospitals and mobilized personnel to serve at Army hospitals in the Zone of the Interior within the United States, including 493 ophthalmologists sent to U.S. military installations. "*In some instances entire army posts were converted into hospitals*," and a total of 44,000 beds were available for use in large camps at home by the fall of 1917. According to the American Journal of Ophthalmology, doctors at overseas base hospitals dealt with everything from optic atrophy to gassing, but those at home initially did ocular operations rarely and found few cases of glaucoma in the healthy young men they saw. At these military facilities, a doctor's primary responsibility was for sight testing recruits, correcting presbyopia in clerical staff, treating minor ailments such as corneal ulcers and iritis, and operating large refraction departments. Domestic military installations, however, later played a major role when the worst cases of eye trauma among the American forces were returned to the United States. Among facilities receiving these casualties, six hospitals initially served as eye centers and a number of auxiliary hospitals went into operation later.

MacPherson, W.G. et al., v. 2: 501;
"Ophthalmology in the American Expeditionary Forces," 659-728;
Military Medical Manual, 347

As the war progressed, American eye specialists became aware of the need to provide more adequate accommodations for special eye injury cases. A suggestion was made to the U.S. Surgeon General that one base hospital be organized and equipped exclusively for care of eye and ear injuries and diseases. The response came in August 1918, when a centralized facility known as Base Hospital No. 115, or the "head hospital," mobilized at General Hospital No. 11, Cape May, New Jersey, embarked for Vichy with 1,000 artificial eyes in the optical unit's equipment, and immediately went into operation. Development of the Head Hospital acknowledged the importance of the specialty and marked a new level of advance in military medicine. The complex operations of this hospital increased the number of specialists returning to the United States since it also trained officers needing advanced instruction in the specialties.

MacPherson, W.G. et al, v. 1, 92

The results of this operation were significant. In addition to the systematic organization of medical personnel on a nationwide scale, the war intensified public interest in specialized medicine. Medical Department performance evaluations later concluded that "*the World War demonstrated that through specialization results had been accomplished which otherwise would have been unattainable.*" Ultimately, training programs at Camp Greenleaf and the Head Hospital provided many American doctors with access to specialty training otherwise unavailable to them.

"Ophthalmology in the American Expeditionary Forces," 659-728

Other significant gains were made in the area of research. Just as doctors treating eye injuries in the Franco-German War (1870-1871) had gained valuable understanding of the condition known as sympathetic ophthalmia from serious ocular injuries that often produced the condition, ophthalmologists handling the injuries and illnesses suffered in World War I also made significant breakthroughs. The use of mustard and other poisonous gases created a class of eye injuries that turned the theaters of World War I into research laboratories. The huge number of "*gassed cases*" requiring treatment broke down into three classes: those caused by pulmonary irritants, lachrymatory gas, or mustard gas. Lachrymatory gas caused no permanent damage, but produced an intense burning pain and inability to keep the eyes open. Mustard gas produced serious effects on the respiratory passages and caused lasting ocular problems such as chronic conjunctivitis and lesions similar to those following burns by ammonia, lime and other caustics. By the war's end, doctors compiled extensive reports detailing the variations in these injuries and best methods for treatment.

MacPherson, W.G. et al., v.2: 360, 529-532;
U.S. War Department, Surgeon General's Office. VII: Training, 514-522, 530-1;
"Ophthalmology in the American Expeditionary Forces," 714;
William C. Lloyd, III, M.D. interview

In recognition of the quantity of valuable medical experience already gained by 1915, the U.S. Surgeon General's Office midway during the war directed the Medical Corps to use the knowledge that doctors had acquired on the battlefield to the benefit of medical science. Their statement read: "*Eye surgeons and ophthalmologists at present on duty in the various American base hospitals should be required to expand their duties beyond the mere details of clinical work along the lines of investigation.*" In the new requirements established for specialists, officials encouraged them to pursue research interests as they treated the injured. More specifically, ophthalmologists were encouraged to investigate pathological and bacteriological conditions and the phenomenon of "*ocular malingering*" that debilitated many soldiers, and to compile systematic records of the ocular investigations they conducted. As a result, eye specialists treating large numbers of cases never before seen began to collect information and pose the kinds of questions that produced innovation and sparked medical research.

"Ophthalmology in the American Expeditionary Forces," 659-669, 714-716; 724-728;
U.S. War Department, Surgeon General's Office. VII: Training, 124-131; 556-559;
MacPherson, W.G. et al, v.2:360

Among the medical accomplishments of World War I, the average time for injured soldiers to reach European field hospitals (roughly five to eight miles from the front line) was reduced to about five hours, and from the front line to evacuation hospitals to about ten hours. The wounded arrived at base hospitals in several train loads of 300 to 500 men each day. The principal British medical history of World War I states that, "*For the purpose of treating injuries and affections of the eye during the war an extensive specialist organization was gradually established.*" Improved procedures were rapidly shared, and one observer noted that, "*Lessons learned regarding recovery of the wounded from the field of battle and then rapid and safe transportation to the hands of surgeons at the rear are now being taught to students for the benefit of the entire American Army.*" Battlefield techniques thus came to influence triage and emergency care everywhere, and the experience of caring for the wounded at clinics such as that run by Colonel Lyster at Boulogne ultimately produced a host of other beneficial changes in medical procedures. According to official reports, "*information concerning new methods of treatment and rare cases was circularized, interest was stimulated and the capacity of and results obtained by the various specialists were gauged.*" Eye surgeons expressed interest in studying "*ocular complications of various infections*," "*systematic complete ocular investigations*," and other subjects of research. In addition to the massive undertaking required to support U.S. forces overseas, however, eye specialists participated in equally substantial activities at home.

MacPherson, W.G. et al, v. 1: 126;
MacPherson, W.G. et al, History of the Great War: Medical Services: Surgery, v. 2, London, His Majesty's Stationery Office, 1922, 499, 503;
"Ophthalmology in the American Expeditionary Forces," 659-728;
Military Medical Manual, 349

## THE WAR REACHES SOUTH TEXAS

World War I became a reality in Texas when the government activated military installations across the state. Between 1884 and 1890, Forts Griffin, McKavitt, Stockton, Davis, and other camps had been abandoned. The closing of Fort Elliott, the last post established in Texas to address the threat from Native-Americans, heralded the end of the frontier. The only posts still occupied in 1890 were Forts Clark, Bliss, Brown, McIntosh, and San Antonio's Fort Sam Houston, the most substantial of the remaining installations. By the time the United States entered World War I, however, new installations were under construction and a massive build up underway. In addition to fighting men, Texas supplied medical units to overseas base hospitals from Camp Travis at Fort Sam Houston, Camp McArthur, and Camp Baker (mobilized at Camp Bowie).

"Centennial Record of the San Antonio Army Service Forces Depot, 1845-1945," 108-9;
Fort Sam Houston Museum, Camp Travis, 35

San Antonio, where the military had enjoyed a strong presence for two centuries already, witnessed a massive build-up of facilities and men. Fort Sam Houston received nearly one-tenth of the money appropriated by a Congressional Act in 1890 to construct new military buildings, and by 1912 was the largest Army post in the United States. Encompassing almost five square miles on the city's northeastern edge, the well-developed military infrastructure made San Antonio a place from which the military could logically expand. When units began to mobilize in World War I, therefore, construction began on a host of new facilities. In June, 1917, the New England firm of Stone and Webster employed 9,100 people to set up a cluster of temporary cantonment buildings on Fort Sam's eastern edge known as Camp Wilson, capable of housing up to 12,000 horses, and additional land was acquired during the war for the construction of Camp Travis, a larger facility that engulfed Camp Wilson and by 1918 housed 12,000 men.

"Centennial Record of the San Antonio Army Service Forces Depot, 1845-1945," 113; Fort Sam Houston Museum, "Camp Travis," 23, 33-35, 62;
Woolford, Sam and Bess, 117-120;
Peyton, Green, San Antonio: City in the Sun, 98;
"Historical Military Data on San Antonio and Fort Sam Houston," Fort Sam Houston archives.

To accommodate massive personnel increases, officials also substantially expanded Fort Sam Houston's medical facilities. In 1882 an 84-bed station hospital had replaced the original primitive log cabin dispensary, and in 1908 building was completed on a 4,382-bed Base Hospital designed to support the camp's medical needs, staffed by 75 officers, 154 nurses, and 697 enlisted men. In 1917 this hospital was organized to form Camp Travis Base Hospital, which treated more than 50,000 patients during the war and provided personnel for the 150th Base Hospital and other units, while Camp Naker supplied the Army Sanitary Train. At the same time, the government began construction of a massive sixty-building hospital complex known as Brooke General Hospital that would eventually occupy the former site of the Camp Travis Base Hospital. The hospital reached its peak patient load a few months before December 1918, when the first wounded men began arriving from overseas. In the course of the war, doctors also treated 13,390 local patients with influenza, measles, and flu. Patients from U.S. General Hospital No. 15 in the Corpus Christi Beach Hotel, a convalescent facility, were transferred to the U.S. Base Hospital at Camp Travis in 1919, and this facility treated 50,000 men before its last patients were transferred to Brooke and it was converted into officers quarters. The medical complex eventually grew to include twenty-four wards, an operating room, laboratory, four isolation wards, seven barracks, and a power plant. San Antonio emerged from the war, therefore, with a new configuration of medical facilities that firmly established its role as a regional medical center.

"Centennial Record of the San Antonio Army Service Forces Depot, 1845-1945," 113-15;
Fort Sam Houston Museum,
"Camp Travis," 33-35, 62;
"Historical Military Data on San Antonio and Fort Sam Houston", typescript, Fort Sam Houston archives, 1-3;
Peyton, Green, San Antonio: City in the Sun, 99

Before the war's end, a total of 208,000 soldiers trained at Fort Sam Houston for overseas duty. Camp John Wise, Camp Stanley, and others saw the arrival of flying cadets and thousands of soldiers, while thousands of civilian workers joined San Antonio's wartime industrial establishment at Kelly Field or worked at general supply depots at Fort Sam Houston and Camp Normoyle on the city's southwest edge. Between 1917 and 1918 alone there were 70,000 soldiers in San Antonio. Breadless days, meatless days, and sugar rationing were necessary, saloons were voted out of existence, and daily life focused on soldiers at home and abroad. Local women not only rolled bandages and nursed the sick, but also took YMCA classes to teach them to replace men on the home front.

Woolford, Sam and Bess, 119; McBride, Donald B., 2

By the war's end, the Medical Corps at the national level grew to 30,591 officers and 281,341 enlisted men. The maximum bed capacity of 91 U.S. hospitals totaled 120,916, and construction of an additional 25,000 beds was in progress at that time. On Armistice Day in November 1918, there were 76,964 patients in base and general hospi-

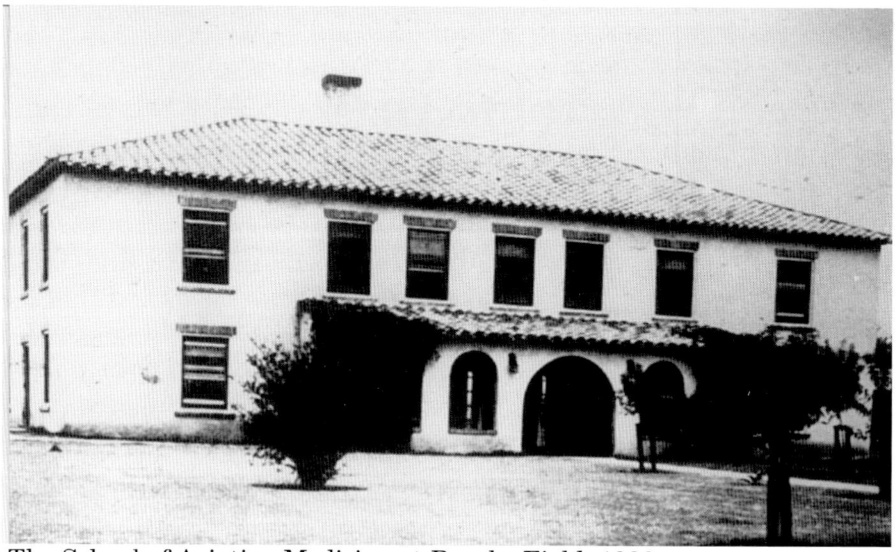

The School of Aviation Medicine at Brooks Field, 1929

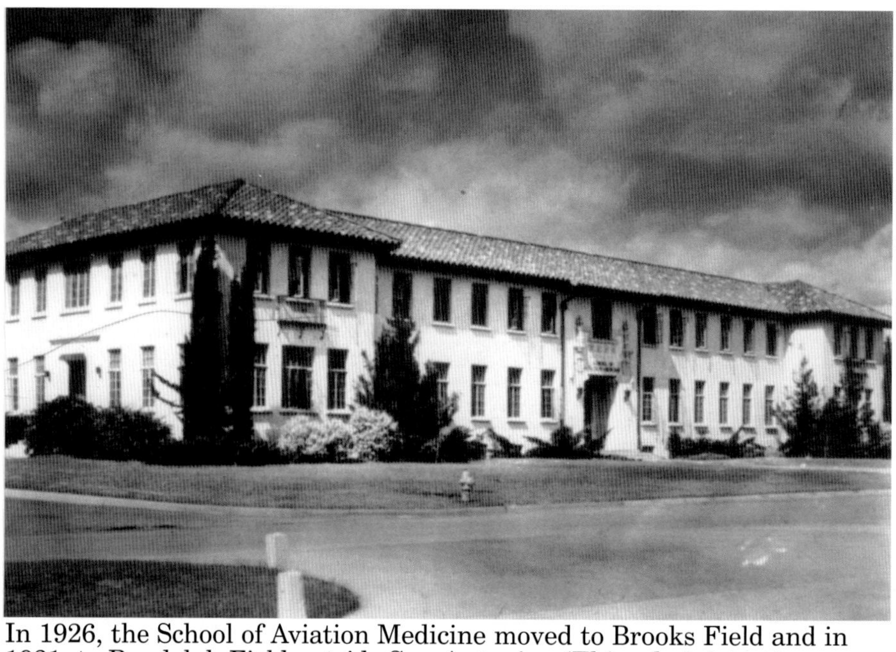

In 1926, the School of Aviation Medicine moved to Brooks Field and in 1931, to Randolph Field outside San Antonio. (This administration building still exists 75 years later.) Then, in 1959, the School of Aviation Medicine moved to Brooks Air Force Base.

tals in the United States and 193,026 patients in hospitals of the American Expeditionary Forces in Europe. There were 153 base hospitals, 66 camp hospitals, and 12 convalescent camps in France alone. Overall, the Medical Department had treated a total of four million sick and wounded men in the course of the conflict. The distribution of overseas patients to general and base hospitals in the United States between July 1, 1918 and June 30, 1919 is represented by the following statistics, showing the scale of that distribution. In Texas, Camp Bowie received 2,908 cases, Fort Sam Houston 1,293, Camp Travis 509, Corpus Christi 95, Camp Logan 65, and Camp McArthur 9 of a total 134,855 cases returned. Of these, a portion of the ophthalmology cases were sent to San Antonio. In addition to general medical support for military personnel, however, San Antonio was involved in activities related to the use of airplanes in combat that produced lasting consequences for ophthalmology.

Peyton, Green, San Antonio: City in the Sun, 104; Military Medical Manual, 346-350;
U.S. War Department, Surgeon General's Office. Report. 1919, 1160, 1180;
Handy, Mary Olivia, 74;
Dammin, 1463;
MacPherson, W.G. et al. History of the Great War Medical Services: Surgery, vol. 2. London, His Majesty's Stationery Office, 1922. 499-500, 530, 543- 44;
Medical Department of the U.S. Army in the World War, 500

## THE AIR WAR

The United States commissioned its first airplane in 1908, but realized the value of this new weapon of war only in World War I when the results of early sorties confirmed that airplanes were effective in battle. By the time General Funston chased Pancho Villa by air along the Mexican border from a base at Fort Sam Houston, the U.S. Air Service had grown to seven aero squadrons. The last large wagon train (125 wagons and over 600 mules) was used to concentrate National Guard troops on the Mexican Border in 1916 and 1917. As large numbers of troops mobilized there, many army medical officers were "in and out of San Antonio." Thereafter, the number of horses and mules decreased steadily. The importance of airplanes to military history is measured by the fact that horses were used for the last time in World

War I, although the U.S. Army owned only 25 trucks in 1914. Military aviation did not truly get underway, however, until the U.S. Army began to expand its pilot training program.

Green, Peyton, San Antonio: City in the Sun, 69, 104;
Nixon, Century of Medicine in San Antonio, 271;
Graeme, 8-9

As the U.S. Army realized the need to bolster its air power, officials decided that existing airfields and support services were inadequate to train pilots and conduct related operations. As early as 1911, officials testing aircraft for effectiveness in reacting to the border crisis acknowledged that Fort Sam Houston's existing airfield was inadequate to operate a full-scale pilot training program. After the U.S. Army Signal Corps authorized its sole Aviation Section at San Antonio in 1914, therefore, plans were made to build two new airfields in the area, Kelly and Gosport (later Brooks Air Force Base). This action represented a first step toward making South Texas a key national center for military aviation activity. At the same time, medical officials realizing that "*a man fit for general military service was not necessarily fit for aviation*" began to devise the first physical standards for flight training. As early as 1912, the U.S. War Department published instructions for conducting physical examinations of candidates for aviation duty that required candidates' "*visual acuity without glasses to be normal. Any error of refraction requiring correction by glasses*" and "*color blindness for red, green, or violet*" was cause for rejection. A special test for night vision soon was also included. Unsuccessful candidates were told, "*No eyes, no wings.*" Physical examination units assembled in 35 major cities to recruit and examine candidates for Army Air Service swiftly grew to 67, and over 100,000 applicants for flight raining were examined during the war.

Armstrong, Harry, 9-11;
McBride, Donald B., 2

When the U.S. entered the war, the nation's first and largest flight training school for pilots opened at Kelly Field with eleven hundred officers, thirty-one thousand men housed in "*tent cities*," and a first class of 593 air cadets. Construction also began on a main hospital and "*flying department hospital*" to handle flight-related accidents. Eye standards swiftly went "*to the head of the list of requirements*." The wartime buildup also produced a school for airplane mechanics along with the first Army bombardier school, navigation school, and air observer school. Student flyers practiced dropping T.N.T. at the nearby bombing range at Camp Bullis. The greatest number of enlisted men at Kelly was 36,898 on December 25, 1917. Approximately 250,000 men were organized into aero squadrons at Kelly between 1917 and 1918, and most American-trained World War I aviators learned to fly here. By 1926 San Antonio was the site of the Air Corps Training Center and Kelly operated an advanced flying school with a Camp Hospital in its Flying Department, equipped with modern operating rooms and a laboratory. Between the two World Wars, most Army aviators trained here.

Greater Kelly Development Corporation, 2-3;
Payne, Brittain F., 488;
Peyton, Green, San Antonio: City in the Sun, 109

In addition to Kelly, Brooks Air Field, a flight center, instructor school, and Army training base located eight miles from Kelly and six miles from the San Antonio city center, further increased the region's aviation resources. Brooks, first known as Gosport Field, originally took its name from a flight training system devised by the Royal Flying Corps at Gosport, England, that allowed instructors to maintain voice communication through a speaking tube with airborne student pilots. Tests of the Gosport system at Gosport Field resulted in its adoption by the War Department and constituted some of the first aviation research in San Antonio. The field was renamed Brooks Air Force Base for Sidney Johnson Brooks, a native of the city who crashed during his qualifying flight. When World War I ended, the Brooks flight instructor school closed and the base became a center for primary flight training. By the war's end, therefore, San Antonio had become a logical place to concentrate activities related to aviation medicine. At the same time, moreover, forces were at work that would soon relocate another institution, the School of Aviation Research, in the Alamo City.

Green, Peyton, San Antonio: City in the Sun, 63-4, 69, 109;
Graeme, 8-9;
Alcott, Edward, Aerospace Medical Division, 130-1;
Alcott, Edward, "A Brief History of Brooks Air Force Base"

## THE AIR SERVICE MEDICAL LABORATORY AND THE SCHOOL OF AVIATION RESEARCH

As the importance of military aviation increased, medical facilities dedicated to the care of injured pilots developed of necessity. The French had established the world's first medical service for aviators in Paris in 1917, and by the end of that year both the Allies and Germany had created medical departments for their air services employing "*the best specialists of the respective countries*." It soon became apparent, however, that a different type of medical service was needed. British analysis of air casualties after the first year of the war attributed two per cent to the enemy, eight per cent to faulty planes, and ninety per cent to pilot error. These reports awakened officials to the need for greater medical knowledge to make pilots fit to fly and treat the victims of air crashes. Early plane crashes often proved fatal because the appropriate treatment for many injuries had simply not yet been determined or was unavailable in most regular clinical settings. Reports also revealed that pilots needed a clearer understanding of the visual aspects of flying and that physical standards such as good vision were essential in selecting pilots. As late as 1910 only a few scattered articles had appeared in the medical literature dealing with the field that would come to be known as aviation medicine.

Remarkably, before World War I and the use of military aviation, the only people interested in medical conditions similar to those experienced by aviators had been balloonists and mountain climbers seeking to better control the effects of altitude on the human body.

Armstrong, Harry, 9-12

Despite San Antonio's emerging role, however the first step in developing a medical service to meet the needs of military aviation had been taken elsewhere. United States medical aviation research began in 1918 with the founding of the Air Service Central Medical Research Laboratory for Aviation Medicine at Hazelhurst Field, Mineola, New York. The first formal course for Flight Surgeons was conducted at Mineola in 1919. The man chosen to become Chief Surgeon of the Air Service Medical Corps, with responsibility for treating members of the Aviation Section, Signal Corps, was Lt. Col. Theodore C. Lyster, who had operated the important clinic at Boulogne earlier. Lyster set out to develop medical standards for pilots and uniform procedures for treating flight-related problems. At the time, three airplane crashes occurred on average for every 721 hours flown, one of which involved a fatality.

Ashcroft, Bruce A., 2;
Military Medical Manual, 348, 511;
Alcott, Edward, Aerospace Medical Division, 2-4;
McBride, Captain Donald B., 2-3;
Fort Sam Houston Museum, "Fort Sam Houston Troop List," 1-4;
Payne, Brittain F., 488

Up until this time, an individuals' average vision on the ground was the only basis for existing medical standards. The notion of "20/20 eyesight," an empirical rubric for measuring visual capacity, meant simply that a person with 20/20 vision could see at a distance of twenty feet what an average normal eye would see. Other measurements, such as 20/10, meant that a person could see at twenty feet what an average eye could see at a distance of ten feet. Similarly, 20/100 meant a person could see at twenty feet what an average eye could see at 100 feet. A pilot with 10/100 vision would have to be 200 feet from earth to see as well as a normal eye at 1,000 feet. Lyster started out with a different idea. All pilots needed three things:

1) to be able to see things at a distance
2) to judge how far away they were
3) to see nearby objects, such as an instrument panel

Dr. Thomas Tredici interview.
For details on post-World War I eye testing, see Payne, Lt. Col. Brittain F., "Aviation Ophthalmology," 488

Lyster set up a research board "*to investigate all conditions affecting the physical efficiency of pilots*," "*to carry out experiments and tests at different flying schools*," and "*to act as a standing organization for instruction in the physiological requirements of aviators*." Members of this board included ophthalmologist William H. Wilmer, for whom the Wilmer Eye Institute was later named. Part of Lyster's plan was to create an eye, ear, nose, and throat department and bring in specialists to explore the visual aspects of flight experience. Lyster's agenda and subsequent research at Mineola, however, were implemented under the direction of Colonel Wilmer, who replaced Lyster and went on to set up six departments, including Ophthalmology, with separate directors for each, and to oversee the growth of the Laboratory to three times its original size by 1918. In that year--with 600 planes in service overseas--U.S. medical officials coined the term "*flight surgeon*" to describe experts in the unique new field of medical practice known as aviation medicine. In addition, 34 medical officers and 15 enlisted men trained in laboratory methods to reorganize the clinical evaluation and care of U.S. aviators embarked for service in Europe with the American Expeditionary Forces. Eventually, branch research laboratories based on the Mineola model would be established at twenty flying fields around the country, and over 100,000 flight training applicants examined at sixty-seven testing centers. Air Service personnel increased from "*65 officers and 1,120 enlisted men in April 1917 to 14,320 officers and 124,726 enlisted men one year later*," when it had become a branch of the Signal Corps.

Jones, Isaac H., 181-254;
Military Medical Manual, 512;
Dammin, 1179, 1456, 1460; "Kelly Field Medical Department;"
Benford, Robert J., 1-8, 11ff., 66;
Peyton, Green, San Antonio, City in the Sun, 98-118.
Alcott, Edward, Aerospace Medical Division, 5;
Payne, Lt. Col. Brittain F., 488).

With new visual standards for flying in place (subsequently adopted by the Civil Aeronautics Administration), the new Research Laboratory for Aviation Medicine expanded its focus to address problems of sustained acceleration, weightlessness, decompression sickness, temperature extremes, oxygen deprivation, vibration, confinement, and radiation encountered primarily in flight. In addition, ophthalmologists began to document visual conditions occurring in flight environments that ultimately expanded the parameters of the science of ophthalmology. No single part of the body or type of function defined aviation medicine as it had other branches of medicine, but rather the atmosphere above the earth where pilots worked. As pilots demanded greater knowledge about human vision, research in aviation medicine was about to create ophthalmology's first sub-specialty field.

Payne, Lt. Col. Brittain F., 488;
Armstrong, Harry, 8-10

One of the first problems to attract attention to ophthalmology and to extend ophthalmological knowledge came from soldiers and especially aviators who complained of an inability to see during nighttime combat. Solving the problem of "*night blindness*" meant extending vision beyond normal capacity. The possibility that use of a specific technology might permit an individual to enjoy improved or even complete night vision transformed the problem into a research question that doctors eagerly addressed and that generated ongoing research when they returned home. Other ophthalmological questions under consideration at the laboratory included whether depth perception and stereopsis were important to flying and how to explain the fact that visual function under hypoxia blurred nearby objects and made pilots cross-eyed and unable to accommodate above a certain altitude. It became clear that pilots not only needed better treatment for flight-related eye injuries, but ways to better adapt their vision to a wider range of flying conditions. At the same time, ophthalmologists sent their accumulated pathological specimens and microscopic sections to skilled artists at the War Office to draw and so produced a research resource of lasting medical and surgical significance. These records later served as the foundation for numerous research projects.

MacPherson, W.G. et al., 527;
Medical Department of the United States in the World War, 506, 530-531

The end of World War I on November 11, 1918, found military aviation resources spread across the country, but the importance of aviation research an unmistakable fact. Officials reviewing research advances at Mineola during the war were so impressed that the Army Medical Department rewrote its mission statement with a new stress on the importance of research. The revised version translated research into conventional military objectives, but expressed a new commitment in the statement that, "*Research can never be relaxed, for the Army's ability to conserve its fighting strength must keep abreast of a potential enemy's ability to cripple it.*" Just as bold, innovative treatments had been developed under wartime conditions, now effective efforts of the first aviation research laboratory would be continued in peacetime by creating a system of organized medical research.

Military Medical Manual, 349;
"Brooke Army Medical Center History"

The War Department next undertook a re-organization with important ramifications for South Texas ophthalmology. In 1919, the Mineola Medical Research Laboratory offered its first eight-week course for flight surgeons. It also moved to a new location at Mitchel Field, Long Island. Thereafter, its efforts shifted increasingly from research to teaching. Officials established a School for Flight Surgeons later that year that linked the Laboratory training course to a more extensive four-month training course for medical personnel who worked with pilots. Recognition of the value of combining the two institutions came in 1921 when the War Department designated the Laboratory and School a special service school of the Army, no longer a purely research facility but an "*integral part of the flight training system*," and changed the name of the Medical Research Laboratory and School for Flight Surgeons in 1922 to the School of Aviation Medicine.

Ashcroft, Bruce, 3; Military Medical Manual, 512

As the original Medical Research Laboratory underwent a major transformation, however, South Texas was becoming the nation's principal training facility for military medical personnel. Extensive medical, military, and aviation connections already existed in Texas. The Lone Star State offered vast open spaces ideal for flying, a suitable climate, and hosts of enthusiasts. One San Antonio woman later captured the excitement by recalling that she had learned to fly before she learned to drive! San Antonio and much of Texas were not only a center for U.S. military aviation operations, but also for amateur flyers, aircraft manufacturers, and airline companies. In 1919 medical officers who had served with aviation units during the war met at Dallas to organize a flight surgeon's association, reinforcing these links. Dallas ophthalmologist and flight surgeon Dr. John O. McReynolds became the first president of another new organization known as the Air Service Medical Association of the United States at the AMA annual meeting later that year, and the creation of the University of Texas at Austin School of Military Aeronautics, though it had no medical component, served to further reinforce the point. These factors no doubt were taken into consideration when military leaders acknowledged that San Antonio had unusual military and medical resources for a community of its size, and orders were approved for major renovations at the Fort Sam Houston Base Hospital. Primary flight training took place at Brooks Field, and advanced training at Kelly. Now all that remained was to bring the military's vital resources together. By placing the School of Aviation Medicine close to these flight training bases, it was thought that more trainees would be graduated. The final step was taken on June 30, 1926, when the War Department transferred the School of Aviation Medicine to Brooks Field at San Antonio.

Green, Peyton, San Antonio: City in the Sun, 88-90;
Alcott, Edward, "Brief History of Brooks Air Force Base;"
Ashcroft, Bruce, 3.

Among Texas eye, ear, nose and throat surgeons and examiners who had served at Mitchel Field was Dr. Henry Louis Hilgartner, who spent much of his later career in Austin, Texas. The first commandant of the School of Aviation Medicine also had ties to Texas. Known as "*Mr. Aviation Medicine*," Major Louis Hopewell Bauer, a Harvard Medical School graduate, had accepted a commission as a first lieutenant in the Army Medical Corps and served in 1913 with the Second Infantry Division on the Texas Border. He then went to the Philippines before returning to Texas in 1917 to join an aviation unit at Kelly Air Field. In 1918 he was promoted to lieutenant colonel, and a year later he succeeded Colonel William Wilmer as director of the Medical Research Laboratory in Long Island. Bauer later served as AMA president, edited the *Journal of Aviation Medicine* for 25 years, became the first director of the Aeronautics Branch of the Department of Commerce, authored a book on aviation medicine, and founded the Aero Medical Association--an organization for physicians working in aviation medicine.

Woolford, Sam and Bess, 120;
"Henry Hilgartner," New Handbook of Texas, 1179;
Texas Medicine 71(March 1975), 101-103;
Dr. Thomas Tredici interview;
Green, Peyton, 50 Years of Aerospace Medicine, 41, 46, 69, 63-4, 109;
Benford, 1-6, 11ff;
Alcott, Edward, Aerospace Medical Division, 5;
"Kelly Field Medical Department;"
Fort Sam Houston Museum, Fort Sam Houston Troop List, 3

The School of Aviation Medicine as originally structured in San Antonio consisted of three components: a Primary Flying School and School of Aviation Medicine, temporarily housed in the hangar meant for the dirigible, Roma, and the Advanced Flying School at Kelly Air Field. Here a professional staff of flight surgeons conducted research and offered 4-month training courses followed by 6 months of practical work at Brooks Field. A decision that allowed military laboratories to engage civilians as research scientists, instructors, and technicians enabled San Antonio community ophthalmologists to take part in activities at the School. Together these men worked with aviators interested in improving the flight experience who gladly joined forces with the school's flight surgeons to produce research advances. According to an Army medical manual, the School of Aviation Medicine functioned "*advantageously as a teaching as well as a research institution.*" In addition, however, the new research facilities were in place at just the moment when important developments in aviation medicine that involved ophthalmologists and advanced ophthal-

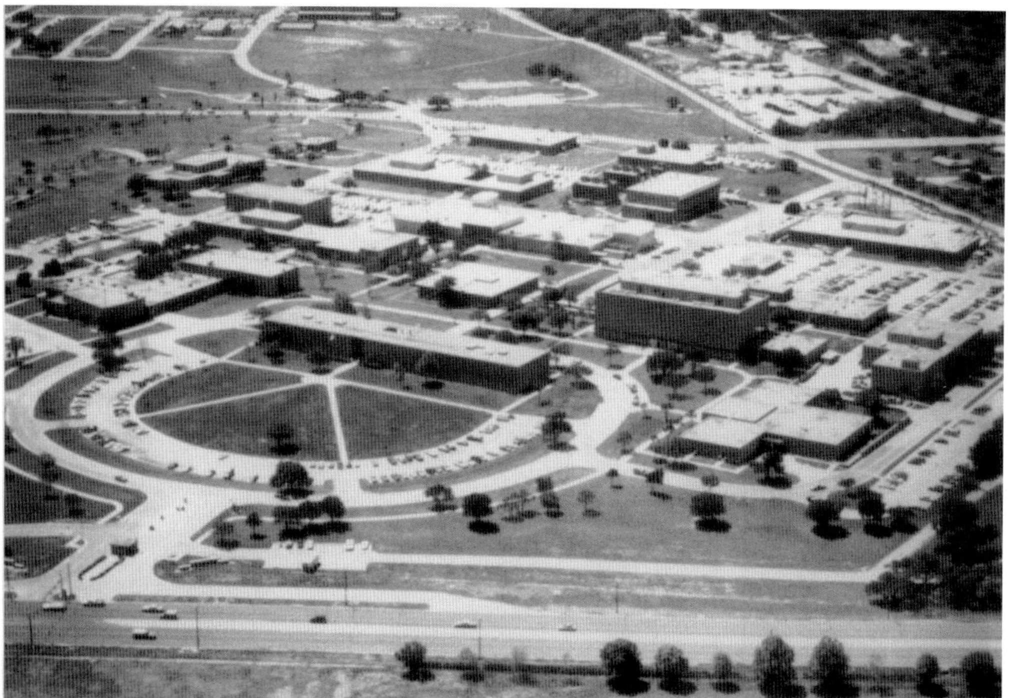

The "campus" of the USAF School of Aviation Medicine, Brooks AFB, Texas. Opened Oct. 1959 and was dedicated on Nov. 2, 1963 by U. S. President John F. Kennedy.

mological knowledge were about to be made. More specifically, military ophthalmologist Dr. Frederick H. Thorne and two aviation researchers named William C. Ocker and Carl Crane were about to plant the roots of a lasting tradition of ophthalmological research in San Antonio.

Military Medical Manual, 512-516;
Isaac H. Jones, Flying Vistas, 58;
Armstrong, Harry, 10;
Graeme, 8-9;
n.a., "A Glimpse Into the Past," 101-3;.
Green, Peyton, San Antonio: City in the Sun, 63, 64, 69, 109;
Link and Coleman, 153.

## WILLIAM C. OCKER AND DR. FREDERICK THORNE

The fact that "*for ten years following the end of World War I aviation medicine almost ceased to exist as a living science and was kept from utter decay only by the efforts of a few individuals who had the foresight to realize that aviation and aviation medicine were more than a freak of necessity of World War I*" only accentuates the importance of contributions to the field by William C. Ocker, Carl Crane, and Dr. Frederick Thorne. The Ocker-Crane system of "*blind flying*" or relying on instruments to fly, the Complex Coordinator used to predict the flying ability of candidates for pilot training, and a number of other devices were developed from medical research at the School of Aviation Medicine directed in part by ophthalmologist Dr. Frederick Thorne. For those who have never flown, the importance of blind flying can be compared to the use of seatbelts in automobiles. Present standard airplane instrumentation capable of compensating for a pilot's physical limitations did not exist before 1914. This was true despite common knowledge that most pilots lacked the flying accuracy required for World War I bombing runs and many aircraft were forced to land when the weather turned bad. People who lost their way tended to go around in circles or tailspins that often led to a crash. The importance of these advances to South Texas ophthalmology, however, lay in introducing ophthalmic research to the region and heightening the level of awareness among local practitioners.

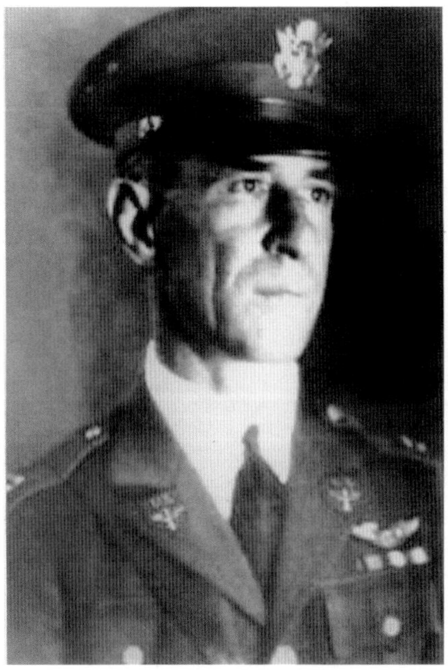

William C. Ocker (1880 – 1942), the father of "Blind Flying," flew from Brooks Field, San Antonio, Texas, to March Field, California in a covered cockpit to prove that a test pilot's instrumentation could be more reliable than his own natural senses.
Flight Captain, 1964. Col. Crane designed and built the Stinson Memorial located at Brooks, which was dedicated on 17 Dec. 1965.

Jones, Isaac, 181, 254;
Green, Peyton, San Antonio: City in the Sun, 67;
Alcott, Edward, Aerospace Medical Division, 4

By 1918 researchers at the Air Service Medical Research Laboratory had shown "*that without vision, disorientation and loss of equilibration*" quickly followed, while others established an association between ocular movement and stimulation of the ear canal that produced vertigo. Few experiments had been done, however, using mechanical substitutes for a pilot's point of reference when clouds or nightfall obscured the landscape. The culture that surrounded fliers and flying acted as a deterrent to instrument development since many pilots believed flying to be an art. A good pilot, they commonly thought, could "*fly by the seat of his pants*."

Air Service Medical, 9;
Armstrong, Harry, 14, 231

William Charles Ocker (1876-1942) was the first person to realize that instrumentation could compensate for pilots' physical limitations and enable them to fly in bad weather. Neither a physician nor a scientist, Ocker lacked formal training but was an experienced Air Corps pilot and something of a self-made man. Ocker's contributions to science came from his first-hand knowledge of physical responses in flight and his insight into how instruments could allow for visual and otological distortions. In working without professional credentials Ocker resembled Helmholtz, who invented the ophthalmoscope but was not an eye specialist. For this reason, validation by qualified investigators such as Dr. Thorne and Carl Crane at the School of Aviation Research, a research institution using procedures that met scientific standards, provided important confirmation of Ocker's advances.

Ocker and Thorne's importance parallels that of Dr. Julius Sichel, who studied with the famed ophthalmologist Beer at Vienna and subsequently had a powerful influence on French ophthalmology as an individual by establishing a private eye clinic in Paris. In both cases, individual efforts foreshadowed a new direction for medical culture throughout an entire region.

Rosen, 41;
"Col. Ocker is Dead;"
Crane, Col. Carl, "Spiral Dive;"
Ocker and Crane, Blind Flight in Theory and Practice, 9

Ocker left grammar school, enlisted in the Cavalry at age sixteen by claiming he was twenty-one, and served in the Spanish-American War and the Philippines before joining the Aviation Section of the Signal Corps as a corporal in aircraft mechanics. After learning to fly while on furlough in San Diego, he entered a small and elite group of pilots and found a job as a test pilot at McCook Field in Washington, D.C., where he joined Billy Mitchell's Signal Corps around 1918. While serving as a commanding officer at Chandler Field in Pennsylvania and a flight instructor at Gerstner Field in Louisiana, he met and became a friend of Orville Wright. Ocker also worked at

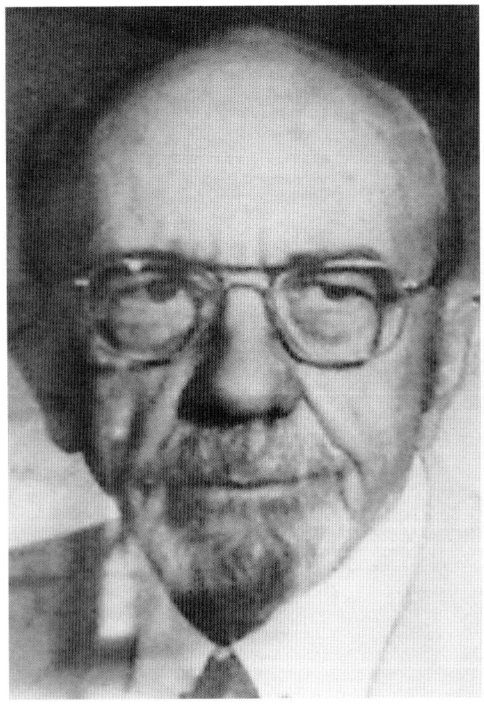

Col. Carl J. Crane, USAF Rt., born Oct. 1900, died 26 April 1982. Graduated from US Army Flying School at Kelly Field, Texas, Sept. 1925. Awarded the Mackay Trophy in 1939, for designing and accomplishing the World's First Automatic Landing at Wright-Patterson AFB on 23 Aug 1937. Was instrumental in founding the Stinsons Flight No. 2 of the Order of Daedalians, and was its' first Flight Captain, 1964. Col. Crane designed and built the Stinson Memorial located here, which was dedicated on 17 Dec. 1965.

Wilbur Wright Field and was commanding officer of the Fifty-sixth Service Squadron at Langley Field.

Ocker biographical materials, Hangar 9, Lackland Air Force Base, San Antonio; "Col. Ocker is Dead"

Using his own experience as data, Ocker wrestled with the problems of vertigo and disorientation in flight that resulted from the lack of visual cues when flying through cloud cover, fog, or at night when pilots could not see the ground. Later he learned that even pigeons are unable to fly blind. The solution emerged from another of his contacts when he became an assistant to pilot Lawrence Sperry of the Sperry Gyroscope Company in Brooklyn, New York, who was later lost while flying over the English Channel. When Sperry asked him to test a company turn indicator for oceangoing ships, Ocker realized that the device could be used successfully to also turn an airplane. He modified the instrument at first only by adding a turn-and-bank feature that enabled him to correct for false impressions. Using this device and a compass for directional control, Ocker managed to fly through fog over the mountains from Washington, D.C., and land successfully in Ohio. He did not yet realize, however, that instruments could entirely compensate for a lack of visual cues, and carried Sperry's device with him for another eight years while he pondered the problems of blind flight.

"Antebellum fledglings;"
Pam Crane interview;
Ocker materials, Hangar 9;
Ocker and Crane, Blind Flight in Theory and Practice, 17

Ocker's most important discovery came in 1926 when he visited a physician for a routine physical examination at Crissy Field in San Francisco, and the exam launched a discussion with the doctor who examined him, a flight surgeon and aviation medicine expert named Captain David A. Myers. Myers introduced Ocker to the Barany Chair, a device named for a Hungarian otologist that eliminated visual references and produced inner ear responses that simulated the effects of blind flight. When rotated in the chair, Ocker discovered he was unable to ascertain the direction in which he was turning. By mounting Sperry's instrument in a box on the Barany chair, however, he was able to pass the test by relying on the instrument for information despite the contradictory data coming from his eyes and ears. The "*Ocker Box*," as the technology came to be known, eventually included a bank and turn indicator and a light that helped to simulate a pilot's sensations during blind instrument flight in zero visibility.

1. David A. Myers, the Army Medical Corps flight surgeon, published a study of the physiologic factors involved in instrument flying and demonstrated the fundamental principles that made blind flying possible in 1936.

2. Training for Flight Surgeon's assistants during World War I included the set up and operation of the Barany Chair.

"Col. Ocker is Dead;"
Crane, Col. Carl, "Spiral Dive;"
Pam Crane interview: Link and Coleman, 156.

Eventually, with the addition of an artificial horizon to restore the pilot's bearings, Ocker obtained a complete, if imaginary, sense of position in the air and a view of the ground as well. Ocker went on to produce a "*flight integrator*" that "*allowed pilots to view an airplane's movements in miniature*" on a moving screen actuated by an electrically driven gyroscope that depicted a sky dotted by clouds. In front of the screen horizon was a miniature airplane that banked in the same manner as the airplane in which the instrument was installed and presented roll, pitch, and yaw in one visual reference frame.

"Col. Ocker is Dead;
Crane, Col. Carl, "Spiral Dive;"
Pam Crane interview;
Benson, Robert, Heritage of Aviation Medicine, 80

Ocker's connection with South Texas developed when he came to the Air Corps Primary Flying School of the Air Corps Training Center in 1927, and began working with researchers at the School of Aviation Medicine. Unfortunately, his Kelly Field contemporaries banned him from teaching instrument flying when he offended his superiors with his zeal. The fact that Ocker was court-martialed for use of "*improper language*" and then acquitted after twelve minutes of deliberation suggests the level of his frustration. He was twice hospitalized for sanity tests, and later joked he was the only Air Corps officer who had two letters to prove he was sane. Despite these setbacks, his position as a flight trainer gave him his first real opportunity to do research. Now at last the aging pilot received the attention he deserved.

Peyton, Green, Fifty Years of Aerospace Medicine, 71;
Crane, Carl, "Spiral Dive," 25-27;
Ocker materials, Hangar 9;
Pam Crane interview.

Carl Crane, a mechanical engineer who met Ocker in 1929, had a distinguished background that offered strong support for Ocker's research and later went on to develop related instruments, including a pre-flight reflex trainer in 1941. Crane was born in San Antonio where he attended St. Mary's College. He went on to attend the Navy program at M.I.T. and work at the Sturdevant Airplane Factory and the Quincy Shipyard in New England. He also worked on railcars outside Michigan and eventually joined the Air Corps, which brought him back to Brooks Field as a flight instructor.

At Brooks and later Randolph Air Force Base, Ocker carried on his experiments with the approval of the Commandant of the Air Corps Training Center, Brigadier General Frank P. Lahm, and worked with Carl Crane, with whom he did many blind-flying tests and other studies. Interest in Ocker's inventions was sufficient that the School of Aviation Medicine assigned a team of medical and aviation specialists to repeat his experiments, including the Chief of the Department of Ophthalmology and Otology, Captain Frederick H. Thorne. Thorne, one of the outstanding ophthalmologists that World War I brought to

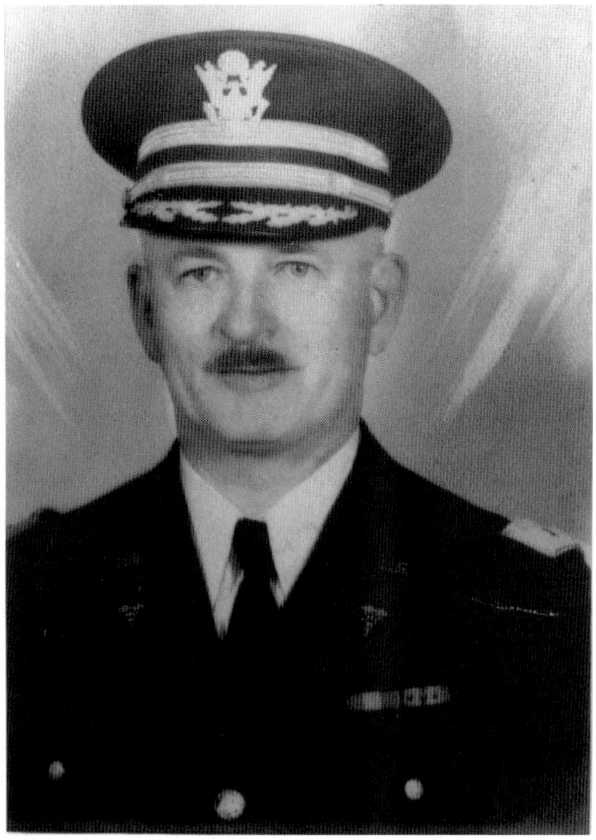

Major Frederick H. Thorne,
Chief of the School of
Aviation Medicine, 1926-1929

San Antonio, was a man like Ocker who had begun his military service in the Spanish-American War. After receiving his medical degree in 1911 and completing an internship at Boston's College of Physicians and Surgeons, Thorne worked as a pathologist at the New Jersey State Hospital and attended the University of Breslau, Germany, for a year of neurology and ocular pathology. He also served in the Panama Canal Zone, on the Mexican Border in 1916, and at the Rockefeller Institute for Medical Research in New York before organizing a mobile field laboratory for overseas service in World War I. He began to practice ophthalmology in 1919 and had conducted research at the Air Service Primary Flying School at Mineola before moving to San Antonio in 1926 to become Post Surgeon and Chief of EENT at the new School of Aviation Medicine. Thorne was a flight surgeon and an expert in plastic surgery with experience in treating aviators injured in airplane crashes. In rebuilding faces, he was among the first to learn that muscles could be successfully attached to artificial eyes to permit movement. When he met Ocker, therefore, Thorne brought to the research effort a wealth of experience and a unique set of skills.

Thorne went on to have a distinguished military medical career that included serv-

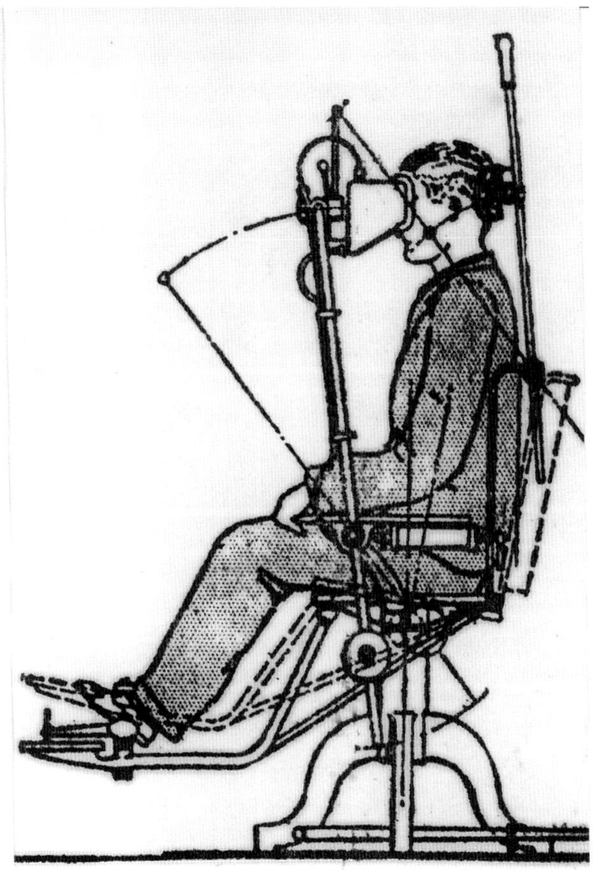

The improved Pilot Test Chair, fitted with eye shield and apparatus for determining the aviator´s ability to fly by instruments only.

ice as personal physician to President Taft. He later worked with the blind and went to England to develop tools for their use. A lifelong collector of clocks, he was typical of many ophthalmologists who enjoy a strong interest in precision of all kinds. In San Antonio he was associated with Dr. Robert Parrish at an office in the Medical Arts Building, served as an associate surgeon in eye, ear, nose and throat at the R.B. Green Hospital, and lived at 950 Grayson Street near Fort Sam Houston in a house known as the Castle. After thirty years service in the U.S. Medical Corps, he went into private practice in the Kerr-Kendall-Gillespie-Bandera area. He is buried in the city's National Cemetery at Fort Sam Houston.

Dorothy Crawford interview;
Peyton, Green, Fifty Years of Aerospace Medicine, 63, 71.

After Thorne and his team of researchers completed their first round of experiments, the School of Aviation Medicine conducted additional blind flying tests with the Mexican Division of Pan American Airlines on flights between Brownsville and Mexico City. These efforts resulted in the publication of Ocker and Crane's Blind Flight in Theory and Practice, the first manual describing how to fly using instruments, in 1932. Thorne also published several articles relating to Ocker's research, including a discussion of the use of a device known as a Prince ruler entitled "*Rule for Measuring Accommodation, Near Point of Convergence, and Interpupillary Distance*." Based on School of Aviation Medicine research, scientists later developed better simulators for night flying, but this was only the beginning.

The manager of the Pan American Airlines office in Brownsville had been a cadet under Ocker and asked for his instruction to learn to fly in bad weather.

Pam Crane interview;
Ocker and Crane, Blind Flight in Theory and Practice, 16-20

In 1930, the year in which *The Journal of Aviation Medicine* began publication, Ocker introduced Crane to Elmer Sperry, who presented them with a Kollsman altimeter, artificial horizon, and directional gyro, and in June of that year Ocker piloted a plane 900 miles from San Antonio to Scott Field in Illinois in a covered cockpit with no view of the outside world. Although he called the trip an "*unofficial test*," the implications of the experiment were clear. According to Crane, the trained engineer who worked as his assistant, Ocker's inventions constituted a "*breakthrough to the understanding of the marked affect of the inner ear apparatus on the pilot's response mechanism during flight when there is no outside visual reference to earth from the airplane cockpit*." What pilots most needed, he claimed, was a "*visual interface within the cockpit that is the full equivalent of outside visual reference during clear weather*."

Ocker met Crane in 1929. "Col. Ocker is Dead;"
Ocker biographical materials, Hangar 9;
Green, Peyton, Fifty Years of Aerospace Medicine, 71;
Benford, Robert, Heritage of Aviation Medicine, 80;
Crane, Carl, Letter to Mrs. T.E. McCray, August 20, 1967; Armstrong, Harry, 231;
Crane, Carl, "Spiral Dive"

Ocker's work coincided with other developments that increased the importance of San Antonio military operations and the School of Aviation Medicine (SAM). In 1931, a year after the Army's principal training center for air cadets moved to Brooks Field, the School of Aviation Medicine moved to San Antonio's Randolph Field next to the hospital on the base's main circle. The "West Point of the Air," as Randolph came to be known, was built to be the largest flying field in the world. Fifteen miles from the city center, it was located on a four-square-mile plot of farmland purchased by the city and presented to the United States government. The new SAM occupied a building complete with lecture halls, offices, laboratories in the basement, and examining rooms on its top two floors. Research was divided into four principal departments, including Ophthalmology and Otology, Aviation Medicine, Psychology, and Neuropsychiatry, to train flight surgeons in:

1) the fundamentals and the basic factors of ophthalmology, including the anatomy, histology, physiology, and pathology of the eye and its adnexa

2) the diagnosis and treatment of common ocular affections

3) special diagnostic methods and instruments utilized in the examination of the eye

4) diagnosis and treatment of the common affections of the ear, nose and throat

5) ophthalmological and otological aspects of the care and maintenance of fliers

6) procedures for conducting the examination of the eye, ear, nose and throat for flying

Green, Peyton, Fifty Years of Aerospace Medicine, 104, 112;
Alcott, Edward, Aerospace Medical Division, 9;
"Minutes of Regular Meeting of March 28, 1918," Medical Annals of Southwest Texas, April 1918, 116ff;
Link and Coleman, 158.

By 1930, a private airline and a school had adopted Ocker's methods of training (though in 1933 Ocker's flight manual fell into the hands of the Soviets, who used it for a time before it was fully accepted in the United States). By 1934 he developed a training simulator and a basic course in instrument flying at Kelly Field that was adopted by the Air Corps, but in that year he was grounded because of his imperfect vision. Ocker tried to obtain patents on the pre-flight reflex trainer he developed with Crane in 1941 and other flying instruments, but lacked the authority to establish the importance of his discoveries, and only later did the U.S. Patents and Design Board award him a $1,000 prize for his inventions. Although Randolph set up classes on instrument training based on his ideas, the United States military establishment failed to adopt his training principles until a year after he died. As late as 1934, however, President Franklin D. Roosevelt cancelled Army Mail contracts because of air crashes. At the beginning of World War II, blind flight training was reactivated by Joe Duckworth at a Mississippi flight school.

Ocker, William C. and Carl J. Crane, 16;
Green, Peyton, Fifty Years of Aerospace Medicine, 71;
Pam Crane interview

Ocker's most enduring legacy lies in setting a challenging agenda for ongoing research at the School of Aviation Medicine on human visual performance in flight. The ability to undertake blind or night flying represented an effort to expand the range of human vision in conditions outside the normal. According to scholars, "*neither advanced terrestrial nor outer-space flight would ever have been possible*" without Ocker's achievements. Orville Wright called him a "*missionary*" of instrument flying who had "*more influence in bringing about the use of instruments than any other person*." Because of the visual elements in Ocker's instrument design, his blind flying research must be seen as a pre-condition or one root of an ophthalmic research tradition in South Texas. For the profession of ophthalmology in this region, Ocker and Thorne's work heightened local interest in research and ultimately added growing enthusiasm for specialty training programs and professional specialty societies. Meanwhile, the School of Aviation Medicine trained all Army pilots for nearly a decade, giving researchers in ophthalmology a unique pool of candidates on which to draw for investigation and experiments. According to Randolph historian Bruce A. Ashcroft, "*the 1930s were a period when aviation medicine began to take shape as a distinct specialty*." In sum, not only the experience and resources that accumulated at the School of Aviation Medicine, but the improved climate for specialization and, to a large degree, today's aerospace research activity in Texas all are, to a large degree, a direct legacy of World War I.

Green, Peyton, Fifty Years of Aerospace Medicine, 70;
Benford, Robert, Heritage of Aviation Medicine, 5-6

## THE GENERATION THAT SERVED

Although only 6,639 specialists (of whom roughly seventy percent focused their practices on the eye, ear, nose and throat) practiced in the United States at the start World War I, the total a decade later had risen significantly. At that time, twenty-three percent (23%) of practicing specialists were ophthalmologists, thirty percent (30%) were eye, ear, nose, and throat specialists, and 47% limited their practices to ear, nose, and throat. These statistics suggest that World War I failed to slow the growth of ophthalmic specialization, and instead acted as a powerful stimulus to professional development by shaping the careers of many youthful practitioners. Eighty-two men, or almost fifty per cent of the 174 members of the Bexar County Medical Society served in the U.S. Medical Corps in World War I. Those who remained at home, however, were no less influenced by wartime experience due to the programs offered at Society meetings. Here community practitioners learned about medical service from the time a soldier was wounded until he arrived at a Base Hospital and became informed about advances made around the world. According to the Medical Annals of Southwest Texas, "a large part of the younger men of the profession" joined the Reserve Corps, but many other practitioners from the region went abroad as well.

Typical of Bexar County Medical Society programs was the one at which Dr. McReynolds sponsored Col. Henry Smith, the general surgeon reported to have done 50,000 Smith-Indian intracapsular cataract extraction operations in India, to visit the region and demonstrate the new technique. Smith was also responsible for creating a procedure used worldwide for removing the sight-destroying growth known as pterygium, prevalent in lands of hot, dry winds and swirling dust such as Texas.

"Minutes of Regular Meeting of March 28, 1918," 115;
Vail, Derrick, 15

Among the South Texas eye, ear, nose and throat specialists who went abroad were Drs. T.B. Askew, F.W. Sorell, and H.O. Wyneken. Captain Thomas J. Walthall, who later practiced ophthalmology at San Antonio, was "*ordered to report to Camp MacArthur*." Other Bexar County Medical Society members, Maj. Newton H. Bowman of Beeville, Lt. J.F. Gibson of Paris, Capt. F.T. McLean of El Paso, Capt. Wallace Ralston of Houston, and Lt. D.C. Compere of Dallas, went overseas in 1918. Charles E. Pinckney, a captain in Army Medical Corps, was stationed in Honolulu, and one Bexar County Medical Society member wrote from a post three miles from Monte Carlo on the Riviera that "*next to Texas, I think it the most beautiful country I have ever seen*." South Texas sent a number of remarkably well-trained and outstanding individuals to the war effort, and saw a quantum leap in the expertise of those who returned.

"War and the Future of Our Societies," 21;
Nixon, P.I., Century of Medicine in San Antonio, 275-6, 279-80.

The importance of the specialists who served becomes apparent with the realization that until 1940 only five San Antonio physicians restricted their practices solely to ophthalmology. Among these few eye specialists who went to war, Dr. Scott Carter Applewhite, a contemporary of Dr. Donald Atkinson, was an Indiana native who came to Texas after graduating from Jefferson Medical College in Philadelphia, practicing and teaching at the University of Pittsburgh, and completing postgraduate ophthalmology work in Philadelphia. Listed in the 1901 *San Antonio City Directory* as an apprentice physician, he may have been pursuing a preceptorship with a local physician at the time. Elsewhere, however, it appears that Dr. Applewhite came to San Antonio in 1911 and had already established a private practice in the Moore Building when he entered the U.S. Naval Academy. Applewhite was eventually stationed at Kelly Field Hospital in San Antonio, no doubt due in part to the importance of his knowledge of ophthalmology to the aviation section there. Records show that he served as Commandant of an Air Force examining unit at the Robert B. Green Hospital, Kelly Field, and the Fort Sam Houston Base Hospital and that he returned to private practice in San Antonio when the war ended. Applewhite later worked with a group of doctors to investigate the feasibility of the San Antonio O&O Society owning a dispensary optical company, a probable reflection of his wartime aviation research on glasses and goggles for pilot use.

Applewhite's wife worked with the local Child Protective Society, county and state level child welfare interests, and the Protestant Orphans Home and Day Nursery Board before they moved to Mexico around 1940. He died in 1944.

Bexar County Medical Society records;
Benford, Robert, Heritage of Aviation Medicine, 5.

At the same time, World War I assembled a host of highly qualified specialists at South Texas military installations. The greatest importance of the war for the region, according to medical historian P.I. Nixon, lay in the fact that "*San Antonio found herself in the heart of one of the greatest military training camps in the world where there were gathered into the military hospitals of these camps many of the most brilliant medical men of the nation.*" The war organized physicians into a national system that heightened communication among practitioners, strengthened local medical associations, and fostered interactions that extended the parameters of medicine. Nowhere did this phenomenon have a greater impact than in South Texas where a rich and ongoing exchange between military and civilian practitioners came to distinguish medicine in the region. Many doctors later recalled that, "*a military motif predominated in medical circles in Bexar County*." Local society programs frequently focused on military medicine and welcomed the participation of visiting military physicians. The *Bexar County Medical Society Minutes* for March 28, 1918, for example, show a scientific program that included discussions of "*Field Hospital Service*," "*Ambulance Service*," and "*Regimental Medical Service*." Many of those who came to San Antonio possessed an advanced level of professional training that enriched the region's medical climate both during and after the war when they entered civilian life in the community. Larger in number than they would have been under normal circumstances, these physicians created a force that enabled the region make a medical leap forward rather than endure the more gradual evolution that might have otherwise occurred.

Nixon, P.I., A Century of Medicine in San Antonio, 276;
The Red Book of Eye, Ear, Nose and Throat Specialists, 1915;
Vail, 15;
"Minutes of Regular Meeting of March 28, 1918," 115.

Of those that World War I brought to San Antonio, none was more distinguished than Dr. Wilfrid Edward Muldoon, another of San Antonio's first strict ophthalmologists. One of seven children born to a family in Youngstown, Ohio, Muldoon joined the Army before beginning his medical training. He first came to Texas when Army officials learned he could drive a car and sent him on assignment to determine whether automobiles could be used for troop conveyance. At a time before adequate highways were fully in place, Muldoon traveled across Texas to the Mexican border, removing fences at ranch borders that impeded his progress. He later realized the trip taught him that competition among doctors was considerably less in Texas than in the East. When the war ended, he took a medical degree at the University of Michigan and interned at Ancon Hospital in the Panama Canal Zone, where he studied tropical diseases and met and worked with American writer Sinclair Lewis. After practicing for two years at the

Tela Railroad Hospital in Honduras and studying ophthalmology at the universities of Paris, Bordeaux, and Vienna, he completed a two-year residency in ophthalmology at the Wills Eye Hospital in Philadelphia and practiced briefly in Washington, D.C., before moving to San Antonio in 1930. Here he joined Dr. John Matthews and eventually became one of the "*premier ophthalmologists*" in the city. An expert ophthalmic surgeon who spoke seven or eight languages fluently and "*had not one medical book in English*," Muldoon was described by his colleagues as "*a prince of a man*" and clearly served as a force for change that enriched the ophthalmological community in the city.

Bexar County Medical Society records.

Like Muldoon, however, there were many other outstanding physicians drawn to the Southwest. Dr. Charles Boehs, a native of London, England, brought both a cosmopolitan background and an extensive military experience to his San Antonio EENT practice. After receiving his medical degree from Georgetown University and interning at the Eastern Dispensary and Casualty Hospital in Washington, D.C., his World War I experience took him to Plattsburg Barracks, Fort Ontario; Fort Banks, Massachusetts; Texas City, Texas, and the Philippine Islands. He also worked at the South Baltimore Eye and Ear Hospital before being assigned to the Fort Sam Houston Base Hospital as Chief of the EENT Service. After the war, Boehs settled in San Antonio, and further specialized in otolaryngology. Dr. Cyrus R. Baker, who practiced for twenty years in New York City before spending three years in the U.S. Army Medical Corps, found his way to San Antonio after the war and set up an EENT practice in 1922.

Bexar County Medical Society Records

Many of those who returned to South Texas as specialists after World War I found that military service added a dimension to their careers. Many individuals who served in Europe had dealt with a concentration of cases that constituted the equivalent of specialty training. Captain D.S. Edwards, somewhere in France, had been "the only eye, ear, nose and throat specialist in a hospital of 500 beds." For these physicians, the intensity of the medical experience often provided the motivation that led to eventual specialization in ophthalmology or otolaryngology. Among them, reports show that Dr. Edwin M. Sykes entered the war with a lieutenant's commission and was stationed at

Fort Sam Houston, Base Hospital No. 1. Here he was "*assigned to do practically all of the eye work*" and later recalled being employed in what he called the "*research laboratory of war*" because, as he put it, "*All kinds of eye conditions and operations have presented themselves.*" After his discharge in 1919, Sykes became an ophthalmologist and established a private practice in San Antonio. His brother, Clarence S. Sykes, who became an ophthalmology professor at the University of Texas Medical Branch in Galveston, served with Battery D in the 19th Field Artillery in France and won a Purple Heart before returning to Europe to complete his studies at Vienna.

Nixon, P.I., Century of Medicine in San Antonio, 275-6, 279-80;
Bexar County Medical Society records.

Dr. William D. Gill, a Dallas-born doctor who later practiced in San Antonio, was another of those who owed their decision to specialize to World War I. Gill attended the University of Cincinnati and Baylor, received his medical degree from Vanderbilt University, and interned at New York Hospital before the war began. It was his military experience, however, that led to his lengthy career in ophthalmology. After training at the Army Medical School in Washington, D.C. and the Medical Field Service School at Carlisle Barracks, Pennsylvania, Gill served as an instructor in eye diseases at the Army Medical School, as head of the Walter Reed General Hospital eye clinic, and as Chief of the Department of Ophthalmology at the Fort Sam Houston Station Hospital in San Antonio, where he learned about the latest research efforts in the field. Gill also trained later at the University of Vienna and spent two years in France and Germany. By the time he resigned from the Army in 1928 to open a San Antonio practice, Gill spoke four languages. One of the first regional specialists to experiment with cornea transplants, Gill was credited with doing the first operation of its kind in the Southwest.

Bexar County Medical Society records

World War I experience also led Dr. Chauncey H. Dolph, Dr. A. Belvin Pritchett, and Dr. Clarence Lucien McClellan to their choice of profession. Dolph made thirty-two trips on a transport ship to pick up the wounded in France, went on to graduate from the University of Oklahoma, and specialized in ophthalmology at the University of Pennsylvania and the Newark Eye and Ear Infirmary. He later taught at the University of Texas and Baylor Medical Schools and practiced at

West Baytown. Pritchett was a San Marcos native who attended Southwestern University and the Galveston Medical Branch and interned at St. Louis City Hospital and the Scott and White Clinic in Temple, Texas. He might never have left the region or specialized had it not been for World War I. Instead, his service as a first lieutenant at an Army field hospital led to postgraduate work at the University of Pennsylvania School of Medicine after the war, and he returned to San Antonio as a specialist in eye, ear, nose, and throat. Pritchett went on to serve as President of the local specialty society and to practice successfully in the community for the next thirty years. Dr. McClellan was a Spanish-American War veteran who entered the Army Medical Corps from New Mexico and served as a first lieutenant at Camp Travis. After the war, he came back to Texas in 1923 and practiced for a year before going to New York to specialize in diseases of the eye, ear, nose and throat. He returned to San Antonio to practice, but later moved to Kerrville where he supervised the EENT division of the local hospital and in 1933 was elected president of the Kerr-Kendall-Gillespie-Bandera County Medical Society. Finally, Dr. John Edwin Manney of Alto, Texas, trained at Tulane, Sewanee University, and the Chicago Eye, Ear, Nose and Throat College and practiced in Falls County, Texas; Tucumcari, New Mexico; and Waco before becoming a captain in the Army Medical Corps. After the war he returned to Waco, but in 1938 chose to relocate to San Antonio, a city with strong military associations, for the remainder of his career.

Bexar County Medical Society records.

No individual life was influenced more by World War I than that of Dr. Spencer Dickerson, an African American graduate of Austin's Tillotson (now Huston-Tillotson) College who received his medical degree from Rush Medical College in Chicago in 1901 and practiced for five years in New Bedford, Massachusetts, before enlisting in the lowest grade of the Sanitary Detachment, Eighth Illinois Infantry National Guard, in 1914. Dickerson was mustered into federal service for Mexican border duty in 1916 and garrisoned at Camp Logan before going to France, where he served with the 370th Infantry in 1917. Promoted a year later to captain in the Medical Corps, he went on to become the first African American Texan to attain the rank of brigadier general and the first African American pathologist at Chicago's Provident Hospital. In Chicago he also served as an ophthalmologist and otolaryngologist from 1920 to 1937, and subsequently became chairman of the department.

Texas Medical Association records.

Dr. Josef H. Kopecky, the son of Moravian immigrants, taught at the Texas School for the Blind in Austin and graduated from the Galveston Medical Branch in 1915 before joining the Army Medical Corps in 1917. Commissioned in 1918, he volunteered for service with the Army's Siberian Expeditionary Forces in Russia, and there found himself in charge of an army hospital. When he returned to Texas in 1920 to enter private practice at El Campo, he brought a depth of experience in medicine and the wisdom of travel. Later, Kopecky taught at the Galveston Medical Branch and served as the first exchange professor to the National University of Mexico.

University of Texas Medical Branch, Galveston. Faculty and Staff, 109

Among the generation influenced by the war at the beginning of their careers or who went as general practitioners and specialized later was Dr. Daniel Abell Russell, a Bexar County native with family links to the Gallagher Ranch near San Antonio. After serving as a Hospital Apprentice with the United States Naval Reserve Force at New Orleans, Russell went on to graduate from Tulane in 1921 and intern at San Antonio's Santa Rosa Hospital. For postgraduate study, he went to the New York Polyclinic Medical School and George Washington University, and also studied with Dr. Chevalier Jackson at Temple University in Philadelphia. On his return to Texas, Russell served as Dr. Donald Atkinson's associate for eleven years, after which he set up his own eye, ear, nose and throat practice. He later served as Chief of Eye, Ear, Nose and Throat services at the Santa Rosa and R.B. Green Hospitals; served as a civilian consultant at Brooke Army Hospital, Kerrville's Peterson Memorial Hospital, and the New Braunfels Hospital; and was elected President of the San Antonio O&O Society. Russell's son, who also attended Tulane, went on to become one of the first strict ophthalmologists in the city.

Dr. Dan Russell interview; Bexar County Medical Society records

Another physician influenced by the war was the colorful eye, ear, nose and throat specialist, Dr. Archibald Fletcher Clark, Sr., whose autobiography provides a rich source for details about medicine in the era. The son of a Confederate war veteran and cowboy who drove cattle to Kansas City, Clark was born to a family of twelve on a Caldwell County farm and attended the Bug-Scuffle country school. Before applying to medical school, Clark picked cotton, learned to speak fluent Spanish, and worked in a general mercantile business at Fentress. His inspiration to go into medicine grew from horse and buggy trips on which he accompanied a local doctor on visits to his patients across the county. With the help of local physicians and his high school teacher, Clark went on to graduate from Tulane University, take a six-weeks course in EENT, and start a general practice at Fentress. After three years during which he referred his difficult eye cases to J.S. Steele at San Antonio, he received a commission as First Lieutenant in the Medical Corps in 1917 and moved his family to the Alamo City while he went off to war. Overseas, Clark organized a gas hospital (Field Hospital #358 of the 90th Division in Europe) where he recalled many men who had received mustard gas, phosgene, or di-phosgene gas sufficient to cause death. Later, his hospital was converted back to a regular field hospital and Triage, and then sent to Germany to take over the Trivollier Hotel in Bern Castle Quiz on the Malta River as a base hospital. Clark's experience interested him in otolaryngology, and he soon found himself working as an assistant to a Major in charge of EENT. When the war ended, he applied to the EENT Hospital in New Orleans for an internship, completed his training, and returned San Antonio to become the partner of J.S. Steele in1921.

Clark, Archibald Fletcher, Sr. "Autobiography"

But what of San Antonio during the long years of World War I? So concentrated had San Antonio been on the war effort that city officials cancelled the city's annual Fiesta celebration for the duration of the conflict, and wartime food shortages forced residents to buy armadillo meat in Haymarket Plaza. The sheer numbers of people who flooded into the city during the war alone might have changed its character, but the population doubled in the decade that followed to an estimated total of 201,308 as many of those engaged in the war effort poured into the region. Wartime hostility toward Germany and the local German-American population had been particularly strong in South Texas. During the conflict, non-German San Antonians destroyed the city's King William German community, named for the King of Prussia, and renamed King William Street in honor of General Pershing. These events produced a lasting effect by changing the city's previously cosmopolitan atmosphere into one more regional in feeling even as it enjoyed greater contact with the world beyond Texas; in the postwar decade, non-Hispanic parts of the city lost their European feeling and adopted an atmosphere more like that of the Southern United States.

Light Years, 6

By 1924, however, San Antonio emerged as a major metropolis of the Southwest with improved transportation, educational, financial, and military facilities. Ray Lambert converted an abandoned rock quarry into a Japanese Garden at Brackenridge Park, giving the community one of the "*most beautiful and extensive park systems of any city in America.*" Amidst this development, the opening of the Robert B. Green Memorial Hospital on January 29, 1917, went largely unnoticed as did the building of a People's Colored Hospital in 1914 and an unsuccessful effort in 1919 to move the University of Texas Medical Branch at Galveston to San Antonio. The addition of the R.B. Green Hospital to the region's permanent medical institutions, however, represented a milestone in South Texas medical history and a foreshadowing of greater things to come.

U.S. War Department, Surgeon General's Office. Report, 1919, 1180;
Fehrenbach, Landmark Years;
Bexar County Medical Society Minutes, 1914;
"Minutes of Regular Meeting of March 28, 1918, 115;
Nixon, Century of Medicine in San Antonio, 278;
Green, Peyton, Fifty Years of Aerospace Medicine, 58, 98, 194, 188-190

# CHAPTER 8

## THE INTERWAR YEARS: PROFESSIONAL DEVELOPMENT AND INFLUENCES OF THE GREAT DEPRESSION, 1919-1939

*. . . ophthalmological history acts as a standard of comparison and frame of reference for current trends. If one is to take a stand in controversial issues, such as . . . public health measures involving ophthalmology as a social force, advance will appear clearly only on the pages of history.*

Arrington, History of Ophthalmology, 8

The period between the two World Wars witnessed extremes that ranged from the exuberance of the Roaring Twenties to the fear and hardship of the Depression. For South Texas eye specialists it was an era characterized by important educational and organizational advances, a surge in professional development measured by the appearance of the region's first local and state level professional societies in branches of specialized medicine, and later by the call for dedicated service in the face of Depression. In addition, the region gained some of its first facilities dedicated exclusively to eye care, new general hospitals, and new institutions for the blind. Before the Depression slowed growth across the nation, a new generation of eye specialists joined those who resumed their practices after the war, enriching local communities and giving San Antonio increased status as a regional medical center. At the same time, military ophthalmologists provided a rich resource for the community by generating interest in research and creating a force for the development of a new form of medical education to prepare specialists. Medical advances were overshadowed in the public mind by the Works Progress Administration effort that produced city's crown jewel, a winding path along the San Antonio River known as the Riverwalk, but, though less visible, advances in ophthalmology constituted milestones along a path that would eventually make the health care industry one of the strongest contributors to the San Antonio economy.

World War I medical mobilization had created a momentum whose benefits for the American medical system were only fully realized in the interwar years. Ophthalmologists and eye, ear, nose, and throat specialists who went to war with a relatively provincial attitude and few contacts in other states returned better trained, in touch with their counterparts around the world, and committed to improving medical practice, having participated in a national effort that demonstrated the effectiveness of specialization. World War I made greater professional organization a necessity and distributed a higher level of professional standards nationwide. In addition, the war heightened public interest in medicine when soldiers reported back home on the specialized care they had received, and this in turn generated social sanction that helped to make ophthalmology an accepted specialty.

As reverberations of the Flexner Report of 1910 circulated through the region demanding improvements in American medical schools, doctors became aware that the preceptorship system had become outdated. Ophthalmologists and other eye specialists recognized the need for a new vehicle for training capable of addressing these issues. In 1932, Sir William Osler's book Aequanimitas articulated the importance of research in training with the statement that: "*Thoroughly equipped laboratories, in charge of men, thoroughly equipped as teachers and investigators, is the most pressing want today in the medical schools of this country*." Houston physicians had formed an Oculists and Aurists Association in 1907 before the medical watershed years of World War I, but their organization clearly represented earlier, more old-fashioned interests. The American Board of Ophthalmology--the first board in any field of medical specialization--

had been active since in 1916, but problems unique to Texas called for a regional equivalent capable of mustering organized professional support for change, conveying the implications of ophthalmic research, communicating new standards, and unifying practitioners to achieve their goals. South Texas, moreover, possessed two uniquely powerful forces for professional development in the Bexar County Medical Society and the School of Aviation Medicine. In the creation of the San Antonio Society of Ophthalmology and Otolaryngology, these institutions played the roles of midwife and mediator.

Goar,82; Osler, 30; Vail, Derrick, "Rise and Fall of EENT," 16

Within a decade after the end of World War I, ophthalmology achieved its full separation from the specialty known as eye, ear, nose and throat. At the war's end ophthalmologists could be found throughout the eastern United States and "eye, ear, nose and throat" practices were well-established in the Southwest, yet only two strict ophthalmologists practiced in San Antonio. In one sense, therefore, the greatest impact of World War I was on medical education, although its effects would not be fully manifested until some years later. European training had declined, but no state educational institution as yet offered an approved ophthalmology residency and most Texans were still forced to seek training outside the state. This fact and the small numbers of practicing ophthalmologists meant that ophthalmology had not yet fully matured in the region. Appearance of the first professional specialty societies during the interwar years, therefore, signified that a foundation had been laid for the development of the first ophthalmology residencies and that these years constituted an important transition period in the growth of the field.

## STATE-OF-THE-ART MEDICINE IN SOUTH TEXAS

While the country experienced the more relaxed, sometimes wild moods of the Roaring Twenties, San Antonio became the Queen City of Texas with a new configuration of hospitals in the 1920s and 1930s that made the medical community for the first time an important part of San Antonio's local economy. One of the period's most notable institutional developments appeared when five physicians established the 35-bed Eye, Ear, Nose and Throat Hospital of San Antonio in 1924 (opened in 1931) in Romana Plaza between the

Jewish Synagogue and Central Christian Church at 728 Main Avenue where the M&S Tower (Medical and Surgical) stands today. In 1925 Dr. Archibald Fletcher Clark, Sr. joined the existing partnership of Drs. J.S. Steele, John Burleson, T.J. Walthall, and J.H. Judkins that oversaw the hospital. Sadly, the Depression killed the enterprise and Clark moved on to work with Dr. Donald Atkinson in the Medical Arts Building, but not before this valuable step had been taken.

Dr. Atkinson may also have been involved in this enterprise, but evidence is inconclusive.

"*Romana Plaza in Evolution*," North San Antonio Times, June 20, 1974;
Clark, Archibald Fletcher, Sr. Autobiography, typescript, Prairie Lee, Caldwell County, December 1978, in Daughters of the Republic of Texas Library, San Antonio;
White, Elizabeth Borst, "Patterns of Development in Texas Hospitals, 1836-1935: preliminary survey," Texas Medicine, 82 (December 1986), 55-60;
White, Elizabeth Borst, "Eye, Ear, Nose and Throat Hospitals in Texas," Historical Research Center, Houston Academy of Medicine-TMS Library typescript;
San Antonio O&O Society Minutes, March 3, 1931.

At the same time, local ophthalmologists practiced at a new Medical Arts Hospital that was completed around 1924, and after 1926 at the new Medical and Surgical Hospital constructed by a group of local surgeons across Camden Street from the Physicians and Surgeons, or P&S Hospital. Capping these developments, construction got underway prior to the Crash of 1929 on the Nix Hospital that eventually opened in 1932 in the downtown area. Military medicine saw considerable growth as well with the replacement of the old Fort Sam Houston Station Hospital with its 668-bed capacity (and emergency capacity of 768) through a two million dollar appropriation that completed construction of the new Brooke General Hospital. Opened in 1937 with 1,000 beds and an emergency capacity of 1,200, this facility with the other recent additions gave the Alamo City new stature as a regional medical center that was reflected in the careers of a new generation of eye specialists who practiced there.

Brooke General Hospital is named for Brigadier General Roger Brooke, a former commanding officer there.

White, "Patterns of Development," 55-60;
Nixon, Century of Medicine in San Antonio, 311-320;
"Medical Arts Hospital," San Antonio Express, June 21, 1927;
"San Antonio Medical Arts Building," Texas State Journal of Medicine, December 1924, 462;
"Towering Nix Building Is Medical Landmark," San Antonio Express, January 25, 1949;
Daughters of the Republic of Texas Library clipping file; Handy, 93.

Despite these improvements, to be sure, many San Antonio and South Texas residents still suffered from inadequate medical care and training in medical specialty fields remained limited. Although physicians at the new Robert B. Green Hospital soon donated over $200,000 to the community in professional services annually and doctors and hospitals produced over twelve million dollars each year, local health conditions remained poor. Renewed interest in public health only now led the Chamber of Commerce Health Committee to bring civic, social and religious organizations together to plan a Board of Health for Bexar County. For many physicians, however, the need for better access to medical training became paramount. For good or ill, World War I had forever ended the practice of obtaining specialty training in the centers of European medical education as had been the custom of earlier generations. The Great War placed all activities associated with Germany in question and interrupted the flow of medical students and others seeking postgraduate education abroad.

Bonnabeau, Raymond C., Jr., "Apprenticeship System and the Development of Early Medical Schools in America," Minnesota Medicine, 68(1985), 765-766.

South Texas outside of Galveston offered few medical training opportunities beyond the preceptorship, although many general practitioners who had worked in specialty fields during the war now decided to specialize. Given the nature and extent of their wartime experience, most rapidly became dissatisfied with the preceptorship system. For one final generation of South Texas medical students the path to the profession of ophthalmology remained long, arduous, and challenging. The old system of training died slowly in Texas. For years, key practitioners such as Drs. Atkinson and Burleson maintained professional continuity by making young physicians obtain their imprimatur. Just as membership in the Bexar County Medical Society had been necessary to join the staffs of local hospitals, a young doctor entering medicine in San Antonio had benefited by linking himself with a man who had already established a successful practice. The preceptorship provided training beyond the fundamentals taught in medical school and served as a conduit in smaller communities for specialization to flow from those trained in distant medical centers to their successors by clearing away the barriers of competition. Ironically, what must have seemed a considerable loss at the time--access to a European medical education--had a positive influence ultimately as American ophthalmologists focused their attention on improving the profession at home. Their efforts not only made ophthalmology the first true specialty in the United States, but also eventually helped American ophthalmology to outdistance European medical practice.

Nixon, P.I., Century of Medicine in San Antonio, 311-320.

The careers of three transitional South Texas eye specialists--Dr. Fred B. Cooper, Dr. Edward Dumas, and Dr. Elizabeth Donaldson--demonstrate how regional ophthalmology developed in the interwar years despite the effects of the Depression. Their stories illustrate how links with local leaders in the profession furthered their careers, and how professional continuity from one generation to the next helped the profession achieve further progress. More specifically, these individuals typify those who negotiated the transition from old-fashioned preceptorship to residency training, and illustrate the kinds of variations that accompanied this transition. Framed by events that touched all walks of life, the careers of these outstanding specialists highlight differences between their time and our own and offer rich details about the period.

## DR. FRED B. COOPER

Like the many others who came to Texas from distant lands, Dr. Fred B. Cooper was an immigrant to the United States. The son of Samuel Kupperman (his original surname), Dr. Cooper was born in the small town of Bardiche in the Russian Ukraine in 1901. In contrast to other immigrants, however, he was already a trained specialist and a representative of the growing strength of American medicine when he arrived in San Antonio. Cooper's father came to America in 1904 to escape the cruelty of the Russian Czars and the massacre of helpless people in the *pogroms* (from a word meaning thunder). Desperate to escape attacks that took place with the approval of officials, he had closed his grocery business and bribed officials with cigarettes to make his way to a ship bound for the United States. Fred remained at home until his father was settled and able to bring the rest of the family to New York. When his father's first grocery business failed, however, the family moved on to join relatives in Chicago.

Dr. Fred B. Cooper Interview, with Sue McDonald, February 5, 1990;
Barnard's Dictionary of Etymology.

Dr. Cooper recalled that his interest in medicine had developed from two events in his youth. In the first, he felt the strong influence of family memories of an older sister who had tried to enter medical school but died before she could do so, leaving him to pursue her goal. The second event occurred when his father severely injured his hand and Fred took him to Chicago's Presbyterian Hospital. Many visits made during his father's recovery instilled a lifelong love of hospitals that ultimately cemented the young man's desire to become a doctor. After receiving his undergraduate education at Crane Junior College and the University of Illinois, Cooper took a medical degree at the Illinois College of Medicine in 1924. His then interned at Mt. Zion Hospital in San Francisco, where he received a prize as the best in his class, and returned to the Midwest just before the Crash of 1929.

Dr. Fred Cooper interview

At the onset of the Depression, Cooper passed the state board exam in Fayette, Missouri, and began to practice general medicine. The looming Depression, however, threatened his future as many families could no longer afford medical care. At a time when a hospital stay commonly cost three dollars a day, Cooper spent much of his time delivering babies, a service for which he received little or no fee. Remarkably, he managed to avoid severe hardships and overcame the limited prospects facing new doctors when his father-in-law convinced him to choose an area of medicine and specialize. An emergency appendectomy kept him from beginning a residency at St. Louis University's Oscar Johnson Hospital, but he applied again and this time received an offer from the University of Chicago's Billings Memorial Hospital, then a "closed" institution much like the Mayo Clinic. By marrying the daughter of a man who operated several Chicago optical shops, he also developed an affiliation that foreshadowed the direction his career would take.

Dr. Fred Cooper interview; Bexar County Medical Society records

Cooper's residency program enabled him to train not only with the head of the Ophthalmology Department, but with German science translator, Dr. E.V.L. Brown, who inspired him to complete a second residency at Rush Medical College and Presbyterian Hospital, Chicago's biggest and the place where he had taken his father as a boy. Among Cooper's advisers there were a physician named Moncrief and his wife, Bertha Klien, a Vienna-trained artist and histopathologist who regularly sectioned eyes to study disease. By supplementing his training, Brown and Klien gave Cooper all the benefits of European training in an American context in the midst of the Depression.

Dr. Fred Cooper interview

His training completed, Cooper considered an offer to teach at the University of Illinois, but began to look for a warmer climate when his wife objected to Chicago's cold winters. He now took the step that brought him to Texas and made him the partner of one of the most important specialists in the state. Donald Atkinson's reputation had reached Chicago, and Cooper was pleased when the renowned ophthalmologist not only agreed to serve as a preceptor, but asked him to join his practice. Atkinson would also serve as a preceptor for several other men who became his partners, including Dr. Dan A. Russell, Sr. and Joe De Gasperi who completed their training in 1922 and after 1950 respectively. Drs. Dan Russell, Sr. and another of Atkinson's trainees, William Riley, eventually established their own EENT practices, but when Cooper arrived in San Antonio the only other strict ophthalmologists besides Atkinson locally were Dr. John Burleson and Dr. Wilfrid E. Muldoon. Atkinson's office on the eighth floor of the Medical Arts Building that today houses the Emily Morgan Hotel lay at the heart of downtown San Antonio.

Dr. Fred Cooper interview

The partnership and preceptorship provided a vehicle for the exchange of knowledge and mutual benefit. Cooper achieved a cultural transfer of medical expertise to the region similar to that which both Dr. Atkinson or Dr. Ferdinand Herff had achieved a generation earlier. As he learned from Atkinson, the young doctor was surprised to learn that his mentor operated in darkened rooms and followed certain outdated practices. When he tried to introduce techniques he had learned in Chicago he met with some resistance, but the cultural transfer of medical knowledge took place anyhow. After Cooper agreed to work at the R.B. Green Hospital without pay, he instituted a day surgery program and did outpatient or ambulatory cataract surgery there with Dr. M. W. McCurdy. Bolstered by the sanction conferred by his association with Atkinson's successful practice, he was able to work over the objections of many who feared complications. The combination of the new and traditional embodied in the two doctors enabled Cooper to successfully introduce new techniques to the region, particularly through his teaching at the R.G. Green. Representing one of the most up-to-date, state-of-the art medical educations available in America at the time, Cooper contributed to the acceptance of ophthalmology in the region by facing the hesitation many felt in consulting someone other than the trusted family doctor. At first, he discovered, younger people were willing to visit an ophthalmologist, while older folks continued to prefer their familiar eye, ear, nose, and throat specialist.

Dr. Fred Cooper interview

Well established by the start of World War II, Cooper left Atkinson in 1941 or 1942 for four years of eye, ear, nose, and throat service at Fort Custer and Fort Sam Houston. Because Army men had few cataracts, he spent most of his time examining new recruits and writing articles for the EENT Monthly and the Digest of Ophthalmology. When Atkinson welcomed him back to the practice after the war, he was considered one of the community's most outstanding specialists. Henceforth, he worked at the Santa Rosa and Baptist Hospitals (then the Medical and Surgical Hospital), treated many patients from Mexico, and enjoyed a practice that reached from San Antonio to Corpus Christi with few physicians in between. When Atkinson died a few years later, Cooper took over the practice and a role as consultant at Brook Army Medical Center. In 1952 he was elected President of the San Antonio O&O Society. Finally, Cooper's long career also enabled him to see the region achieve a new level of medical service with the opening of the University of Texas Health Science Center at San Antonio, where he briefly served as a consultant. Although in him San Antonio ophthalmology equaled that to be found elsewhere in the country, however, several steps remained before the profession in the region would become fully mature.

Dr. Fred Cooper interview, Bexar County Medical Society records

## DR. EDWARD De VAN DUMAS

Dr. Edward DeVan Dumas was among the city's first eye, ear, nose and throat specialists to intern in San Antonio. Born in 1898 in Mobile, Alabama, Dumas took a job as a dockworker unloading boats

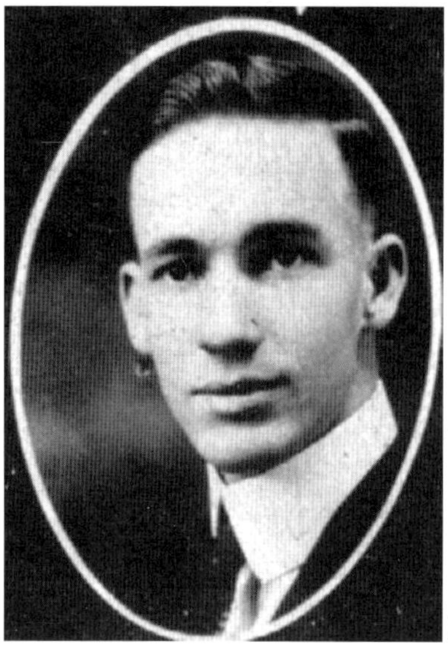
Dr. Edward De Van Dumas (1898-1992)

arriving from Central America to earn money for college at the University of Alabama. In 1921, he graduated from Tulane University Medical School in New Orleans at the gateway to the Southwest at twenty-two years of age, for which he was dubbed the "*boy doctor*."

Bexar County Medical Society Auxiliary Research Committee, "Anecdotes and Memoirs of Bexar County Doctors," typescript, 1984, 15.

In July 1921, Dumas set out for San Antonio to begin an internship at the R.B. Green Hospital. Living at the hospital, he worked with two fellow interns who became outstanding regional physicians--Dr. Reuss of Cuero and Dr. Arthur Carroll Scott, founder of the Scott and White Hospital with Dr. Raleigh R. White in East Texas. At a time when diphtheria ran riot on the floor that housed contagious diseases such as typhoid, leprosy and consumption and the great flood of 1921 brought numbers of emergency injuries, Dumas assisted with operations, did laboratory work, wrote up patient histories, and ran the emergency room. So impressed was Dr. Reuss with the young man that he invited him to join his general practice, an act of professional support that would shape the young man's future.

"Anecdotes and Memoirs," 10-15

Unfortunately, two years later Dumas fell ill with tuberculosis. He spent the next year recuperating on the screened porch of a house behind the Alamo Heights Church where his grandmother came to care for him. When he regained his health, the young doctor was unable to return to a general practice surrounded by contagious diseases, and chose instead to pursue a career in eye, ear, nose and throat. For postgraduate work, Dumas enrolled at the New York Polyclinic and then spent a month in 1929 in Vienna "*working mostly in the morgue under those wonderful Viennese doctors*." He also made a trip down the Rhine and visits to Darmstadt, Prague, and Nuremberg before returning to the Southwest.

"Anecdotes and Memoirs," 15-17

Back in San Antonio, Dumas established a successful eye, ear, nose and throat practice working in a suite in the Hotel St. Anthony and then in the Medical Arts Building. Like more traditional physicians, he also augmented this local practice by serving as a railroad physician for the Missouri Pacific and Southern Pacific Railroads. Whenever his family passed through Palestine, Texas, where the company hospital was located, railroad officials came down for a visit while the train stopped over. In San Antonio, Dumas took an active role in the Conopus Club, Christ Church, and Bexar County Medical Society, and in 1950 served as President of the Texas Ophthalmological and Otolaryngological Society. His fifty-year practice may be best remembered for his habit of seeing patients without scheduling appointments. If a wait was necessary, the good doctor referred to by a colleague as a true "*Southern gentleman*" instructed his patient to spend the time shopping at Joske's.

Elaine Hoffman Wagener, comp. and ed., George C. Vaughan: Early Entrepreneur, San Antonio, Watercress Press, 1984, 126;
Curtis Vaughan, Jr. interview;
Bexar County Medical Society records. Dumas married George C. Vaughan's daughter, Cornelia, a San Antonio girl from a distinguished family from St. Johnsbury, Vermont, and moved into a house on French Place built by Mr. Albert Steves, Sr., of the local building firm.

## DR. ELIZABETH DONALDSON

Just as Dr. Donald Atkinson aided Dr. Fred Cooper in establishing himself in the community, Dr. John Burleson served as a preceptor for a group of physicians including Dr. Elizabeth Donaldson, one of the earliest women to practice ophthalmology in Texas. Revolutionary in her time simply by being a female physician, Donaldson was born in Bexar County in 1894 and received her inspiration to enter medicine from an uncle who was a physician in Uvalde. After studying at the Galveston Medical Branch and graduating from Baylor University in 1924, she began a preceptorship with Dr. Burleson and then set up a general practice in San Antonio. Eventually, Donaldson completed postgraduate training at the Barnes Hospital in St. Louis, the Chicago EENT Hospital, and the New York Eye and Ear Infirmary, but the preceptorship shaped her future.

Mrs. Bell Louise Stevenson interview, May 14, 1991;
Bexar County Medical Society records

As part of her training under Dr. Burleson, Dr. Donaldson accompanied a group of physicians to the small community of 5,000 people at Del Rio to do "*wholesale*" tonsillectomies at the "*Lying In*" or "*Home*" Hospital. Seeing the need for a specialist there, she went back after completing her training and established an eye, ear, nose and throat practice in 1931 in the town's Ross Drug Store Building. One of the region's most colorful specialists, Donaldson managed to overcome the community's reluctance to abandon its family doctors by joining the ladies club and singing in the Methodist Church choir. She later recalled frontier conditions in places where she practiced in a poem about making a house call one moonlit night on the Mexican border. Donaldson, like Dr. Dor Brown, sent patients with cases too complicated for care in the hinterland on to her mentor, Dr. Burleson, in San Antonio for much of her career.

Mrs. Bell Louise Stevenson interview, May 14, 1991;
Bexar County Medical Society records

## MILITARY RESEARCH AND THE ROLE OF PROFESSIONAL SOCIETIES

As South Texas began to draw larger numbers of specialists, military research performed a key role in San Antonio ophthalmology during the interwar years by raising awareness about the importance of research across the community. Dr. Fred Cooper and other local practitioners were invited to serve as consultants at local military installations, but military medicine had an equally powerful influence when community and military medical professionals came together at the Bexar County Medical Society. For the handful of specialists in the region there were few opportunities for professional communication at medical meetings still geared chiefly to general practitioners. Doctors looked to local medical societies to keep them on the cutting edge, but no specialty society as yet had been established. Bexar County Medical Society meetings, however, opened a channel of communication that allowed community specialists and their more highly specialized counterparts in ophthalmic research at the School of Aviation Medicine to meet together to discuss problems under investigation at the School, allowing new knowledge to filter out through the community to specialists across the region. P.I. Nixon's recollection that "*a survey of the list of speakers at the Bexar County Medical Society*" would show "*how much we have relied on the Army*" bears witness to the important professional stimulus provided by the Bexar County Medical Society.

Nixon, Century of Medicine, 226

The individual who established a tradition of communication between military and civilian practitioners that continues down to the present by setting up joint meetings at the Bexar County Medical Society was Eye, Ear, Nose, and Throat specialist Dr. Robert E. Moss. According to Daniels' 1892 Texas Medical Journal, Moss had:

*removed from Mexia to San Antonio and having fitted himself by two special courses on the eye, ear, etc.--one with the celebrated Knapp-in addition to his general knowledge, has abandoned the general practice, and will devote himself exclusively in future to diseases of the eye, ear, nose and throat. The doctor is a courteous gentleman, and has a statewide reputation as a surgeon and physician.*

A transitional figure like Drs. Cooper and McCurdy, Moss was a graduate of Jefferson Medical College at Philadelphia in 1883, who went on to complete postgraduate training at the New York Polyclinic in 1891 and at one of the earliest United States centers for specialty training, Knapp's Ophthalmic and Aural Institute in 1892. After a preceptorship with the "*celebrated Knapp*," he practiced for a time at Mexia. By 1905 Moss was in San Antonio and offering specialist care to the military, as confirmed by his official report that in May a "*Dr. F. of Fort Sam Houston consulted me about acute conjunctivitis of the right eye.*" Although the city directory listed him as an oculist and aurist, Ross was not the old-fashioned doctor the terms described, but a clear voice for specialization. As early as 1913 his clinical research interests appear in an article entitled, "*Observation of the Effects of Salvarsan from the Standpoint of a Specialist in Eye and Ear*

*Diseases*," published in a Texas medical journal. He also served as Associate Chief of EENT at the R. B. Green Hospital. As President of the Bexar County Medical Society during World War I, Moss set up the first joint professional meetings between military and civilian practitioners. Through this channel, news of Ocker and Thorne would have reached the local medical community. The event, therefore, constitutes a milestone in the development of community interest in ophthalmic research.

Bexar County Medical Society Records; Nixon, Century of Medicine, 312; Daniel's Texas Medical Journal, 1892; San Antonio City Directory, 1905. In 1926, however, Moss moved further into the hinterland, locating at LaGrange.

The School of Aviation Medicine in effect added a research component to the local medical community that served as a source of enrichment from moment it arrived. When the U.S. Army established an Ophthalmology Department at Walter Reed General Hospital in 1923 and began sending medical officers to the clinic there for ophthalmological training, the event would have likely emphasized the need for training programs in San Antonio. Local specialists also learned, for example, that in 1933 Major R. Keith Simpson, a School of Aviation faculty member, was discussing aviation goggles containing corrective lenses for errors of refraction and accommodation being developed at SAM at a meeting of the Aero Medical Association in Chicago, suggesting a need for the creation of a local medical specialty society.

Benford, Robert J., Doctors in the Sky, 48.

Some of the community excitement surrounding ophthalmic research is captured by records of eye, ear, nose and throat specialist Dr. Scott Bronson's effort to employ a galvanic current in removal of the lens in cataract operations. Using dry cells and applying one electrode to the body and another to the lens, Bronson discovered that current caused the loop to adhere to the lens capsule and the lens to be lifted from its bed. Bausch and Lomb investigated his instrument for studying the contour of the anterior surface of the lens in 1935 with the thought of putting the device on market. Together with the arrival of new specialists and growing professionalism, this type of activity soon combined with other forces to provide the impulse that developed the first specialty societies in the region.

San Antonio O&O Minutes, March 7, 1934

## THE SAN ANTONIO OPHTHALMO-OTOLARYNGOLOGICAL SOCIETY, 1921-1982

By organizing the San Antonio Ophthalmo-Otolaryngological Society, eye, ear, nose and throat specialists and ophthalmologists strengthened the work of the Texas Medical Association and Bexar County Medical Society and furthered the goals of scientific medicine in the region. The founding of the Society commonly referred to as the "O&O Society" and later renamed the San Antonio Society of Ophthalmology and Otolaryngology, was a product of World War I and a logical outgrowth of military activities and research. Community practitioners, who had looked to the Bexar County Medical Society to keep them on the cutting edge of new advances, now saw the value of a society for specialists. According to E.H. Cary, the men who came to Texas to practice in the early part of the twentieth century "*had the advantage of some hospital training, and this brought a growing interest in the segregation of men interested in the eye, ear, nose, and throat.*" Although few specialists were as yet board certified, most were no longer interested in the needs of general practitioners as an audience. Instead, they became "*interested in their own knowledge and in the interchange with fellow practitioners.*"

San Antonio O&O Society Minutes, E.H. Cary, "Eye, Ear, Nose, and Throat as a Specialty," 299;
Dr. Bland Schwarting interview.

The Society was first proposed at a luncheon at San Antonio's Menger Hotel in 1921. For leadership, the San Antonio Society combined the charisma of an ex-military man, Dr. Edwin M. Sykes, as its first President with the political wisdom and tradition represented by Dr. John H. Burleson as Vice President. This order reflected the shift within the profession from the older generation to the new and corresponding changes in its focus. As Secretary-Treasurer, the membership chose Dr. James S. Steele, who had been educated at Vanderbilt University, worked for fifteen years in Monterrey, Mexico, as an oculist for the Mexican National Railways, and in 1911 spent a year in Vienna, Austria, learning from, among others, Ernst Fuchs. Eye specialists from the community in attendance at the luncheon included Drs. Scott C. Applewhite, Charles J. Boehs, A. Fletcher Clark, Wesley Dallas Hicks (then serving as associate chief at the R. B. Green Hospital), George E. Gwinn, and John Wesley Ellis (who arrived in San Antonio in 1919 and later practiced EENT at Lampasas).

Representatives of the military community included ophthalmologists Majors Trinder and Dewey from Fort Sam Houston. Houston physicians also created their first ophthalmo-otolaryngological society that year, although it was the older Harris County Oculists and Aurists Association that invited Dr. Ernest Fuchs, the distinguished professor of Ophthalmology at University of Vienna, to give a two-week course at Houston's Rice Hotel in the 1920s.

O&O Society Minutes, October 27, 1921;
Moursund, Walter H., Sr., M.D., "Medicine in Greater Houston," 442

Membership in the new society was initially limited to one hundred individuals whose practices dealt exclusively with "*disease and surgery of the eye, ear, nose and throat*." The organization's mission was to "*further the study and intensive research pertaining to diseases*" of the same, but its meetings were also seen as important occasions for socializing to promote the exchange of information and ideas. Strict orders were given for ladies to be invited and for the convened physicians to have time for a game of golf. By 1923 Dr. Burleson noted reassuringly that the last meeting of the season included "*a good meal, a good smoke, and a good attendance*," and that the Society had both done "*good deeds*" and "*promoted good fellowship among the specialists of San Antonio*." In the beginning, meetings were sometimes held at the home of Dr. Ed Dumas on West French Place, but at other times meetings were held at the Bexar County Medical Society, the San Antonio Country Club, the Mitrovich Cafe, the St. Anthony Hotel, the Plaza Hotel, and the Casino Club in the center of downtown San Antonio as well as a number of local military sites.

Society Minutes; Dr. Jack Lee interview

In 1926, the San Antonio O&O Society became a truly regional organization when the decision was made to broaden the membership. At the annual banquet held at the French Cafe on Garden Street in San Antonio, the members invited "*physicians in the surrounding territory who limit their practice to diseases of the EENT*" to join. A year later, Dr. John Burleson made a motion to make "*all those men who limit their service to treating diseases of the EENT automatically (honorary) members of the society*." In 1927 the O&O Society acknowledged the relationship between military and community by adding an amendment that elected all those in the Medical Corps of the U.S. Army, Navy and Public Health service residing in San Antonio to honorary fellowship, many of whom continued as members when they made the transition from active service to community practice. Many of those who dominated local ophthalmology for years to come, including Drs. Ed Dumas, P.I. Nixon, and T.B. Askew, joined the new organization along with others who enriched the postwar medical "climate of creativity" such as EENT specialist, Dr. Virgil S. Steele, a graduate of the University of Georgia in 1933 who had joined the U.S. Army Medical Corps and came to Brooke General Hospital at Fort Sam Houston in 1935.

San Antonio O&O Minutes, October 22, 1926;
The concept of a "climate of creativity" is attributed to Dr. William Goetzmann of the University of Texas at Austin

Society records reveal that the membership was highly interested in what had been learned in World War I and that the civilian medical community was aware of local developments in aviation research. The first program meeting, held at Kelly Field Hospital on November 17, 1922, and attended by civilian physicians and military specialists from Fort Sam Houston, Kelly, and Brooks Field, illustrates the link between community and military interests. On this occasion, Major A.M. Brailsford gave a paper on the "*Duties of the Flight Surgeon*," and with Captain S.E. Brown and C.T.C. Buckner presented an "*Explanation of Past-Pointing with Demonstration of the Barany Chair and the Henderson Rebreathing Apparatus*," followed by a demonstration of the use of the chair.

Society Minutes, November 17, 1922; May 29, 1923

Subsequent meetings offered presentations on injury, disease, and equipment innovations, but military topics as often as more general medical subjects dominated the discussions. Dr. O.H. Judkin's 1923 discussion of an "*Intracapsular Cataract Extraction*" technique developed by Dr. Burleson, Dr. L.K. Back's paper on "*Cases of Detached Retina*" in 1925, and Burleson's account of "*Fundus Hemorrhage*" in 1925 represented community interests. Papers given in 1925 and 1926 at the Fort Sam Houston Medical Library and other military locations dealt with fractures about the orbit, enucleation, and fat transplant, but there were other talks by Captain W.D. Gill on plastic surgery and by others on new techniques in ophthalmic surgery. In 1928 the Society met at the School of Aviation Medicine at Brooks Field to hear Major G.C. Greene of the U.S. Army Medical Corps welcome the members and Capt. C.F. Snell, M.C. give a history of aviation medicine. In addition, a demonstration was made of depth perception apparatus used in Air Corps examinations and the special rule devised by Captain Frederick H. Thorne for "*determining the amplitude of accommodation and near point of convergence.*" Refreshments were served in the Officers Club. Military and civilian practitioners together reported on aspects of glaucoma in 1931, and Drs. William D. Gill, J.H. Burleson, G.W. Johnson, Scott C. Applewhite, and Major Frederick Thorne discussed various aspects of the disease. In 1934 medical officers at the new School of Aviation Medicine at Randolph Field, like those at Fort Sam Houston had done earlier, invited the Society's entire membership out for dinner and a program. Evidence of postwar scientific ferment could also be found in the *American Journal of Ophthalmology* and other journals where Society members who had served in the military contributed information about discoveries on matters such as "*optic atrophy due to gassing.*"

Dr. Judkins predicted that "twenty years hence" this would be operation of choice by American ophthalmologists in the Texas State Journal of Medicine, 20 (1920-23), 27; Society Minutes, 1923, 1925, November 7, 1928.

Over time the O&O Society advanced the science of ophthalmology and strengthened the profession, exerting control over it in several important ways. In 1927, the Society adopted a constitution stating the organization's purpose as "the study and interchange of views, the elevation of this branch of the profession to a high standard, and the maintenance of a close fellowship between its members." Entry into the local marketplace was controlled by the provision that all applicants be endorsed by two members of the society and voted into membership. By facilitating professional communication within the membership, however, it established a network that rapidly unified practitioners across the state. Society dues were one dollar per year. After 1936 women were excluded from membership and the society's rejection of Jewish practitioners caused Dr. Lyle M. Sellen to resign. Finally, in 1948 the by-laws were amended to require applicants for membership to write a thesis, a provision that emphasized the importance of scientific contribution as part of the profession.

Society Minutes, January 4, 1927.

Although the membership increased from twenty-three to only twenty-nine by 1928, the Society provided a framework for the exchange of ideas, a forum for discussion, and a place for socializing important to the still relatively-isolated specialists. By 1932 O&O Society members talked about the possibility of establishing a dispensing optical company to be owned and operated by the membership. *Society Minutes* for 1931-1932 record that Dr. John Burleson spoke on registering doctors and the relationship between optometrists and eye doctors in his ongoing effort to improve the quality of Texas medicine, while other members made recommendations concerning broadcasting by optometrists. In spite of the Depression, scientific progress continued. In 1935, Dr. John Crockett of Harlingen presented a paper entitled, "*Interesting Cases of a Valley Specialist*," on a case of a feather in the Stenson duct and three cases of gumma of the iris that were resistant to treatment but cured by relieving the tension in the eye by paracentisis. Eventually, these beginnings would foster interest in and the necessary momentum to create the first statewide professional organization for specialists in ophthalmology.

Society Minutes, 1931-32; November 13, 1935

## THE TEXAS SOCIETY OF OPHTHALMOLOGY AND OTOLARYNGOLOGY, 1926

While other major Texas cities such as Houston developed organizations at the local level in the 1920s similar to the San Antonio O&O, members of this organization were among the leaders who laid the groundwork for the first statewide specialty organization in Texas. As one might expect, the motivation behind the creation of a state level organization came from the man who had been instrumental in developing early medical legislation and the San Antonio O&O society. Dr. John Burleson apparently began thinking about the possibility as early as 1910. Finding his section at the Texas Medical Association meeting poorly attended that year, Burleson suggested that a special society for eye, ear, nose, and throat practitioners across Texas would serve a useful purpose. Eleven years later, however, the only specialty meeting an ophthalmologist could attend hadn't changed.

Goar, 82-4;
Harris, Herbert H., M.D. "A Fifty Year History of the Texas Society of Ophthalmology and Otolaryngology," Houston, n.d., typescript;
Harris, Herbert, M.D., "Historical Notes of the Texas Society of O&O, n.d. typescript.

The 1920s gave rise to two important national professional organizations--the American Board of Ophthalmology in 1921 and the American Board of Otolaryngology in 1925. It took a golf game on a spring day in Dallas, however, for the opportunity to arise that brought Burleson's dream to fruition. Between golf shots in a game played with Drs. Wallace Ralston, John H. Foster or Claude Cody, and Dr. E.H. Cary of Dallas, Burleson convinced Cary to serve as chairman of a meeting to organize a Texas society for the "*advancement of ophthalmology and otolaryngology*." The group also promptly arranged for letters to be sent to twenty or thirty leading eye, ear, nose and throat men across Texas inviting them to a meeting in the Medical Arts Building at Dallas. At the time, according to Burleson, there were only six strict ophthalmologists in the state of Texas and EENT specialists numbered approximately forty. Plans were also made for an organizational meeting to be called later that occurred in Dallas on September 26, 1926, with thirty physicians proposed for membership and Drs. Robert E. Moss (the former Bexar County Medical Society President who had helped to create the San Antonio O&O Society), T.J. Walthall, A.F. Clark, F.H. Rosebrough, S.C. Applewhite, O.H. Judkins, and John Burleson in attendance.

Letter from Dr. John Burleson to Dr. August J. Streit, June 18, 1956;
Burleson, Dr. John H., "The Texas O&O Society In the Beginning," typescript, Texas Ophthalmological Association Archives;
E.H. Cary, "Eye, Ear, Nose and Throat as a Specialty," 300;
"Minutes of the Meeting of the Pre-Organization for the Formation of a Texas State Eye, Ear, Nose and Throat Society," Dallas, typescript, Texas Ophthalmological Association Archives;
Texas O&O Minutes, September 26, 1926.

The first meeting of the Texas Society of Ophthalmology and Otolaryngology (or the Texas Ophthalmological and Oto-Laryngological Society, according to Dr. E.H. Cary) attended by specialists from across the state took place in Houston in December 1926, with scientific meetings including a clinic on "*The Management of Acute and Chronic Glaucoma*" in the Medical Arts Building and a reception and banquet at the Rice Hotel. Candidates were required to present a thesis in order to qualify for active membership, thus assuring that the Society would maintain a serious scientific interest. Membership originally was limited to 100, and a motion from Dr. John Burleson at the first meeting initiated the practice of including members from the military. Among them was Captain Frederick Thorne of Brooks Field in San Antonio. In its first year, the society met at Fort Sam Houston and Major Sherman offered the use of Brooke Army Hospital facilities to society members for the purpose of holding a clinic and demonstrating the use of a slit lamp corneal microscope.

Texas O&O Minutes, December 10-11, 1926;
E.H. Cary, "Eye, Ear, Nose and Throat as a Specialty," 300.

A year later, Dr. John Burleson was elected president and the Texas Society's second annual meeting was held in San Antonio. Among local practitioners in attendance were Drs. Steele, Beck, Sykes, Sorell, Adams, Applewhite, Judkins, Hicks, Clark, Rosenbaugh, and Walthall. Members arriving at the station were met with carriages and driven about town to visit Fort Sam Houston and other places of interest. The following evening members listened to a Mexican orchestra while enjoying cocktails and tamales in a room decorated to resemble a Mexican village at the Gunter Hotel.

Minutes of the Second Annual Meeting, December 9-10, 1927

By the 1930s, the Society's menu of programs was filled with scientific presentations on a wide range of ophthalmological topics. At Houston Dr. Lewis M. Helfer spoke on "*the Differential Diagnosis of Lesions about the Optic Chiasm*" and Dr. Conrad Behrens of New York discussed "*Newer Work in Ophthalmology*." Dr. Alfred Nisbet spoke on "*Some Observations regarding Contact Lenses*" and Frank Roseborough on "*A Chart for Recording Visual Fields taken with the Tangent Screen and a Chart for Recording Intra Cellular Tension*." In 1946 at the end of World War II, women were admitted to a membership that had expanded to 150, and in 1952, by which time the Society became an active advocate for ophthalmologists across Texas, it incorporated and established its headquarters in Austin.

Moursund, Walter H., Medicine in Greater Houston, 1836-1956, 443

Finally, in addition to the valuable exchange of ideas provided by the new state and local professional societies, community ophthalmologists and eye, ear, nose, and throat specialists in San Antonio also participated in other events held at local military installations. When the School of Aviation Medicine hosted the Aero Medical Association's seventh annual meeting at San Antonio, senior officers at the air base were honored guests at the Gunter Hotel but it was local ophthalmologist, Dr. Tamisiea, who entertained the members with Texas stories. Speakers at the meeting included the man who had had a hand in almost every regional development of the twentieth century, Dr. John H. Burleson, then serving as president of the Texas Medical Association and one of the city's foremost ophthalmologists. At this meeting, a resolution was developed to urge Congress and the War and Navy Departments to place flight surgeons on flying status to allow them to work more closely with pilots.

Benford, Doctors in the Sky, 63-64

## THE DEPRESSION ERA

Post-World War I growth and the Texas oil boom cushioned the effects of the Depression such that, before conditions worsened, San Antonians were not only able to build a new post office, courthouse, and a public library on the grounds of the old Carnegie Library but to create the first San Antonio Symphony Society. In the interwar years, the city boasted the first air-conditioned hotel in the world, the St. Anthony, and undertook restoration efforts on the old village in the city center known as La Villita. Midway during the Depression in 1935, however, San Antonio encompassed an area far smaller than today's sprawling metropolis, with a northern boundary reaching only to Olmos Drive. As the Depression deepened, San Antonians began to suffer and doctors shifted their attention away from research and professional development back to public service. One San Antonio resident recalled a phrase that summed up the fear many people felt about their inability to pay doctor's fees. For new families during the Depression, she claimed, it was "*send money or send the baby*."

Fehrenbach, Landmark Years;
quote from Eleanor Johnson, long-time San Antonio resident, December 16, 1997

For much of the 1930s, local doctors found the competition strong, and resources few. Charges for office calls were generally $2, and for house calls between $3 and $5 dollars. Operating rooms in San Antonio were hot by 5:30 a.m., and windows in the Nix were generally kept closed. San Antonio native Dr. Thomas Walthall Folbre managed to complete his medical training in the midst of the Depression, graduating from the Galveston Medical Branch in 1934, completing an internship at Philadelphia's Temple University and two years of eye, ear, nose and throat training at Long Island College Hospital in Brooklyn, New York, before setting up an ear, nose, and throat practice in his hometown in 1938. Later he recalled that when he began his practice, doctors took care not to visit friends in the hospital for fear other doctors would accuse them of trying to steal their patients. Another competitor, he remembered, was put on probation for sending boxes of candy to other doctors' receptionists in an effort to get patient referrals. He also recalled being paid in the Depression with farm produce, including one occasion on which he received a "*live hen in a paper sack*." Eventually, an agreement was reached between the Texas Medical Association and the Texas Relief Commission that established contracts to provide doctors with compensation for service to the indigent at roughly half the usual medical fees, but many doctors experienced difficult times, indeed.

Bexar County Medical Society Records;
Dr. Tom Folbre interview.

## FOUNDING OF THE SAN ANTONIO ASSOCIATION FOR THE BLIND

As the effects of the Depression reached Texas, professional development in San Antonio helped the community to acquire another eye-related institution when Dr. William Gill announced to the San Antonio O&O Society in 1932 that The San Antonio Lions Club had become interested in the establishment of a Lighthouse for the Blind. Earlier state-level services for blind and visually disabled Texans had been limited to the Texas School for the Blind, where educational programs were offered primarily for school-aged blind children. In 1931, the Texas Legislature had created the Texas Commission for the Blind to address the needs of blind adults, acknowledging that "*the most beneficial, necessary, and pertinent service to be provided to a disabled person is that service that makes it possible for the individual to help himself*," but little direct support was available in San Antonio.

Texas Commission for the Blind, "First Fifty Years in Review," brochure; San Antonio O&O Society Minutes, November 8, 1932;
Texas State Journal of Medicine, 34(1938), 583-4; San Antonio Association for the Blind, The Assembler, vol. 1-2 (1980-1981);
San Antonio Association for the Blind publicity materials.

The man responsible for creating the San Antonio Association for the Blind was World War I veteran, Dr. Henry O. Wyneken, whose mother had been blinded by glaucoma. Wyneken invited doctors and prominent community members to organize a program to train the blind in marketable skills and to educate the public about their needs. Initially, arrangements were made for twenty people to do part-time work at a local sewing plant. By October 15, 1935, the San Antonio O&O Society noted Wyneken's progress with a record of his talk on "*Sight Preservation in Schools with Reference to the San Antonio Association of the Blind*" and recorded that Wyneken had asked the Society "*to endorse this work*." During World War II, local blind individuals worked at local factories producing pillowcases, laundry bags, mops and brooms. Working with the local Lions Club where Wyneken served as president in 1935, the Association later expanded its services into the San Antonio Lighthouse and Lighthouse Industries. Wyneken and the Association also secured the passage of an ordinance authorizing white canes for the blind of the city and obtained passage of a 1937 state constitutional amendment granting blind adults a $15 a month pension. As new technology and vocational rehabilitation programs appeared, the Texas Commission went on to provide home teaching, sheltered workshop employment, selective placement and medical assistance to Texans, and in 1936 initiated a Business Enterprises Program that established blind-operated vending stands in public buildings. When Helen Keller visited Austin on April 7, 1941, the State Commission received additional support and public attention, and by 1996 the agency served a population of more than 150,000 blind and visually disabled Texans.

Texas Commission for the Blind, "First Fifty Years in Review," brochure;
San Antonio O&O Society Minutes, November 8, 1932;
Texas State Journal of Medicine, 34(1938), 583-4;
San Antonio Association for the Blind, The Assembler, vol. 1-2 (1980-1981);
San Antonio Association for the Blind publicity materials.

## THE INTERNATIONAL POSTGRADUATE MEDICAL ASSEMBLY

Although progress was made through professional societies and accommodations for the blind, however, advances in medical education in the interwar period were limited by the Depression. A last vestige of links with Vienna and European science flourished in the period, however, through the efforts of the American Medical Association of Vienna, founded in 1903 with the aim of helping American physicians studying there. This institution enjoyed a golden era after the first World War, when international postgraduate courses were organized that formed the basis for the present Academy of Postgraduate Medical Education.

At home, specialists perceived a need for some type of training that would facilitate and exchange of information between themselves and non-specialists and provide an opportunity to help them in educating the public and referring patients for specialized care. In response, Drs. James L. Mims, Jr., A.F. Clark, Jr. and Sr., J.H. Burleson, John Matthews,

E.M. Sykes, D.A. Russell, Jr., and Jack Lee cooperated with others in the region to design an event that would bring primarily general practitioners together for a scientific program at which specialists could "talk about things which the family physician encountered every day." Dr. Sam E. Thompson of Kerrville, who appointed Dr. W. B. Russ chairman of an organization with authority to organize and develop the symposium, conceived the program in 1930. Growth of the annual clinical conference known as the International Postgraduate Medical Assembly of Southwest Texas, held each fall or spring at San Antonio, represented a response to the comment by Dr. Herbert Hill that San Antonio was "*not where it should be in taking care of physicians of the surrounding counties*" so far as clinics were concerned. Another participant observed that the event also strengthened the regional medical center with the comment that "*one of the main reasons behind the meeting was to promote San Antonio medicine.*" Programs eventually included talks by representatives of the military, films, exhibits, and a social program.

Lesky, 445-6;
"Postgraduate Assembly Now 19 Years Old," January 25, 1949, DRT clipping file;
International Medical Assembly of Southwest Texas, Minutes, November 1955-December 1976, in Bexar County Medical Society;
Nixon, P.I., Medicine in San Antonio, 340-1

The first Assembly was held January 10-12, 1933, with 510 physicians attending, including ophthalmologist Dr. W.T. Davis from Washington, D.C. Also invited were representatives from Mexico whose presence, P.I. Nixon noted, was "*not mere accident or coincidence. The medical problems of the two regions are much the same and the health interests are closely interrelated. San Antonio is the physical gateway to Mexico. Why should it not be the medical gateway?*" Henceforth, the network of South Texas physicians created by the Assembly stretched into Mexico and focused new attention on problems of the area's large Hispanic population, a foreshadowing of current interests in San Antonio. By 1956, 674 physicians from Texas and Mexico attended the annual event. (Houston and Dallas also drew up organizations to provide a voice for postgraduate medical education in the period).

IMA Minutes, November 1955-December 1976;
Nixon, Medicine in San Antonio, 340, 342;
Drs. Matthews, Russell, Mims, and Lee interviews

The Assembly offered special benefits for ophthalmology because of the large number of eye and EENT military specialists in the area, many of whom served as speakers, and by 1946 the San Antonio O&O invited speakers from the Assembly to participate in a separate symposium for its membership. By the 1970s, interns and residents of the new University of Texas Health Science Center Medical School were encouraged to attend and medical school faculty members were heavily utilized. The institution lasted until 1976, when air travel made attending distant meetings feasible for most practitioners and the Texas Association of Family Practitioners established a separate meeting in the Valley. As annual attendance dwindled, members voted to disband it. In 1980, the Assembly was transformed to become the annual Alamo City Residents Conference, sponsored every March by ACORA, the University of Texas Health Science Center, and the three local residency training programs in San Antonio.

IMA Minutes

## DEPRESSION ERA PRACTITIONERS

For many Texans, the most significant development of the interwar period took the form in many smaller South Texas towns of the appearance of their first specialist. Perhaps the most well known of these was Dr. Earl King Gill, Dallas-born in 1902 and a graduate of Texas A & M, where he earned eight letters in football, basketball and baseball and was voted into the school's athletic Hall of Fame. After graduating in engineering in 1924, Dr. Gill coached for a year before entering the Baylor School of Medicine and then setting up a general practice at San Antonio in 1929. He went on to complete his training as an ophthalmologist, however, and in the depths of the Depression in 1935 moved to Corpus Christi where he practiced until 1972.

With Gill at Corpus Christi was Dr. Clarence B. Collins, born in Clay City, Indiana, in 1896 and graduated from Indianapolis College of Pharmacy in 1919 and Indiana University School of Medicine in 1931. Collins practiced at Corpus from 1931 to 1934, went back to Indiana for six years, and then returned to Corpus, where he retired in 1948. Dr. Sanders Key Stroud, who graduated from the University of Texas Medical Branch and completed his residency at Marcy Soniat Hospital in New Orleans, an eye, ear, nose, and throat specialist, practiced at Boling, Robstown and Corpus Christi after 1932. Dr. Bernard B. Friedman, a

1927 graduate of the University of Buffalo, brought specialized medicine a step further in the hinterland when he established himself as an ophthalmologist at Corpus Christi soon after graduation.

Bexar County Medical Society Records

Dr. Walton E. Douthit graduated from the University of Texas in 1925 and chose to set up his practice at the old medical center in Cuero rather than in one of Texas' larger cities, and Dr. J.O. Hicks specialized in EENT and treated cases at Victoria. Others reached even more remote parts of Texas. Dr. Charles A.D. Langer, Jr., a graduate of Johns Hopkins University, opened his eye, ear, nose, and throat practice at Knippa in central Uvalde County deep in South Texas. In Atascosa County, Dr. Robert E. Mann, a Baylor University graduate, practiced eye, ear, nose and throat at Pleasanton, and Dr. John Crockett, who was born some time in the 1890s, practiced EENT at Harlingen before moving in 1946 to serve the Student Health Center at the University of Texas at Austin.

Grimes, Roy, 300 Years in Victoria County, 534-5;
Texas Medical Association records

Dr. Owen R. O'Neill negotiated both World War I and the Depression before retreating to the Texas hinterland. Born in Clarksville, Texas, and graduated from the Galveston Medical Branch, he spent a year on the founding staff of the Sanitarium of Paris (now McCuistion Regional Medical Center) when it opened in 1914 and then set out for specialty training in Philadelphia, Chicago, Washington, D.C., and the New York Eye and Ear Infirmary. He completed his education just in time for World War I, serving at Base Hospital 54 in France before he returned to Red River County to set up his practice at the onset of the Depression. Nonetheless, he practiced successfully for the next thirty years and was elected chairman of the EENT section of the American Medical Association and President of the Texas Society of Ophthalmology and Otolaryngology.

Bexar County Medical Society Records;
Texas Medical Society records

Only a fraction of the EENT specialists who practiced in South Texas during the interwar years, however, trained or practiced entirely in the Southwest. In addition to Dr. Edward Dumas, Dr. W. .H. Cooley, who came from Memphis, graduated from Baylor in 1913 and practiced in Oklahoma before taking up an office in San Antonio's Maverick Building. Dr. Douglas Edwards, who was born at Bonham and attended the Coronal Institute at San Marcos, practiced at San Antonio during the war years and served as a consultant at the American Hospital in Mexico City from 1921 to 1926 before returning to the Alamo City. Records also show that Dr. Newton Bowman practiced EENT in Bee County after 1914, but later moved to Mercedes, and a Dr. Schultz practiced there during the 1920s. But these career paths were rare. Goar, 82; Lois Chestnutt, Bee County Families, 72; Bexar County Medical Society Records

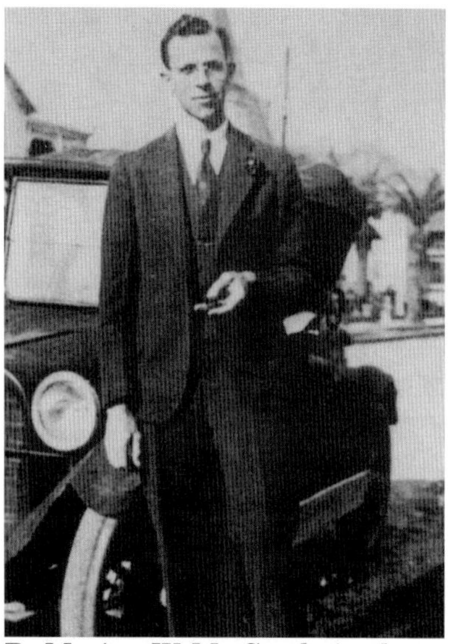

Dr.Marion W. Mc.Curdy in the 1930´s, when Dr. Burleson asked him to join his practice.

Progress was registered by the fact that the training pattern most common to South Texas eye specialists now involved some time both at home and at one of the country's best medical schools. Dr. James P. Aderhold, a native of Del Rio, attended Rice University and Tulane, interned at San Antonio's Santa Rosa Hospital, and studied EENT at the University of Rochester Medical School for two years before settling in San Antonio. Setting up an office around 1933 in the Medical Arts Building, Aderhold

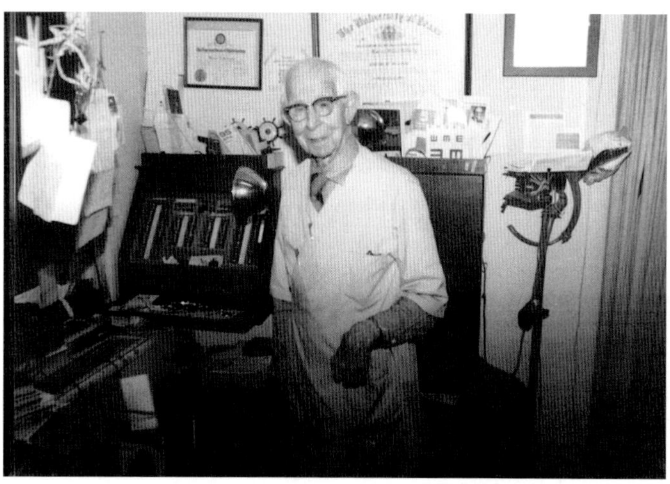

Dr. Marion W. McCurdy, in his office during the 1990's in the Nix Building in downtown San Antonio. His preceptorship was at the Robert B.Green Memorial Hospital under Dr. John H. Burleson, one of the city's early ophthalmologists, from 1933-1935, some 25 years before the UT Medical School was established.

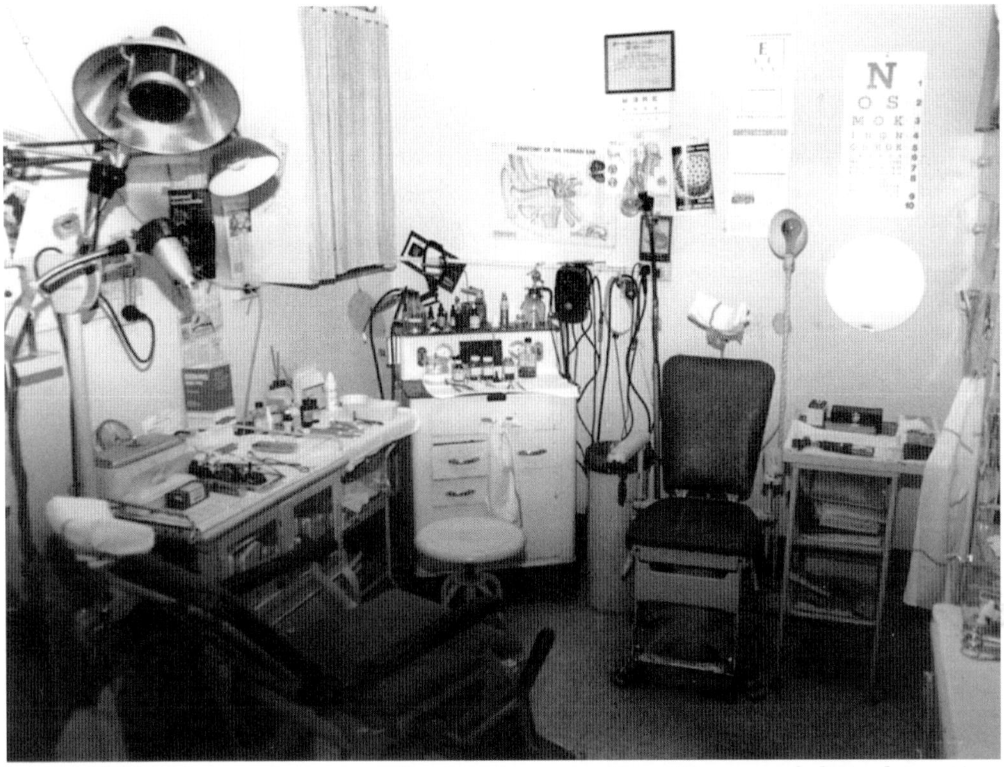

During the more than 60 years of clinical practice,
Dr. McCurdy's office changed little

began a lengthy and successful practice that endured both the Depression and World War II. Dr. Franklin Pinckney Steed went from Arkansas to the Universities of Arizona, New Mexico, and Tulane as well as Emory before he established a local EENT practice in 1931. Finally, Dr. Raymer C. Jewell received his medical degree at the Pacific College of Medicine in 1916 and worked for at time at Massachusetts General Hospital, Boston Eye and Ear, and in Chicago before coming to Texas. These individual careers were a product of a unique period in South Texas medical history, a composite of knowledge, training, and experience with the promise of greater advances to come.

Bexar County Medical Society Records

## DR. MARION WALLACE McCURDY

The generation who entered the profession in the years between the wars was transitional. As Dr. Marion Wallace McCurdy, reflecting on his 58-year career dispensing medical care, noted, he was "*one of the last of the eye, ear, nose, and throat specialists."* After his generation, ophthalmology would be practiced predominantly by those who specialized exclusively in the eye. Eye boards were first given in 1916 as hospitals began to require specialized training, and many early physicians chose eye, ear, nose and throat for economic reasons rather than a more highly specialized ophthalmology practice. According to one San Antonio specialist, the custom had been "*to do eyes in the summer*" and "*ear, nose, and throat*" in the winter. McCurdy enjoyed the unique experience of witnessing the growth of ophthalmology all the way from Dr. John Burleson and the first eye specialists in San Antonio to the latest in modern ophthalmology. His career illustrates both the beginnings of formal ophthalmology training in South Texas and the importance of that training to the community.

Nix Health Care System, "The Nix News," June 1993, 1;
Dr. Dan Russell, Jr. interview

Born in deep South Texas at Brownwood in 1906, McCurdy came to San Antonio with his family in 1914 at the beginning of World War I. While his father, the Rev. Dr. A.H.P. McCurdy, served as the minister at the Pine Street Presbyterian Church, McCurdy graduated from Brackenridge High School at such a young age, not yet 17, that his parents had him take extra courses at Western Texas Military Institute (later the San Antonio Academy and Texas Military Institute). He also worked as a meter reader for the Light and Power Company and delivered potato chips for a local company and, before he graduated in 1928 from the University of Texas at Austin, helped build many of the buildings on that campus in order to pay for his education. His timing was unfortunate, however, because he graduated from the Galveston Medical Branch in the early 1930s in the depths of the Depression.

Dr. Marion W. McCurdy Interview with Sue McDonald, January 25, 1990;
Biographical materials supplied by Mrs. (Anne) McCurdy;
McCurdy, Anne Ayers Lide, "Pleasant Places: A Goodly Heritage," 1982.

When Dr. Mac, as he was commonly called, looked to his home town for formal medical training to supplement his basic program, he found little at hand. At the new county charity hospital, the R.B. Green Memorial Hospital, however, he discovered a patient population up to ninety percent Hispanic and a place where a young doctor might observe the wide range of cases necessary to a good education. Since the strong family tradition among Hispanics tended to produce more normal outcomes from treatment than common in most indigent populations, novices here, it seemed, might even experience a considerable amount of success. McCurdy interned in general medicine at the Green in 1933, and then began an informal eye, ear, nose and throat residency. Along the way he also worked as a physician for the San Antonio Independent Schools, received a contract to treat the men of the Missouri Pacific, Southern Pacific and MKT Railroads, and worked with the Warm Springs Foundation at Gonzales, positions in which he eventually learned to speak Spanish.

Drs. Joseph De Gasperi, James Mims, and McCurdy Interviews;
Biographical material from Mrs. (Anne) McCurdy;
"Pleasant Places"

McCurdy's training at the R.B. Green Hospital, however, did not qualify him as a specialist. As one observer put it, "*eye training was still recognized on an individual basis*." To fully qualify as an ophthalmologist, the young doctor still needed to fulfill the traditional requirement of a preceptorship under one of the community's outstanding specialists. Fortunately, McCurdy's father had been a hunting buddy of Dr. John Burleson until the doctor moved to San Antonio in 1905. When Dr. Burleson met the young Dr. McCurdy, he found him to be a worthy son of his old friend and took an interest. Burleson invited the young man to become his associate in 1935 in the new eye, ear, nose and throat partnership with Drs. Steele, M.O. Judson, and T.J. Walthall that began in an old boarding house and eventually became the Eye, Ear, Nose and Throat clinic at the new Nix Memorial Hospital. Initially, McCurdy arranged a preceptorship that, as it had for his predecessors, conveyed the necessary professional blessings on him. By opening a place for him to fit into the community, moreover, it extended Burleson's influence to another generation and ensured continuity and an orderly process in passing on vital professional information.

Dr. Burleson also insisted that McCurdy spend part of 1935 working with the eminent eye physician, Dr. Everett Goar, in Houston, and in succeeding summers studying at the New Orleans Charity Hospital under the guidance of Dr. Buffington, in St. Louis, Chicago, and Washington, D.C. Burleson and McCurdy became close friends, and the older doctor, referred to by McCurdy as Dr. B, Uncle John, or "*Teo*," in time presented his associate and his young wife with gifts of china, crystal, and more as they set up their household and entertained friends with dinners of "*pinto beans and biscuits with an occasional tomato*." On October 7, 1939, McCurdy passed his American Board of Ophthalmology examination.

Bexar County Medical Society clipping file;
Dr. Dan Russell, McCurdy Interviews;
"Pleasant Places," 147-49

Although McCurdy lacked a formal appointment, he went on to spend four or five days at the R.B. Green Hospital, going each morning before his other duties to see patients. There he learned Tex-Mex Spanish and eventually built up a practice that made him one of the community's most beloved practitioners. As the fortunes of his charity patients improved, they did not forget him. McCurdy developed a love for his Mexican-American clientele and found it mutual and enduring. At the end of his life his memorial gifts were designated for their use. Among his patients were many who came to San Antonio and stayed with relatives because they could not afford hospitalization, and others for whom local hospital care was poor and recovery better at home. To meet the needs of this clientele, McCurdy did ambulatory cataract operations that constituted some of the first outpatient cataract surgery in the region. Before World War II began, he found time to author a paper with Dr. John Burleson entitled "*Is the Operation for Senile Cataract on an Ambulatory Patient Justifiable*?" discussing the pre and post operative care of patients unable to afford hospital care, that he read at the Section on Public Health, State Medical Associate of Texas, Dallas, May 15, 1940. Before writing the paper, McCurdy had operated on at least 60 patients in his office and allowed them to recover on the day bed in the back of the office for the rest of the day. He continued the practice until the AMA made him desist; an innovator, decades ahead of his time.

Biographical material from Mrs. (Anne) McCurdy

As late as 1943, McCurdy extended the old form of training to another generation and another community by serving as a preceptor for Dr. Dor Brown and for Dr. William Alvalais of Mexico City, who later returned to that city. Brown received his medical degree at the Galveston Medical Branch and discovered ophthalmology in World War II when he joined the Navy and became a flight surgeon. After completing the preceptorship, Brown took over the Fredericksburg practice of a retired colonel a few miles north of San Antonio, but continued to send complex cases to his mentor in San Antonio throughout his career. Brown's accomplishment was to extend the influence of

McCurdy's training still further, reaching patients from as far away as El Paso, Brownsville, Amarillo, and East Texas. During World War II McCurdy left his joint practice with the seventy-three year old John Burleson, who came out of semi-retirement, and went off to serve as a Lieutenant and Lieutenant Commander at the Corpus Christi Naval Hospital. Burleson, meanwhile, maintained the practice, and later shifted from EENT to strictly the eye. McCurdy returned in 1947, and when Burleson retired in his nineties McCurdy assumed his practice, but did not remove Burleson's nameplate from the office door for twelve years out of respect for his mentor.

BCMS Records;
"Pleasant Places"

McCurdy remained in the same office suite until the 1980s and, at eighty-three, was still working and making San Antonio headlines by taking trips to treat patients in a jungle village near Cancun, Mexico. Nearing the end of his Nix building career, he explained his work as "*taking care of the people who come to town on the bus*" and being "*easily available to those people who need me*." With McCurdy, an era in the history of Southwest ophthalmology came to an end, but not before he had seen the significant new advances in the profession that resulted from World War II.

McCurdy Interview;
"47 Years and Going Strong," "Dr. McCurdy Celebrates 50 Years of Practicing in the Nix;"
McCurdy obit, October 10, 1995;
"The Nix News," June 1993

The path to competence as an ophthalmologist during the inter-war years remained difficult, particularly for native Texans since no local institution as yet offered residency training in the field. In the transitional period before approved residencies could be established, not only were most forced to seek training outside the state, but a number completed both some type of informal residency training and preceptorships as well.

# CHAPTER 9

# WORLD WAR II<br>AND<br>THE EMERGENCE OF A TRUE SPECIALTY, 1939-55

*It is the breadth of health activities that distinguishes the Army from the civilian hospital.*

Gustave J. Dammin, M.D.,
"*Military Medicine and Its Influence on Medicine*," 1457

The second great conflict of the twentieth century interrupted the orderly growth of medicine, but, like its predecessor, generated a flood of positive change in the medical profession both during the war and after. In Ophthalmology, World War II was instrumental in generating the essential public recognition required for the field to at last fully differentiate itself from the broader specialty of Eye, Ear, Nose, and Throat. For many aspiring physicians, military service once more provided access to learning opportunities they would not have had otherwise and ultimately determined the direction of their careers. The war facilitated increased networking between doctors that stimulated innovation and created a new medical leadership to oversee further medical progress. While it caused a crisis of global proportions for a generation, World War II produced a new agenda for ophthalmological research, further professional development, and the spread of ophthalmologists across South Texas.

For "advances in ophthalmology" from World War II, *see* Tidy, Sir Henry Letheby, 500.

The era in which the story of South Texas ophthalmology truly begins and the first "*Golden Age of Ophthalmology*" in the region coincide with the events of World War II. When the war began, there were only five practicing ophthalmologists in San Antonio--Drs. John Burleson, Donald Atkinson, Frank Rosebrough, Wilfred Muldoon, and Scott Applewhite--and few others across the region. By the time it was over, stellar ophthalmologists with impressive military backgrounds from elsewhere joined these men and the local Texas EENT practitioners who had served in distant places such as New Guinea and the Philippines. In 1939, two-thirds of the 1487 ophthalmologists certified by the American Board of Ophthalmology practiced in 9 states (primarily in the East and California). Within a decade, however, the total number of ophthalmologists in San Antonio increased to nine, including Drs. Jack Lee, John Matthews, Alfred Nisbet, and Harmon Brunner, and by the 1950s the pioneer specialists were joined by Drs. Marion Wallace McCurdy and Fred Cooper, Frank Weixel, James Mims, Jr., Dan Russell, and others with successful practices in many smaller communities. The war also produced increased demand for higher standards, better medical education, and new institutions for training that gave rise to techniques including the first successful use of steroids and lasers and the first successful treatment of detached retinas. In San Antonio, it strengthened existing relationships between community practitioners and their military counterparts and led to the founding of the region's first professional organizations devoted exclusively to ophthalmology. Finally, the generation of ophthalmologists who participated in World War II continues to exert an influence today, and evidence of their military background can still be detected in a certain military tone heard in the voices of many San Antonio practitioners.

George Rosen, 81;
Dr. Stephen G. Waller interview

The greatest impact of World War II on South Texas medicine, however, lay in advances in aviation and related medical research made largely in the decade that followed. School of Aviation Medicine research teams, including many men who eventually became community practitioners, laid the foundation for today's U.S. space program in this period. Their efforts produced a host of discoveries that served as a powerful influence on regional and national medical development alike. The stories of two distinguished ophthalmologists, Drs. John L. Matthews and Victor Byrnes, emphasize the importance of aviation-related activity to the advance of ophthalmic specialization in the region and important connections between ophthalmology and aviation that eventually led to the growth of the American space program. In a sense, everything up until this time had been a prelude.

Huesinger, Fort Sam Houston Papers; "History of the Medical Training Center, Brooke Army Medical Center, Fort Sam Houston," typescript.

## THE BEGINNING OF THE WAR IN EUROPE

In World War II as in World War I, the United States entered the conflict some time after it began. In this case, Americans went to war after the bombing of Pearl Harbor. Conditions in Europe at the start of World War II, however, help to explain the medical conditions that American ophthalmologists, including those from South Texas, faced on their arrival overseas. When it began, Great Britain had engaged Sir Stewart Duke-Elder to serve as Consulting Ophthalmologist to the Army, and he promptly set to work to create a system capable of meeting the complex needs emerging from the conflict. The efficient ophthalmic service assembled in World War I had largely disintegrated by this time, and Duke-Elder and a new group of physicians had to begin all over again. Images of blinded men sent to St. Dunstan's linger in the memory as portraits of wartime despair, but most casualties were rapidly evacuated by sea, air, or rail to care facilities that were highly effective in treating patients and returning them to active duty or productive lives. By 1941, fifty-one English ophthalmic centers, 138 subcenters, and a staff of seventy-three ophthalmologists answered the call to action. The British medical service swiftly developed the capability to return almost eighty per cent of the wounded to duty and a special military component distributed over 282,000 pairs of spectacles to the troops. English soldiers obtained the most up-to-date antibiotic treatments even at mobile ophthalmic units in North Africa.

Link and Coleman, 305-315; Crew, F.A.E., 514-17

In the intervening period before the U.S. entered the war, the Army Medical Center at Walter Reed General Hospital, where medical officers had been sent for ophthalmology training between the wars, organized the American response. American military doctors devised new plans for handling casualties and preparing doctors for combat and mobilized medical forces that included a significant number of eye, ear, nose and throat specialists and ophthalmologists, most initially from the Eastern United States. The new approach employed a system for handling casualties similar to that devised in World War I, but with capabilities improved by the accumulated knowledge garnered in that conflict. The Great War taught that grouping eye casualties at centers improved the rate of success, hence cases routinely were categorized and labeled to allow for an orderly workflow. Patients with intraocular foreign bodies, orbital or intraocular neoplasms, and others with enucleations, retinal detachments, glaucoma, cataracts, or problems requiring surgery of the lids were assigned to general hospitals or specialized eye centers as needed. Standard equipment at most centers included "*small Lancaster hand electromagnets, lensometers, Brombach perimeters, stereocampimeters, ophthalmoscopes, phorometers, and instruments for corneal transplantation as well as more usual instruments*." In addition to handling a heavy caseload, moreover, some ophthalmologists collected pathologic materials and others developed a new type of acrylic artificial eye.

Dr. Stephen G. Waller interview; Crew, F.A.E., 514-523.

The ophthalmologists' first duty in this war, as in other wars, was to treat casualties and provide soldiers with general eye care. According to official medical histories, Axis troops in World War II wounded 598,000 United States soldiers, sailors and Marines, of whom roughly twelve to seventeen per cent received head or neck injuries, including wounds to the eyes. It was later observed that "*an inordinately high rate of ocular injury*" occurred "*relative to the amount of surface area exposed to injury*," given that the eyes comprise "*as little as 0.10% of total body surface and only 0.27% of the erect frontal silhouette.*" Even remote ophthalmologic services in distant theaters of operations including the 6th General Hospital in the Mediterranean that operated as a "*special eye center*" "*at the end of an evacuation chain*" handled eye injuries and diseases representing seven per cent of total injuries. Response to the needs of these patients provided long lasting benefits as doctors expanded on knowledge gained in the first

World War to develop new systems of caring for the injured both on the battlefield and at home.

"History of the Medical Training Center, Brooke Army Medical Center," typescript, Ft. Sam Houston archives;
U.S. Department of Defense, 310

During the course of the war, ophthalmologists at overseas medical centers commonly treated everything from burns, vehicular accidents, fist fights, sports, mines and grenades, shell blasts, gunshot wounds, aircraft accidents and explosions to keratoconjunctivitis, chorioretinitis, macular degeneration, iritis, optic atrophy, and macular edema, and evacuated only the worst cases to the Zone of the Interior (the military term for the United States). The idea of sending wounded Americans with severe eye injuries back to the United States for treatment originated with the Ophthalmology Branch of the Surgeon General's Office, activated in 1944 to establish policies and procedures to care for the blind men of the Army. This proved possible when doctors learned that what came to be known as the "*golden hour*," the first hour after trauma in which immediate treatment might make a difference in a patient's recovery, was less critical for eye injuries than others. As a result, five specialized ophthalmic-plastic centers went into operation, including one at El Paso where the patient load was constantly high and others at Letterman, San Francisco; Valley Forge, Pennsylvania; O'Reilly, Missouri; and Bushnell, Utah. World War II increased activity at both Fort Sam Houston and its hospital. By 1945 there were 10,000 patients hospitalized at Brooke Hospital Center, which established a special hospital unit for eye, ear, nose and throat cases. An ophthalmology center was established in 1950.

Link and Coleman, 305-313;
Wiener, Meyer, 45;
"Brooke Army Hospital and Brooke Army Medical Center"

Surgeons in World War II continued to cherish Grieshaber needles made in Europe and carried their own sutures--first made of silk, later, nylon--and eventually a substance that could be absorbed by the body. Ophthalmologists performed cataract surgery under Zeiss hammerlights hand-held by their assistants. The success rate in handling eye problems further improved with the introduction of new instruments that included slit lamps, electro-magnets for removal of foreign bodies within the globe, and the first corneal grafts.

Phospholine iodide and cortisone, considered more valuable than gold and kept in vials in locked storage rooms, became available and ophthalmologists first used penicillin to reduce bacterial infections from eye injuries. After the war, Diamox was added to the ophthalmologist's formulary around 1955.

Drs. James Mims, William C. Lloyd, III interviews

In the continental United States, aviation personnel were treated at "*regional hospitals, station hospitals and dispensaries by medical officers assigned to the Air Forces*." For the majority of Texas eye specialists and other physicians, the typical World War II experience either took this form or meant stateside training followed by service at an overseas medical facility or caring for the wounded at a U.S. military base. In one typical experience, Dr. June Yates, a Grapevine, Texas, native who had graduated from North Texas State University, received his medical degree from Baylor in 1933, and completed a New York Polyclinic residency and study at the Newark Eye and Ear Infirmary before the war began. He also practiced for three years in Ada, Oklahoma, and for a brief time at Corpus Christi before entering the service in 1940. Yates spent his first years of service during World War II at the Camp Bowie Station Hospital near Brownwood, assigned to the Eye, Ear, Nose and Throat Service. There he was promoted from Captain in the Reserve Officer's Corps to Major and later in 1942 to Chief of the Service. In 1944, he was sent to the European Theater of Operations assigned to the 180th General Hospital as Chief of the EENT Section and spent almost two years in England, France, and Germany before being discharged when the war ended. The experience increased his knowledge and improved his skills as was true for most doctors who served, to the ultimate benefit of local communities in Texas and elsewhere. Returned to civilian life, Yates went back to Corpus Christi, resumed his practice, and spent the next thirty-two years serving South Texas residents. For others, however, the experience of World War II was defined by aviation.

Payne, Brittain F., 495; Bexar County Medical Society records

## WORLD WAR II AVIATION AND DR. JACK BENNETT LEE

Physicians working in the context of military aviation, in contrast to Dr. June Yates, had a different kind of experience. World War II expanded new aviation operations in South Texas that stimulated corresponding advances in medicine. While Texans along the Gulf Coast prided themselves on shipyards that turned out Liberty Ships in under 200 days by the war's end, the state's feats in aviation were even greater. Across Texas, the war made the defense industry a permanent part of the economy and aircraft manufacture one of that industry's most important components. When Franklin D. Roosevelt asked for 50,000 airplanes in 1940, the Defense Plant Corporation and the Reconstruction Finance Corporation headed by Texan Jesse Jones converted the region into a major producer for the long term. Dallas, in particular, found itself in a position to benefit from millions of dollars in defense contracts since it had recently modernized, already possessed a skilled work force, and had numbers of manufactories ready for retooling to produce military materials of all kinds. Artisans and craftsmen who had started in business producing wagon wheels for pioneer settlers now converted their machine shops from making farm machinery to the manufacture of aircraft parts and equipment. Between 1941 and 1945 the North American Aviation plant at Grand Prairie produced over 20,000 airplanes, delivering 728 in one month alone.

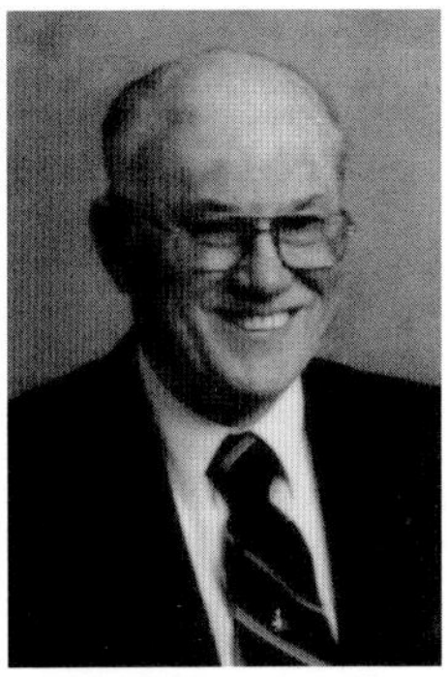

Dr.Jack Bennett Lee

Barksdale, 1-3;
"World War II," "Aviation in Texas," New Handbook of Texas, 50

The Texas climate and terrain were ideal for Air Force operations and they concentrated in South Texas at a host of military air bases. The presence of so much aviation activity in turn necessitated medical facilities capable of preparing pilots for the physical stress of flying and treating also injury and disease that occurred in this highly specialized population. In addition Bergstrom in Austin, Corpus Christi and Kingsville Naval Air Stations, Foster Air Force Base at Victoria, Gary at San Marcos, Goodfellow at San Angelo, Ft. Hood at Killeen, Laughlin at Del Rio, and Webb at Big Spring, other bases included those at Bryan, Harlingen, Hondo, and Laredo in addition to the airfields at Brooks, Kelly, and Lackland in San Antonio. In 1939, after

Congress authorized $300 million for the Air Corps, hundreds of new airplanes, officers, and enlisted men arrived at Kelly, turning the base into a huge industrial complex. Training components and corresponding medical activities grew correspondingly. With the addition of night flying to the school program alone, the amount of training time needed to prepare pilots had doubled. The experience of San Antonio's ninth strict ophthalmologist, Dr. Jack Bennett Lee, provides an example of how World War II brought higher standards and new skills to South Texas ophthalmologists and reflects the importance of military aviation to the city both during and after the war.

Greater Kelly Development Corporation
website: www.gkdc.org;
Greater Kelly Development Corporation, 1995, 5.

Had it not been for World War II, Jack Lee might have settled in Texas as did his father, who was a railroad clerk for the Missouri, Kansas and Texas Railroad. It is likely he would have become a surgeon rather than an ophthalmologist, since the demand was higher for surgeons in most Texas towns. After a combined internship and residency at Dallas' Parkland Hospital in 1938, Lee had, in fact, intended to become a surgeon. Instead, as war loomed he signed up for the Army Reserve and became a general medical officer at the Air Corps Center at Lowry Field in Denver, Colorado. The link with aviation was significant, and set the tone for his subsequent career in ophthalmology.

Bexar County Medical Society membership records;
Dr. Jack Lee interview

As the war deepened, the country faced a growing need for the new medical officers known as a "*flight surgeons*," whose expertise was employed in selecting candidates for flight training and dealing with the unique problems of aviators. Lee's career began when he left Colorado on orders to take a six weeks course for "*aviation medical examiners*" at Randolph Air Force Base in San Antonio to prepare him to test cadets for their potential to complete flight training. Part of the training for aviation medical examiners consisted of an introduction to the basics of ophthalmology that included instruction on how to use the ophthalmoscope, do refractions, examine the eyes and ears, and test for depth perception, muscle balance, color vision and hearing. Along with use of the Flying Adaptability Rating Test his companions humorously referred to by its acronym, Lee also learned to conduct tests in psychology and cardiology to select the best candidates. Given the standards of the day, these fundamental techniques were enough to qualify him for the position and he soon found himself on the road in charge of a "*traveling flying cadet examining board*." With help from a lieutenant who placed newspaper and radio advertisements to attract potential flyers, Lee traveled across the country, meeting in the basements of churches, post offices, schools and lodge halls in places like Cedar Rapids and Sioux City, Iowa, with enthusiastic young men hoping to become pilots. Selecting some for further testing and rejecting others based primarily on his assessment of their visual responses, Lee had a powerful influence on many individual careers. In the process, he became a flight surgeon.

Dr. Jack Lee interview

His adventures, however, had only just begun. When the Army decided to issue two pairs of glasses to every serviceman after Japan bombed Pearl Harbor and the draft began, Lee was put in charge of doing refractions with the help of several optometrists. At Deritter, Louisiana, he next worked with pilots and aircrews, training artillery observers for the small aircraft used by observation squadrons. He then moved on to Rapid City, South Dakota, where he served as the flight surgeon for a B-17 group engaged to train bombing crews. In addition to medical examinations, pilot immunization, sick call, and treating the survivors of airplane crashes (a not-uncommon phenomenon at the time), he also spent four hours each month flying to build rapport with the pilots. In the process, he developed a strong respect for the courage of the flyers he treated. He eventually became a "*Ribbon Rider*," one of a group of non-pilots who received Air Medals for completing bombing missions. Armed with a number of special skills, he was now ready for service overseas.

Bexar County Medical Society membership records;
Dr. Jack Lee interview

Lee left South Dakota to join a B-17 group forming at Geiger Field in Spokane, Washington, and followed these men to Florida and Savannah, Georgia, before they were all shipped out to Italy. The long voyage to Europe took him on a route through Puerto Rico, Trinidad, British New Guinea, Brazil, Natal (the coaling station for British ships at Ascención Island), Accra on Africa's west coast, and Casablanca in Morocco before he finally arrived in Italy. There at Foggia and Camosa he worked to set up a thirty-six-bed hospital and dispensary with four flight surgeons under him assigned to treat cases and handle the victims of air crashes. Major injuries were sent on to a large general hospital at Naples. Lee served in Italy for a year and a half before the European war ended, and then returned to the United States. On the way home, he passed through Trinidad and Belem, Brazil, where he helped to process returning flight crews and handle air crashes on the edge of the jungle. As a result, he arrived in Florida just after the bombing of Hiroshima, leaving the war behind only when he was finally placed in charge of a troop train bound for San Antonio.

Dr. Jack Lee interview

World War II not only gave Lee a chance to improve his medical skills, but an opportunity to travel, compare his knowledge with others, and learn skills in the new field of aviation medicine that had become the equivalent of a medical sub-specialty. Returning home, he carried with him the motivation to further his career, and simply took the next logical step. When the railroads offered cent-a-mile rates to travel anywhere in the nation, Lee boarded a train for Iowa City hoping to begin an ophthalmology residency there. No openings were available when he arrived, so he got back on the train with the idea of seeing the Mayo Clinic at Rochester, Minnesota, before returning to Texas. Arriving almost on Armistice Day, he was welcomed to begin his training at one of the nation's premiere institutions, becoming part of the first generation to use the phoropters, tenonometers, slit lamps, and perimeters now considered essential instruments of the field. A few years later, he returned to San Antonio a full-fledged specialist with extensive military experience, a world traveler's sophistication, and one of the best medical educations in the country. Lee became the seventh ophthalmologist in San Antonio and joined the Bexar County Medical Society in 1949 to become one of its 400 members. Over the next twenty-five years he practiced in San Antonio, slowly building up his practice through referrals, and later expanded his knowledge in the emerging field of medical law. Today, as an active member of the medical community, he continues to serve as a resource for local ophthalmologists and an influence for higher standards and improvements in medical education.

Dr. Jack Lee interview

## WARTIME AND POSTWAR SCHOOL OF AVIATION MEDICAL RESEARCH

While Dr. Jack Lee and other flight surgeons prepared pilots and eventually went overseas themselves, ophthalmologists at the School of Aviation Medicine in San Antonio spent the war conducting research on a wide range of visual and other aviation-related problems, treating and preparing aviators, and training and assisting flight surgeons. Here ophthalmology constituted a particularly important component of most activity. Special appeals were made early in the war to induce ophthalmologists of good standing to "*align themselves*" with the Army Air Forces, and some of the best came to San Antonio. Under Brig. Gen. Eugen G. Reinartz, Commandant of the School, the course in ophthalmology was expanded to 129 hours of didactic clinical and laboratory work as part of the eight-week course in Aviation Medicine. "*The time devoted to ophthalmology exceeded that of any other course*," and resulted in a growing interest in ophthalmology that many followed up on when the war ended.

For details on the Course in Ophthalmology at the AAF School of Aviation Medicine, see Payne, Lt. Col. Brittain F., 493

With the arrival of a new Director of Research, Dr. Harry George Armstrong, near the end of the war in 1941, SAM researchers went to work for a man who had assisted in setting up the first aeromedical laboratory at the original School of Aviation Medicine at Wright Field in Dayton, Ohio. In addition to his research on aviation-related physiological problems, Armstrong also had vivid accounts of the German blitzes on London from his assignment as the first aeromedical observer with the Royal Air Force in World War II and was among the world's experts on the problems of aviation. Aviation warfare had become ever more sophisticated as giant factories and airports called for better illumination, blackout regulations forced pilots to conduct night bombing raids, and new questions arose about the properties of "*night vision*." As scientific interest in vision shifted away from basic physiology toward adaptation, ophthalmic research under Armstrong's leadership took a new direction. Flight surgeons realized that goggles could help pilots withstand the glare of reflected sunlight on cloudbanks and might significantly improve night flying. Ophthalmologists seeking to further the war effort studied conditions relating to skybrightness, wartime street lighting, visual signals and codes, and camouflage that made it difficult to distinguish between object and background. Another group investigated flying accidents that called attention to the structural design of windshields and other aircraft parts and equipment. Devices were needed to adapt pilots' flying skills to more advanced aircraft that were capable of expanding vision beyond normal limits and adapting it to extremes of environmental change. Given the implications of discoveries for civilian applications, moreover, research was scarcely interrupted when the conflict ended.

Armstrong, Harry, 8-17, 231-234; Benford, 250-254

After World War II, the nation resumed its domestic agenda and most military operations returned to peacetime status. All but twelve of thirty-four Army Air Force installations in Texas were deactivated, and most training sites reverted to the communities or counties from which they had been purchased or leased. In an effort to consolidate facilities around the nation's capital, components such as Fort Worth's Flying Training Command moved to Washington, D.C. As the Cold War began after 1947, however, the United States Air Force became a separate military service. This important reorganization made Texas Army air fields into air force bases and Randolph, Kelly and Brooks Air Force Bases in San Antonio into Pilot Training Centers. The old Aviation Cadet Center adjoining Kelly Field, renamed Lackland Air Force Base in that year, became the receiving and training center for all incoming enlisted personnel and the new location of the Air Force Officer Candidate School. The fact that 6,804 aircraft and 20,700 licensed pilots were active in Texas in 1948 further reflected the state's strong interest in aviation.

"Aviation in Texas," Handbook of Texas, 50;
"History of the Medical Training Center, Brooke Army Medical Center," typescript, Ft. Sam Houston archives;
"ASF Medical Training to Occupy All of Fort Sam," San Antonio Light, November 2, 1945, 10-A;
"Army Plans for Fort Sam Big Question," October 21, 1945, n.p.;
Aerospace Medical Division, 10-15

Military reorganization and downsizing only increased the importance of the School of Aviation Medicine, and aviation research there not only continued, but expanded. Since its transfer from Long Island in 1926 and throughout World War II, the School had proven to be an important component of military operations. By reassigning it from the Air Training Command to Air University, the Army now made SAM the Air University's postgraduate medical college and institutionalized its wartime role in training specialists. "*Patterned after a civilian university*," the School of Aviation Medicine henceforth focused its efforts on professional education "*as distinguished from technical skills*." This action freed its staff of researchers, including ophthalmologists, to adopt a new role. Henceforth, SAM researchers would dedicate their efforts "*to concentrate on exploring new medical aspects in the flight environment*" and to offer "*specialized clinical services on a limited basis and only for exceptional cases*." In conjunction with these developments, Army officials also noted that the nearby San Antonio flying school would serve as "*an excellent source for research in aviation medicine*."

Barksdale, 1-3;
"Aviation in Texas," Handbook of Texas, 50;
Link and Coleman, 313- 340

In the late 1940s, only two military institutions conducted organized studies of the effects of flight on human beings. All aeromedical research was done at either Wright Field in Dayton, Ohio, or at SAM on San Antonio's Randolph Air Force Base. Ever since 1918, moreover, when Major Conrad Behrens began studying the effects of hypoxia on visual functions at SAM's laboratory predecessor in Mineola, the ophthalmology branch had worked at the forefront of School of Aviation Medicine research. Making "*the aviator's task more visually effective*" became particularly important when doctors realized that "*eighty-five percent of the neurosensory input into flying is through the visual apparatus*." Groups of SAM researchers devoted solely to eye-related problems now concentrated the talent and expertise of military ophthalmologists and flight surgeons to produce new synergies, building on the work of William Ocker and Dr. Frederick Thorne. Aircraft design that allowed an unhampered field of vision was essential, windscreens and canopies needed good optical properties, and the reduction of cockpit light so as to not impair the pilot's vision required the study of aircraft enclosures with high optical qualities. Other research projects focused on developing visual standards, requirements for occupational categories in the AAF, constructing tests for personnel selection, and designing specialized visual equipment to train aviators. Efforts also focused on the use of penicillin to treat eye infections and the effects of altitude, drugs, and fatigue on visual efficiency. Research teams now moved away from the purely clinical settings where most previous discoveries in ophthalmology had been made to the laboratory and concentrated their efforts on a selective population of those with the highest visual potential--no longer sick patients, but healthy individuals in whom fundamental conditions could be studied. Part of their attention also focused on the discovery of information about visual reaction in extreme conditions. Dr. John Paul Stapp, whose rocket sled tests at Holloman AFB, New Mexico, had caused his macula (retina) to hemorrhage was among the new type of patients seen by SAM ophthalmologists during this period.

Benford, 258; Link and Coleman, 310-11

Research conducted during the war and in the decade that followed produced a new type of equipment commonly referred to as "*visual appliances*," along with a variety of treatments and surgical techniques to help aviators better adapt to the flight environment. Among the most important advances made in World War II had been the discovery that pilots, whose eyes had been pierced by shrapnel or pieces of plastic from airplane windshields, often suffered no discomfort or loss of vision. The material remained inert within the eye and seemed to cause little or no immune reaction. This gave an English physician, Dr. Harold Ridley, the idea of producing intraocular lenses or lens implants from a plastic material that could be made to correct for aphakia following cataract surgery. Ridley's discovery eventually led to the manufacture of the first intraocular lenses for general use. Flight surgeons such as Drs. Mark Coffman and Dean Carlson made other discoveries by accompanying pilots in combat, and their efforts spawned research on movement detection, vision improvements using ultraviolet light, and a host of other visual reactions that concentrated research on developing new adaptive technologies. From the Howard and Dolman depth perception testing apparatus developed at Mineola to test stereoscopic vision (still in use over seventy-five years later) to a host of other devices, SAM developed products that eventually aided civilians and generated new parameters for human performance.

Alcott, Edward, Aerospace Medical Division, 150-200;
Alcott, Edward, "Brief History of Brooks Air Force Base"

In November 1948, under Commander Harry Armstrong's direction, the School of Aviation Medicine also set a new agenda for medical research, and ophthalmology in particular, when it sponsored a meeting of authorities to discuss "*Aero Medical Problems of Space*

*Medicine*." This meeting not only produced the list of problems that was published in the *Journal of Aviation Medicine*, but intensified interest in a field about which few scientists had substantial knowledge. By 1949, as the Air Force gained increasing autonomy from the other armed services, research efforts were directed to a range of questions broad enough to lay a foundation for space research. When the School of Aviation Medicine resumed its original identity as part of the Air Training Command in 1959 to participate in the emerging United States space flight program, its educational and research roles were both firmly established and it had begun to move the cutting edge of research forward at a more rapid pace. In the years ahead, SAM researchers and San Antonio community practitioners through what had become strong professional links began to consider aspects of vision that took ophthalmology in new directions. These activities also placed the region for the first time in the forefront of the field.

Alcott, Edward, Aerospace Medical Division, 150-200;
Alcott, Edward, "Brief History of Brooks Air Force Base"

## DR. VICTOR BYRNES

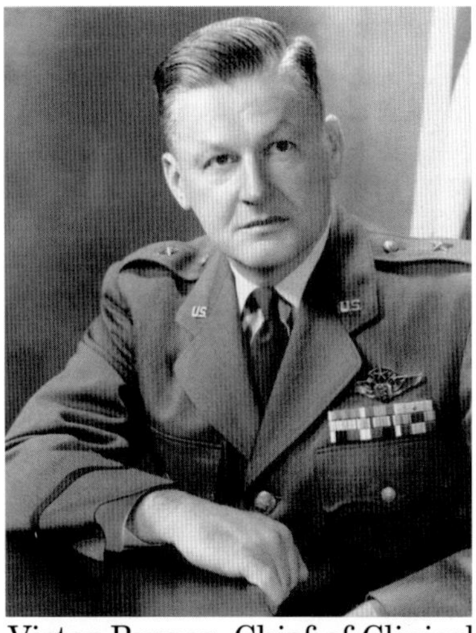

Victor Byrnes, Chief of Clinical Medicine and Head of the Eye Department at the School of Aviation Medicine after World War II

The man in charge of School of Aviation Medicine ophthalmological researchers after the war ended was Dr. Victor Byrnes, a transitional figure whose work influenced both military and civilian medicine and helped to stabilize and expand the foundations of ophthalmic research. Unlike many senior ophthalmologists who returned to private practice, Byrnes went to the School of Aviation Medicine as Chief of Clinical Medicine and head of the Eye Department when the war ended. Under his direction, SAM research now proceeded along three main lines: 1) studies of visibility and field of vision from aircraft; 2) efforts to design and develop goggles and sun glasses; and 3) night vision studies or, according to another observer, aviator and pilot selection problems, general vision problems, visual standards, and spectacles and goggles. In addition, Cold War concerns about problems of defense and weaponry sparked

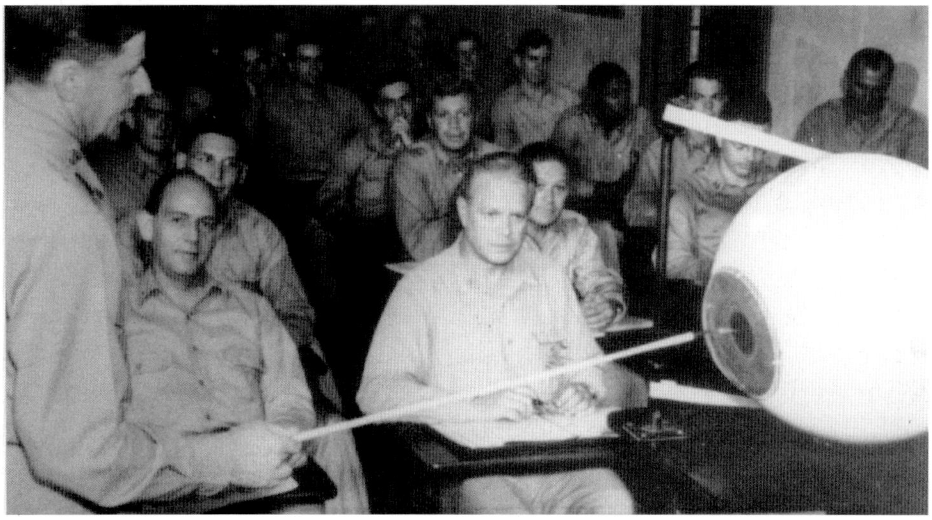

1950- Dr. V. Byrnes lecturing flight surgeons on ophthalmology

research efforts by a group of SAM ophthalmologists who focused their investigations on the possibilities of thermonuclear warfare. With oversight for the Eye Department, Dr. Byrnes participated in some way in each of these efforts.

Benford, 207;
Link and Coleman, 305

Byrnes came from a medical family with important national military and medical connections. His grandfather, the son of an Irish immigrant, not only served as a hospital steward in the Civil War but also took care of Mrs. Lincoln after President Lincoln was shot. Graduated in 1865 from Georgetown College Medical School, Byrnes' grandfather went on to practice medicine in a small Iowa farming community and raised five sons who became doctors and two daughters who married doctors. One son was Byrnes' father, Victor Warren; another was Walter L. Bierring, who became President of the American Medical Association. Vic Byrnes' future became clear at the age of twelve when his father took him to a Davenport, Iowa, Eye, Ear, Nose, and Throat specialist named Dr. Gordon F. Harkness. So impressed was the boy with this gentleman that he determined to become an ophthalmologist.

Byrnes interview and biographical sketch

Byrnes graduated in 1922 from the University of Iowa College of Medicine, the youngest man in a class of eighty-four. After an EENT residency at Letterman General Hospital in San Francisco and Army Medical School training in Washington, D.C., he spent part of 1934 at the School of Aviation Medicine concentrating on ophthalmology. Prior to the bombing of Pearl Harbor, he also served as head of the Eye, Ear, Nose and Throat service at Los Angeles' Barksdale Field and Honolulu's Tripler General Hospital. During World War II, Byrnes worked at convalescent hospitals in Nashville and New York and served as a surgeon for the Fifth Air Force stationed on Okinawa, arriving in Japan the day after McArthur. In 1947, he completed a six-month ophthalmology residency at Washington University in St. Louis, and generated his first research papers on subjects that reveal a treatment then on the frontier of ophthalmic research. Byrnes later presented a discussion of a new treatment for "*Delayed Post-Operative Formation of the Anterior Chamber*" that involved a process to stop the loss of aqueous by cauterizing the corneal incision with a hot muscle hook, or electrocoagulation to the San Antonio O&O Society. Among his other papers were discussion of an "*Eyelash Buried in Clear Lens Substance*" and "*A Case of Self-Mutilation Involving Both Eyes*." Ten years later, the focus of his investigations would testify to the quantum leap of change that SAM research had brought to the field.

Byrnes interview and biographical sketch

At the School of Aviation Medicine, Byrnes oversaw dozens of research projects on subjects ranging from night vision and blind flying to color vision and defectiveness, muscle disorders, and pilot reaction time (the need for pilots to perceive objects rapidly when in flight, a phenomenon based on the relationship between a pilot's psychological and visual levels of perception). Because visual research applications could be employed anywhere from mountaintops to sea bottoms and everywhere in between, the School also answered inquiries from visual scientists in a range of non-military agencies and institutions.

Byrnes interview and biographical sketch;
Dr. Thomas Tredici interview

Among other activities, Byrnes and his team assisted by the National Research Council established the criteria for automated vision screening in 1948 that led to today's Bausch and Lomb Orthorater. From investigations of ultraviolet effects on the eye, SAM researchers also developed blue blocker sunglasses with a neutral density that did not alter colors. Another 1948 project took Byrnes to the

Industrial Home for the Blind in Brooklyn, New York, to do color vision testing on patients with reduced visual efficiency. A year later he discussed the use of colored glass in windshields, windows, and the backlights of motor vehicles with the National Bureau of Standards. In the early 1950s he worked with the Joint Committee on Industrial Ophthalmology to develop reflecting, polarizing and absorbing filters for windshields. He also did considerable work on the selection of filter lenses for railroad engineers, sent advice on how to test railroad brakemen with a history of night blindness, and developed other tests and sunglasses for railroad employees.

Byrnes interview and biographical sketch;
Dr. Thomas Tredici interview

A sample of the research projects carried out under Byrnes' administration conveys a sense of the excitement that School of Aviation Medicine researchers must have felt in pursuing their new research agenda. Byrnes and his team corresponded with colleagues at the Wilmer Eye Institute about the use of ophthalmic filters in the Arctic and made recommendations to the medical director of North Atlantic Construction in Thule, Greenland, on visual problems there. They also worked with a Stanford University geography professor on the proper use of color in relief maps, evaluated other chromatostereoscopic cartography, and discussed the best choice of visual factors to create an impression of height in flat maps. Assistance given to the Massachusetts Institute of Technology improved submarine visual detection, and cooperation with Polaroid Corporation led to polarizing devices that could eliminate reflections from radar scope faces. Byrnes also directed retinal burn studies in 1952 that paved the way for the photocoagulators used to treat retinal disease., Finally, he helped develop plans to broaden educational facilities for postgraduate training in aviation medicine at both military and civilian institutions at a 1952 meeting at the School of Aviation Medicine attended by groups such as the American Board of Preventive Medicine and Public Health. In addition to studies on "*the relationship of visual capabilities to flight performance, eye injuries incurred in a flying environment, and the use of data and models for student training*," Byrnes ultimately produced over 100 publications and presentations ranging from "*Eye Problems in Combat Aviation*," to "*Visual Problems of Supersonic Speeds*" and "*Recent Advances in Military Ophthalmology*."

Dammin, 1464;
Byrnes interview and biographical sketch;
Benford, 208

Byrnes' later career demonstrates how news of this research at reached the international scientific community. Acting as Deputy Surgeon of the United States Air Forces in Europe in 1953 and as Consultant to the Eye Service of the United States hospital at Wiesbaden, Germany, he gave talks on "*Retinal Burns Produced by Atomic Flash*" to officers of the Norwegian Air Force in Oslo, Norway, and to the German-American Medical Conference. He also addressed "*Visual Aspects of Night Driving*" at Burderop Park and London, England, and "*Effects of Atomic Flash on the Retina*" at the Supreme Headquarters of the Allied Powers in Europe at Paris, France. During this period he also remained active in ophthalmological organizations at home, and so became a conduit for information flowing from Texas to the wider world. Byrnes' connections with South Texas were far from over, however.

Byrnes interview and biographical sketch

In 1955, Byrnes returned to the United States to become the Director of Professional Services for the Office of the Surgeon General of the U.S. Air Force in Washington, D.C. and a Brigadier General a year later. The appointment allowed him to work on a thesis at the Armed Forces Institute of Pathology that won him a membership in the American Ophthalmological Society in 1959. With help of John Paul Stapp, who contributed animal eyes from his Holloman deceleration experiments, Byrnes produced a work entitled "*Elevated Intravascular Pressure as an Etiological Mechanism in the Production of Eye Injuries*" that he considered the best research of his career. After thirty years of active duty, Byrnes requested retirement in 1959 to begin a new career, spending two years running an intern and residency training program in Florida and then practicing privately for the next thirteen years. He retired again in 1974, took a five-year vacation, and in 1979 went to work as a Medical Adjudicator for the regional office of the Veterans Administration at St. Petersburg, Florida. Finally, at the age of eighty, his career came full circle when he retired for good in 1986 and moved back to San Antonio with his wife to live at the Air Force Village "*in tranquility*."

Byrnes interview and biographical sketch

## A FEW OF BYRNES' CONTEMPORARIES

Although official records seldom mention School of Aviation Medicine researchers by name, several of Byrnes' contemporaries are worthy of note for their contributions to ophthalmology or the breadth of experience they brought to San Antonio. As the developer of motility standards for flight training and retention in 1942 and author of numerous articles on ocular motility, Dr. Richard Scobee became one of the nation's first authorities on an emerging ophthalmic sub-specialty field through his research on strabismus. Scobee published the first American textbook on the subject, *The Ocular Rotary Muscles*, based on his Randolph experience in 1947, and went on to head the low-vision service at the Wilmer Eye Institute of Johns Hopkins Medical School.

Dr. Thomas Tredici interview

Another SAM researcher, Dr. Louise Sloan, developed a color vision testing lantern (CTT) in 1943 that expanded the pool of available candidates for flight training, and other Randolph staff produced a night vision trainer. In 1948, in cooperation with the National Research Council Committee on Vision, researchers invented a vision screen subsequently manufactured by Bausch and Lomb and still used today for testing the visual function of entering candidates and aircrew. Dr. Howard N. Rose, a Chicago native, conducted research on effects of atomic radiation on the eye at Randolph beginning in 1957, while Drs. Ray Milton Balyeat and William Bruce Clark studied the electromygraphy of extraocular muscles.

Green, 99, 112;
Dr. Thomas Tredici interview;
"Dr. Howard N. Rose," New Handbook of Texas.

Dr. Richard Fixott, who trained pilots in ophthalmology and was an active researcher at the School of Aviation Medicine after the war, represents the varied backgrounds of many of those who served there. Fixott came from a French Huguenot heritage and a family of doctors from the Channel Islands, including a practitioner licensed in Nova Scotia in 1840 who somehow found his way to the Far West. Fixott was born in Portland, Oregon, graduated from Stanford University and the Oregon Medical School, and practiced locally until Pearl Harbor changed his destiny. Ordered to active duty, he took a correspondence course in aviation medicine, studied Eye, Ear, Nose, and Throat, and completed a preceptorship with outstanding Portland ophthalmologist,

Dr. Ralph Davis. His subsequent military experiences in Panama and in China with the 14th Air Force Flying Tigers were an outgrowth of his San Antonio experience.

Dr. Richard Fixott interview;
Bexar County Medical Society records

## THE REMARKABLE CAREER OF DR. JOHN L. MATTHEWS

Of all those associated with the School of Aviation Medicine during and after World War II, however, none was a more powerful force for growth in South Texas ophthalmology than Byrnes' contemporary, Dr. John Larkin Matthews, known to the San Antonio community as "*Jack*," who practiced in San Antonio for sixty years. Matthews'

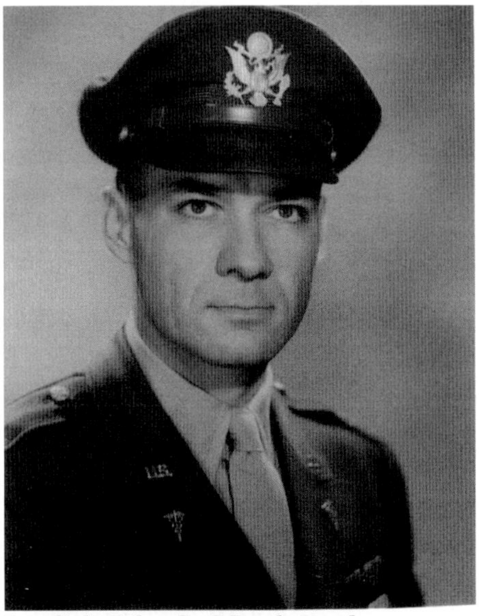

Lt. Col. John L. Matthews became Chief of the Department of Ophthalmology at the School of Aviation Medicine in 1943

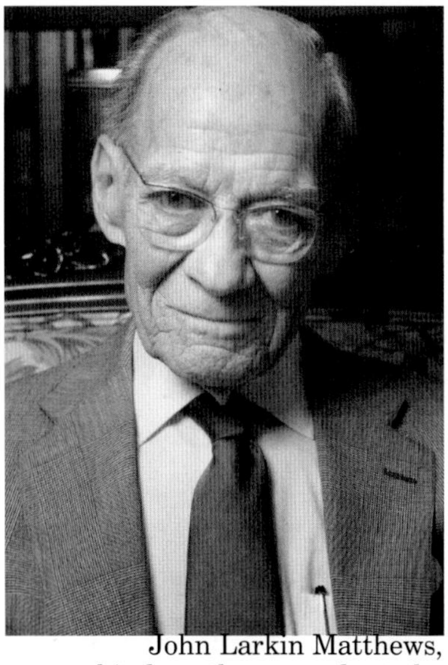

John Larkin Matthews, a kind gentleman and yet the most influential ophthalmologist in South Texas during the 20th century.

career at the School of Aviation Medicine was merely the first step in a lifetime of contributions to ophthalmology that influenced the growth of medical facilities and practices in the region.

Good, Pat, "Dr. John L. (Jack) Matthews"

Matthews' military experience, family connections in South and West Texas, and personal wealth of strengths and abilities combined to make him a medical leader and, in many ways, the heir of Dr. John Burleson's legacy, as well as a successful practitioner. His grandfather, D.S. Combs, fought with Terry's Texas Rangers in the Civil War, trailed cattle for a number of years, and later established the Combs Cattle Company Ranch near the West Texas town of Marathon in 1881. As in the case of Dr. Jack Lee, Combs' grandson might have become a general practitioner or a surgeon had it not been for World War II. Instead, the war altered Jack Matthews' professional development, added a dimension to his career, and ultimately made him one of the most outstanding ophthalmologists in all of South Texas.

Bexar County Medical Society membership records;
Dr. John Matthews, Mrs. John Matthews interviews;
Good, Pat, "Dr. John L. (Jack) Matthews"

Born in San Antonio in 1908, Matthews spent his first two years at Eagle Pass and Laredo while his father cashiered at the Border National Bank and conducted an import business with Mexico. In 1910, the family returned to San Antonio where Jack attended Stephen F. Austin, Travis and the Main Avenue High School before beginning pre-med courses at the University of Texas. The inspiration to become a doctor apparently also came from his other grandfather, James A. Matthews, who had graduated from Tulane and become a general practitioner, serving in several small Texas towns including Kosse, Hondo, Pearsall, Cotulla, and Eden before he turned to farming. Another mentor was the family doctor, Homer T. Wilson.

Bexar County Medical Society membership records; Dr. John Matthews, Mrs. John Matthews interviews; Good, Pat, "Dr. John L. (Jack) Matthews"

After graduating from the Galveston Medical Branch in 1933 and completing an internship at Philadelphia's Episcopal Hospital, Matthews returned to San Antonio and joined eye, ear, nose and throat specialist, Dr. W.E. Muldoon, in his Nix Building practice, expecting to begin a successful career in the place of his birth. With Muldoon, Matthews did surgery in tandem and discussed cases much as would the collaborators in an old-fashioned preceptorship. Muldoon had invented an instrument to simplify tear-duct surgery, was something of an innovator, and no doubt added an important component to the young man's education. Along the way, Matthews also learned to speak a passable Spanish. His first link to the war came from a German refugee at the Nix who introduced him to a remarkable new drug he had brought with him called sulfanilamide. Matthews' decision to specialize in ophthalmology, however, came from his connections with the School of Aviation Medicine. While serving in the Army Reserves, he took the ophthalmology correspondence course offered by the School to attract needed personnel and decided to pursue the specialty. In 1939 he returned to Philadelphia to begin a residency at the Wills Eye Hospital.

Bexar County Medical Society membership records;
Dr. John Matthews, Mrs. John Matthews, Dr. James Mims, Dr. William C. Lloyd, III interviews;
Matthews archival materials, Briscoe Library

Although Matthews opened his first ophthalmology practice in 1940, the young specialist was about to be transformed from a traditional EENT into a flight surgeon and research ophthalmologist. Later that year he entered military service with the 36th Division of the Texas National Guard and was sent to join the 111th Observation Squadron at Camp Bowie in Brownwood. When officials learned he was the only Guardsman with a flight surgeon's credentials, Matthews found himself transferred out of the infantry and back to San Antonio to examine servicemen at the Lackland AFB Aviation Cadet Center. A month later he was ordered to the School of Aviation Medicine to teach flight surgeon trainees the basics in aviation medicine required to treat working pilots and select candidates for flight training. Among other instructors were Drs. Brittain F. Payne, P. Robb McDonald, Albert Ruedeman, Jr., David V.L. Brown, Richard G. Scobee, Gustav Bahn, Louise Sloan and her husband William Rowland. Matthews spent the rest of the war at the School of Aviation Medicine, becoming Chief of the Department of Ophthalmology in 1943. In that year he also became a Diplomate of the American Board of Ophthalmology and was accepted into the American College of Surgeons. (In 1940, to supply a sufficient number of well-trained Flight Surgeons, the length of the training course was increased to 6 weeks and then 9 weeks, after being cut back to only 3 weeks, and class size increased from 100 to about 320. "*In 1941 instruction in ophthalmology included: the proper technique of eye examination; visual pathways; perimetry; use of the tangent screen; plotting of he red lens test; the field of binocular vision; the field of binocular fixation; heterophoria; concomitant and paralytic squint; optical effects of lenses; lens neutralization; retinoscopy; ophthalmoscopy; tonometry; the use of the large and hand slit lamp; the use of the binocular loupe; the method of instillation of mydriatics and myotics; the removal of corneal foreign bodies; color-vision testing; the use of the spectacle fitting set; and the properties of antiglare glasses.*" As the war developed, training included the "*treatment of burns of the eyes and eyelids; treatment of gas injuries to the eyes; immediate treatment of trauma of the face, eye, and eyelids; and night vision and dark adaptation,*" and more. Expanded facilities included a 7-lane darkroom with 13 eye lanes.

Dr. John Matthews, Mrs. John Matthews, Dr. James Mims, Dr. William C. Lloyd, III interviews;
Matthews archival materials, Briscoe Library;
Link and Coleman, 158-60, 177-78

Matthews now found himself in a place where he could perfect his skills in ophthalmology and widen his knowledge. Medical school students commonly received little ophthalmology training unless they elected it, and many schools taught little ophthalmology of any kind. In response to the need for trained flight surgeons, therefore, the School of Aviation Medicine at Randolph Air Force Base offered more extensive ophthalmological training than any medical school or residency program in the country! According to Dr. Victor Byrnes, "*Many doctors were introduced to ophthalmology through the School of Aviation and, later, Aerospace Medicine, through our ophthalmology portion of the Aerospace Medicine course.*" In fact, more people were introduced to ophthalmology in SAM's forty-hour flight surgeon's course in this period than at any other single institution in America. Given the importance of good vision to flying and the imperative that flight surgeons be proficient in eye examination, however, the School ordered the design of new classrooms, developed new training aids and teaching methods, and increased teaching personnel with outstanding practitioners from the San Antonio community, expanding SAM's achievement from ten graduates every six months to 330 every six weeks. As knowledge of this activity spread, moreover, the demand for and interest in civilian medical education in the specialty increased as well. A San Antonio military historian later quoted a statement recognizing the impact of the training program as follows: "*Evidently, the brief course at the School of Aviation Medicine stimulated an interest in ophthalmology, which is being followed up in civilian life.*"

Dr. John Matthews, Mrs. John Matthews, Dr. Victor Byrnes, Dr. Joseph De Gasperi, Dr. Thomas Tredici interviews;
Matthews archival materials, Briscoe Library;
Payne, Brittain F., 493

While his assignment lasted, Matthews taught aviation medicine, including the rudiments of ophthalmology, to three or four thousand medical officers who passed through the school. In this way, a single individual produced a generation of specialists. Three to four hundred doctors educated in San Antonio every year became flight surgeons, each with nearly sixty hours in ophthalmology, and over 5,000 physicians completed the course between January 1942 and September 1944. Departments within the Research Division grew to include ophthalmology as well as aviation medicine and other medical specialties. While his initial job dealt with training, however, Matthews was uniquely positioned when the war ended as Commander of the Eye Department to participate in aviation-related research.

Over the six years of its wartime service, the school graduated 4,672 physicians.

Ashcroft, Bruce, 5;
Drs. John Matthews, Thomas Tredici interviews;
Alcott, Edward, Aerospace Medical Division, 10-15

In 1944, Matthews delivered a paper at the George Washington School of Medicine on the "*Ophthalmic Injuries Incident to War*" caused by blasts of high explosives that produced retrobulbar hemorrhages, retinal and choroidal ruptures, cataracts, and dislocation of the lens in addition to traumatic keratitis, rupture of Descemet's membrane, transient opacification of the substantia propria of the cornea, and other injuries. Before the war ended, however, he also worked with SAM research teams studying improved signaling using colored VERY flares, color vision, color blindness, and the effects of weapons such as radar on the human body and assisting in projects to develop night vision and color vision testers. This experience set an important precedent for his subsequent career, involving him in cutting edge ophthalmological research.

"*Research in ophthalmology at SAM was concerned with the development of vision standards and the construction of tests for personnel selection. Emphasis was also placed on developing specialized visual equipment to train aviators. Important problems studied included color vision, night vision, pioneering in the use of penicillin in treating eye infections, and the effects of altitude, drugs, and fatigue on visual efficiency.*" It should also be noted that research funding more than doubled between 1940 and 1941.

Matthews, Dr. John, "Ophthalmic Injuries of War," 247-61;
Matthews archival materials, Briscoe Library;
Drs. John Matthews, Thomas Tredici interviews;
For the subjects and results of SAM research in the early 1940s, see Link and Coleman, 305-13;
Dammin, 1461

After retiring from the military in 1944, Matthews published or spoke about the research he had conducted or been part of at the School of Aviation Medicine. Later, he described the use of metallic filters made of platinum, gold, silver, chrome, or nickel alloy deposited on lenses to shut out infrared rays and allow pilots to scan around the sun for hostile aircraft, an innovation that also proved useful for skeet-shooting sportsmen. In 1946, he wrote about "*The Use of Goggles and Protective Lenses by Flying Personnel*" and on "*Observations of the Effects of Diisopropyl Fluorophosphate (DFD).*" Two years later, he was one of the world's leading experts among the distinguished ophthalmologists chosen to attend the Third Pan-American Congress of Ophthalmology at Havana, Cuba, along with Ernst Fuchs and others. In that year, he described the "*Effects of Ophthalmic Filers on Color Vision*," in 1949 the "*Use of Absorptive Lenses: Facts for the Profession*" and "*Some Considerations in the Selection of Flying Sunglasses*," and in 1952 he published a paper on "*Tinted Optical Media.*"

Matthews archival materials, Briscoe Library

Matthews also pursued several separate lines of research on his own, including a study of the genetically transmitted condition known as choroideremia, and, after renewing his ties with the cattle ranchers of West Texas, on the cure of bovine cancer eye and links between eye problems in humans and cattle. This important work, however, was only the first of his extensive accomplishments in a multi-faceted career that in the 1950s turned his attention to building permanent medical institutions and other efforts to strengthen medicine in the region. The first glimmer of that activity came in 1949 when he joined the Board of Directors of the San Antonio Association for the Blind. At the time he was Chairman of the Eye Clinic at the Robert B. Green Hospital, performing cataract operations for indigent patients at a cost of only ten dollars for the operating room. In 1950 he became President of the San Antonio Society of Ophthalmology and Otolaryngology, and in 1956 he was chosen as President of the Bexar County Medical Society. From this post he was ready to lead the community toward objectives that would change the scope of medicine in the region.

Program, Highland Hereford Breeders Association Conference, Marfa, Texas, August 24-25, 1951, Briscoe Library Archives;
Good, Pat, "Dr. John L. (Jack) Matthews"

## POSTWAR SAN ANTONIO

With his Texas background and wartime research experience, Matthews was uniquely positioned when he returned to private practice in 1944 to become the "*Dean of San Antonio Ophthalmologists*." Because he had already established a local practice, he not only had important contacts with the School of Aviation Medicine but was familiar with the community. With the significant changes caused by the war and those that followed, Matthews was perfectly positioned to negotiate for advances in both military and civilian medicine. In the postwar climate of recovery, it was natural that men who enjoyed comfortable relationships with both military and local society would gain prominence.

South Texas culture at the start of World War II had been a blend of Southern manners and the cowboy traditions of area ranchers. Long before doctors advertised, they received referrals from fellow practitioners and satisfied patients with whom they maintained lifetime ties, often reaching back to family pioneers in the region. Ranch families still used Sunday houses when they came to town for church, and most people were as reticent and formal as their parents' generation about health matters. It was considered more proper for Texans to refer to "*limbs*" than "*legs*," and modesty about the human body and its frailties remained the norm. Many doctors saw Afro-American or Hispanic patients at different times than whites, and often required them to use a separate entrance for office visits. These practices declined as the harsh realities of war increased human awareness and necessitated a new frankness, but old customs died hard. A physician's ability to negotiate traditional social relations could still be essential to his success, but now there were new standards as well.

Cary, E.H., 298-300

Matthews' family roots and the lasting friendships he made at the Galveston Medical Branch and in Philadelphia nurtured a practice based as much on personal ties as technology. His wife later recalled that many of his Galveston classmates dined at their house when he taught at the School of Aviation Medicine, and some lent her their cars for a trip downtown when gas and tires were rationed. Because of his West Texas heritage, Matthews' patients in time included many wealthy Texas ranching families, some of whom he would later marshal to the cause of supporting a South Texas medical school. After the war, he became a fixture in the community, treating cases at the Medical and Surgical Hospital (now the Baptist), the Physicians and Surgeons (later absorbed by the M &S), and the Nix, Santa Rosa, and R.B. Green Hospitals before most had a Division of Ophthalmology. Ultimately, his spirit of mutual cooperation and friendship, coupled with his knowledge of the city's cutting-edge research facilities, created social sanction that made him a force for professional development in specialized medicine.

Mrs. John Matthews, Dr. Joseph De Gasperi interviews

The scale of change in San Antonio that greeted physicians and soldiers returning from World War II was profound. The war had shut down civilian construction projects in San Antonio for almost five years, but worked like a magnet in drawing population and stimulating the growth of new business. An urban landscape had sprung up out of the old ranches beyond the city center, including the Essar Ranch on Culebra Road that oil producer and philanthropist Tom Slick would later convert into the Foundation for Applied Research. Suburbs had been created, and now the population flowed outward from the city center. Terrell Hills and Olmos Park were strong enough to incorporate as municipalities in 1939, and, as the city's population increased, another 9,000 residents settled in those communities. Although in 1946 retired police and firemen still drove ambulances, cases of leprosy continued to appear from time to time at the R.B. Green Hospital, and hospital rooms cost only $8 a day, by 1950 San Antonio boasted a population of 406,811 and was among the fastest-growing cities in the nation. The construction of the San Antonio Municipal Airport gave Texas natives easier access to other states and brought in visitors, while Trinity University's relocation from Waxahachie enriched the city's educational and cultural offerings. In 1947 the Texas Legislature had authorized the creation of a medical branch at San Antonio; nothing would come of this first effort, but it would foreshadow developments to in the not-too-distant future.

Green, Peyton, San Antonio: City in the Sun, 68-103;
Nixon, History of the Texas Medical Association, 411;
Dr. Jack Lee interview;
"San Antonio," "World War II," New Handbook of Texas.

In 1937 the San Antonio Light observed that the Alamo City was now second only to Washington, D.C., as the permanent home of retired Army officers. At that time, *"the total army payroll at fields and camps around San Antonio was eleven million dollars a year*" and the peacetime Army produced an estimated nineteen million dollars a year for San Antonio merchants. During the war, San Antonio military installations had a population of over 100,000 soldiers, and many men left their families behind in the community when they went off to war. In 1945 about 300 retired officers, including sixty generals, resided near military sites. As one observer put it, "*The city that was founded by a soldier and a priest, populated by men who went to bed with their boots on and their guns under the pillow, is still a soldier's city.*" General Thomas T. Handy, Commanding General of the Fourth Army at Fort Sam Houston, observed in 1948 that, "*I know of no other large city with such close integration between the civilian population and the military establishment as San Antonio has had in the past and maintains today.*" Fort Sam Houston sat adjacent to the city's upscale Alamo Heights neighborhood, and military officers frequently socialized with community leaders.

By the 1950s, Fort Sam Houston employed 10,000 military and 1500 civilian personnel; Lackland AFB, with the Air Force's largest hospital, handled 30,000 inpatients and 280,000 outpatients annually.

McBride, 3-8; Green, 68, 97, 101, 103

In the postwar years, military personnel remained in large numbers at local installations, and expansion continued. With the creation of Brooke Army Medical Center in 1946, Brooke General Hospital was enlarged into "*a sprawling mass of bright brick buildings at the end of the long parade ground, and the Army's main rehabilitation center for men damaged by war.*" A state-of-the-art medical center was created by converting the Medical Detachment Barracks next to the hospital, the post barracks north of the HQ, and parts of the mobilization cantonment into hospital wards and a Convalescent Center at a cost of 6.5 million dollars. The Medical Field Service School established to train military personnel at Carlisle Barracks, Pennsylvania, and other medical training facilities across the country were transferred to San Antonio, concentrating resources here in a new Medical Training Center. Instruction increased in "*scope and degree of specialization,*" including residency training for ophthalmologists and 22 other specialties by the 1970s. Brooke was designated a Hospital Center on its way to becoming the world's largest military medical installation.

The Medical Department Field School at Carlisle, Pennsylvania, created in 1920, had long offered courses in eye, ear, nose, and throat. Ireland, M.W.; "Courses of Instruction at USA MFSS"; "History of the Medical Training Center; "Brooke Army Medical Center Training Activities"

With the onset of the Korean War in 1950, "*World War II installations at Del Rio, Harlingen, Victoria, Bryan and Laredo*" were "*reactivated*" and medical support services were organized to handle over 80,000 members of the American Army who received injuries. Major General George E. Armstrong, Surgeon General of the Army, activated the Medical Replacement Training Center at Brooke Army Medical Center in 1954 and expanded facilities there to 400 buildings covering 874 acres. Anticipating casualties from air force bases around the world, BAMC officials also assembled an outstanding array of ophthalmologists and EENT specialists to handle wounded fliers and others. Elsewhere in Texas, a Medical Replacement Training Center at Camp Barkeley provided fourteen weeks of training in the basic principles of emergency treatment, ward management, and patient evacuation.

"ASF Medical Training to Occupy All of Fort Sam," San Antonio Light, November 2, 1945, 10-A;
"Army Plans for Fort Sam Big Question, San Antonio Light, October 21, 1945;
"Aviation in Texas," Handbook of Texas, 50;
Green Peyton, San Antonio, City in the Sun, 99; 112;
Benford, 257

As these events occurred, Dr. Harry George Armstrong at the School of Aviation Medicine undertook new efforts to reinforce the close ties between military and community medicine formed during World War II. Beginning in 1946, when he became Commander of the School of Aviation Medicine, Armstrong articulated the desire to maintain the high level of cooperation that had existed during the war between military and civilian research, believing that "*a medical center must embrace all fields of science related to human biology and medicine, and that it should have close association with other civilian and military scientific, engineering, and medical-research centers.*" This idea came closer to a national reality in 1949 when the Society of Medical Consultants to the Armed Forces, a "civilian medical consultant program" drawing members from the clinical disciplines, "*developed in a way that made for progressively closer cooperation between the military and civilian participants in clinical, preventive medicine, and research programs.*" Henceforth, military research enjoyed the participation of community practitioners with benefit for both civilian and military constituencies, an idea with important ramifications for the San Antonio medical community and Jack Matthews.

Aerospace Medical Division, 75-100

By the time Dr. Matthews joined the Texas O&O Society in 1945, he not only possessed administrative, clinical, and research skills equal to those of the nation's best-qualified ophthalmologists, but had begun to assume a role much like that of John Burleson as a spokesman for state-of-the-art medicine with interests in research and a commitment to professional development and further specialization. With deep roots in the community, he had returned to civilian practice, but in 1946 renewed his military ties when Commander Dr. James A. Bethea invited him to become a Brooke Army Medical Center eye consultant. Matthews served as the only board-certified BAMC ophthalmologist until the Korean War and later became the first visiting eye consultant at the city's Lackland Air Force Base. A man in whom synergies coalesced, Matthews was now ready to draw upon the civilian-military network that placed him at the center of the regional medical community in the transitional role of building the communication necessary for professional medicine to expand its foothold in South Texas. Among his initial acts on behalf of the profession, Matthews suggested that associate membership in the San Antonio O&O Society be extended to practitioners in surrounding towns, thereby conveying a new level of medical standard across the region. At the same time, however, the San Antonio professional community had grown large enough to support a host of other new developments.

Fulton, Hoff and Perkins, vi-viii;
Dr. Marion McCurdy interview; Dammin, 1464

## POSTWAR OPHTHALMOLOGY IN THE COMMUNITY

By the 1950s, Dr. John Matthews practiced in a professional, highly qualified, and diverse community of ophthalmologists. If World War II had created global crisis for a generation, it also proved to be a stimulus for progress in ophthalmology by helping to create a new agenda for research, fostering professional development, and spreading ophthalmologists across South Texas. For specialists who had remained in the community, World War II generally meant an active, successful career, and the majority continued to practice eye, ear, nose and throat without further specialization. Among them, Drs. Dan Russell, Sr., James and William Gill, Moore, Parrish, Ed Dumas, A. Belvin Pritchett, Cantor, and Frank Steed were poised for post-war prosperity resulting from the defense industry build-up and the major influx of population that accompanied it, but there were newcomers as well.

Bexar County Medical Society records;
San Antonio City Directories, 1940-46

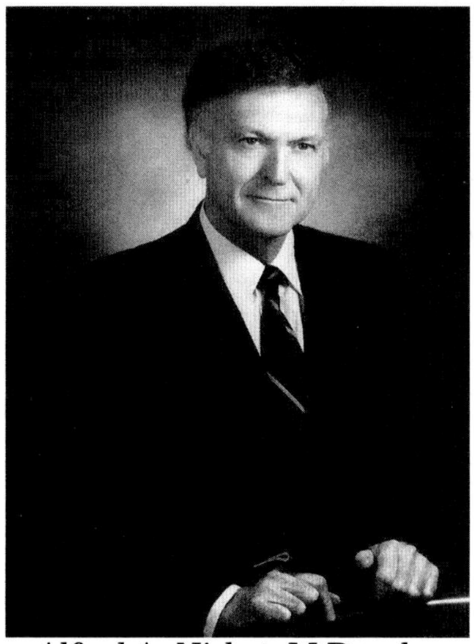

Alfred A. Nisbet, M.D., whose son, R. Michael Nisbet, also became an ophthalmologist in Corpus Christi.

One of nine strict ophthalmologists who practiced in the city in 1948, Dr. Alfred Alan Nisbet joined Drs. Muldoon, John Matthews, John Burleson, Donald Atkinson, and Scott Applewhite and became a close friend of Dr. James Roseborough. After first settling in Georgia, Nisbet's family had gone to California to escape the hardships of Reconstruction after the Civil War, and he was born there in 1909, the son of an oil wildcatter. A San Francisco job selling insurance and plans to become a lawyer did not suit him, and Nisbet decided instead to seek a medical degree after graduation from Stanford University in 1931 despite the Depression. Having met his wife at Stanford and married, he moved to Norman, Oklahoma, to complete his master's degree and an M.D. degree at the University of Oklahoma. While he and his wife lived with in-laws, he met Dr. Tullos Costen, who had just returned from ophthalmology training at the Johns Hopkins Hospital in Baltimore. Costen encouraged Nisbet to apply to the Wilmer Eye Institute, and he did so, completing his residency under the mentoring of Alan C. Woods and going on to study ophthalmology at Washington University in St. Louis while teaching at the Barnes University Medical School and working at St. Louis City Hospital. Finished with his training, Nisbet and his wife decided to leave the cold St. Louis winters when he learned that San Antonio needed ophthalmologists. In the process of working for the Petty Geophysical Engineering Company office in Norman, Oklahoma, he had come to know the Petty family, who came from San Antonio. Nisbet set out from Baltimore the fine needles, sutures, and rubber gloves that had become the norm for cataract surgery, opened his first private ophthalmology practice in the Nix Building in 1940, and slowly built up his practice.

Nisbet typescript;
Bexar County Medical Society records

Nisbet volunteered for service after Pearl Harbor, and spent many hours with Dr. John Matthews at Fort Sam Houston's Dodd Field examining recruits for the Flight Surgeon School. In 1942 he joined the Army Medical Corps attached to the Air Force and spent three consecutive years at the Bombardier School in Big Spring, Texas, working with flight surgeons at Nashville, Tennessee, and doing a variety of medical tasks at Maxwell Field in Alabama. When he returned to San Antonio, he brought extensive experience and important military affiliations. Among the neighbors in his office on the seventeenth floor of the Nix Building was the "*patriarch of San Antonio medicine*," Dr. Ferdinand Herff. To join the Texas Society of Ophthalmology and Otolaryngology, he chose for his thesis a subject appropriate to his Texas identity, "*Recurrent Pterygiums*." Beta radiation had just become a popular treatment to prevent recurrences, and Nisbet possessed one of the early instruments for administering the treatment. Later, in 1960, by which time he had become an expert in the repair of retinal detachments, he was elected President of the society, an accomplishment of which he was proud.

Nisbet typescript

An interesting story about Dr. Nisbet tells of the daughter of a wealthy family in Monterrey, Mexico, who became his patient. This girl, the oldest of three, was extremely near sighted and required thick glasses, making it difficult for her to find a husband. Because oldest daughters were required to marry before their younger siblings, the parents brought their child to San Antonio to see Dr. Nisbet, who fitted her with contact lenses. According to Nisbet's son, the girl soon became engaged and invited the doctor and his family to her wedding, which included a high Catholic mass and sit-down dinner for over a thousand people. Nisbet soon got referrals of patients from "*all over South Texas and Northern Mexico*."

Nisbet typescript

In addition to his practice, Nisbet volunteered many hours caring for the poor at the Robert B. Green Clinic and Brooke Army Medical Center, where he worked as a civilian consultant for twenty-five years. Later he served as a consultant at Lackland Air Force Base and the School of Aerospace Medicine and Chief of Staff at San Rosa Hospital. In the 1950s, as contact lenses became popular for the correction of refractive errors, but before suppliers could provide precise technology, Nisbet spent many hours with a small, automated drill and buffer modifying lenses for patients who needed them, using only a loupe for magnification. He also developed an extensive service treating Catholic nuns and priests and Hispanic patients with whom he

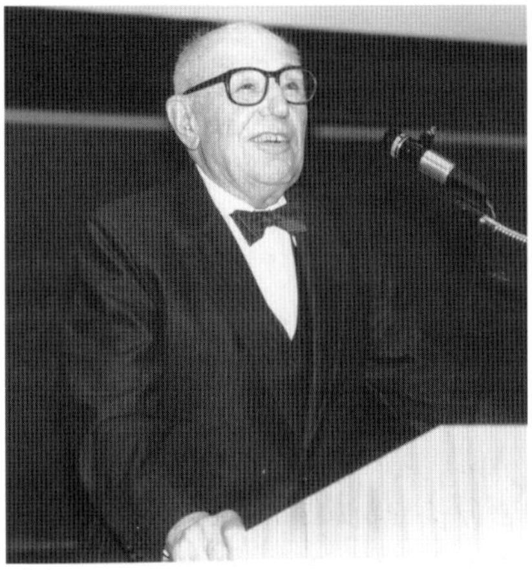

Major General Elbert DeCoursey on his 83rd birthday delivering a speech after receiving the A.C.O.R.A. award at The University of Texas Health Science Center for outstanding contributions to ophthalmology in South Texas. The citation read:

*"Major General Elbert DeCoursey, you, after graduating with a Bachelor of Arts from the University of Kentucky and an M.D. degree from Johns Hopkins University School of Medicine, developed parallel careers, one in the Army and one in pathology. The expertise you developed made both these careers blossom. Soon, you had the vision and wisdom to become particularly interested in the pathology of the eye, which became the subject of the first true atlas of ophthalmic pathology, published in 1938.*

*We in ophthalmology are particularly grateful for your foresight in helping to establish the registry of pathology at the Armed Forces Institute of Pathology as a repository of pathologic specimens from all over the world. Thanks to your efforts, the AFIP became a center of learning, a gathering place for individuals who subsequently made major contributions to the field of ophthalmic pathology. Persons who benefited from your enthusiastic teaching include such names as Helenor Wilder and Lorenz Zimmerman, individuals who have subsequently trained many others in this field. Very few ophthalmic pathologists practicing today have not spent some time at the AFIP.*

*We in San Antonio are particularly grateful that, having trained here, you returned to share you interest and commitment to pathology and research. Most of the educational institutions in this city have received the benefits of your teaching and leadership.*

*We at The University of Texas Health Science Center are grateful for your role in resolving the controversy over the proposed site for this institution. Clearly, this location has proved to be a fruitful choice, as our subsequent growth has indicated. In addition, we recognize your service as consultant in eye pathology to the Bexar County Hospital district and as clinical professor of both ophthalmology and pathology at our medical school from 1970 – 1983.*

*The world has recognized you as a leader and innovator. On this, your 83rd birthday, it is a pleasure on behalf of the departments of ophthalmology at Wilford Hall, Brooke Army Medical Center, and The University of Texas to award you the Alamo City Ophthalmology Resident's Association Award. May you continue your active life of contributions for many years to come."*

spoke Spanish, and made occasional trips to Del Rio and Kerrville to perform surgery.

(Nisbet typescript)

Another outstanding individual who had come to San Antonio, pathologist Dr. Elbert (Frenchy) DeCoursey, trained at Johns Hopkins University, published an important Atlas of Ophthalmic Pathology in 1938 and later established the Registry of Pathology at the Armed Forces Institute of Pathology to serve as a repository for pathologic specimens from around the world. During World War II he had organized and directed the 18th Medical General Laboratory that served the Army in the Pacific Ocean Area, and later he participated as part of the Joint Commission for the Investigation of the Effects of the Atomic Bomb in Japan. Before coming to San Antonio, DeCoursey served as Commandant of the Army Medical Research and Graduate School (Walter Reed Institute of Research) and directed the Armed Forces Institute of Pathology. As Chancellor of the Army Medical Service School at Fort Sam, he had established close ties with community ophthalmologists. When he retired, Brigadier General DeCoursey became the first Director of Research at Trinity University in San Antonio, served as a consultant in eye pathology to the Bexar County Hospital District, and, like Matthews, played a role in establishing the University of Texas Medical School, for which he served as clinical professor of Pathology and Ophthalmology.

Bexar County Medical Society records;
Texas Medical Association membership files

Dr. Dan A. Russell, Jr. was the son of Dr. Donald Atkinson's partner, Dr. Daniel Abell Russell, a Bexar County native with family links to the Gallagher Ranch near San Antonio. The elder Russell completed his premedical studies at the University of Texas, worked as a Hospital Apprentice with the United States Naval Reserve Force at New Orleans while he was a medical student, graduated from Tulane in 1921, and interned at the Santa Rosa Hospital in San Antonio in 1922 in preparation to become an EENT specialist. He was associated with Dr. Donald Atkinson for eleven years before setting up a successful ear, nose, and throat practice at San Antonio, and included among his patients Mrs. John Nance Garner. His son and associate, Dr. Dan A. Russell, Jr., studied at the University of Texas Medical Branch at Galveston, the University of Virginia, and did postgraduate study at the New York Polyclinic Medical School and Hospital, Washington University Medical School in St. Louis, and George

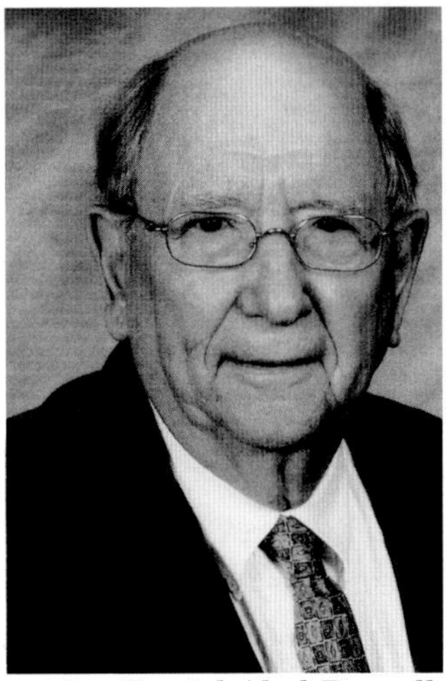

Dr. Daniel Abel Russell, Jr., who together with Dr. Frank X. Weixel was co-Chief of Ophthalmology at The Brady Green Hospital from 1958 to 1970, before the U. T. Medical School existed. Russell and Weixel started a civilian ophthalmology residency program sponsored by the Bexar County Hospital District, which later became a University of Texas residency.

Washington University School of Medicine in Washington, D.C., and at the Wilmer Eye Institute. The younger Russell also studied with Dr. Chevalier Jackson at Temple University in Philadelphia and went on to become one of the first strict ophthalmologists in the city of San Antonio--with a practice that extended to Beeville, Crystal City and other parts of the South Texas Rio Grande Valley--and served as Chief of Ophthalmology at the R.G. Green Hospital from 1958 to 1970. When he began his practice in the 1950s, Russell indicated that about 60-70% of the physicians in San Antonio came from outside of Texas.

Bexar County Medical Society records; Dr. Dan A. Russell obituary, Texas State Journal of Medicine, April1957, 301-2; Dr. Dan A. Russell, Jr. interview, April 25, 1997.

Dr. Graham B. Milburn, the son of a prominent San Antonio physician, received his medical degree at the University of Pennsylvania before entering the service and developed his interest in ophthalmology as a Captain in the Army Air Force Medical Corps in Japan. After the war, he completed a Mayo Clinic ophthalmology fellowship and then returned to San Antonio to begin his career as John Matthews had done, starting out with W.E. Muldoon. Milburn went on to practice the specialty for the next thirty years.

Bexar County Medical Society records

Dr. George Harmon Brunner, one of the community's older members, was a strict ophthalmologist originally from Colorado who had served in the infantry in World War I and arrived in the 1940s. After a residency at the Illinois Eye and Ear Infirmary in Chicago and postgraduate work at the University of Pennsylvania, Brunner practiced briefly in the Midwest and then moved to San Antonio for the remainder of his career. Working with Frederick Bieberdorff at the Foundation of Applied Research, he later published an investigation of the "Effects of the Mesquite Thorn on the Human Eye," based on Dr. John Burleson's description of six cases he had treated in which blindness had resulted from the condition.

Bexar County Medical Society records;
Dr. John Matthews materials, Briscoe Library

Dr. James P. Gill, who was the son of EENT specialist W.D. Gill and a member of one of San Antonio's traditional Southern families, belonged to an older generation that was not greatly influenced by World War II despite his service experience. A graduate of Vanderbilt University, Gill served as a commanding officer at Ft. McIntosh Station Hospital, interned at the Fort Sam Houston Station Hospital, and graduated from the Army Medical and Field Service Schools, but resigned in 1931 to enter private practice at San Antonio all before World War II began. In 1941 he reentered the Army as a colonel and was put in charge of a Medical Supply Depot at Honolulu. When he returned to San Antonio in 1946, Gill resumed his EENT practice without further specializing in ophthalmology.

Dr. Victor Mozersky, a Galveston Medical Branch graduate in 1938 who had been in a partnership with Gill's father, W.D. Gill, joined the Army in 1941.

Bexar County Medical Society records

Also worthy of mention for the quality of their training is Dr. Karl Michael Aijain, a Tulane graduate who had trained at Gorgas Hospital in the Panama Canal Zone, the Wills Eye Hospital, and Harvard University, came to San Antonio from Fort Worth, where he served as director for clinical investigation at Alcon Labs. Aijian's interests lay in clinical research on infections of the eye and eyelids. Finally, Dr. Tuttle Culver Warren trained at the New York Eye and Ear Infirmary and came to San Antonio in 1947.

Bexar County Medical Society records

According to Dr. Fred Cooper, "*no one practiced in the little towns of Texas until after World War II.*" Among ophthalmologists who moved to larger cities in the hinterland, the largest number of strict ophthalmologists worked at Corpus Christi where the new Ghormley Clinic opened as a general hospital in 1947 and in 1949 Dr. J.H. Thomas and Dr. Thomas Spann founded the Thomas-Spann

Clinic and Hospital in 1949. Drs. Clarence B. Collins, Bernard B. Friedman, and Sanders K. Stroud practiced along with EENT specialists Drs. Alfred W. Davisson, Earl King Gill, Edgar G. Mathis, Clarence N. Meador, Arthur Padilla, Oscar H. Peterson, and William L. Rhodes. Dr. Collins had trained in Indiana and at Johns Hopkins before opening his practice in 1931. Although he left and spent six years in Indiana, he later returned to Corpus Christi where he continued to practice until 1948. Dr. Levon David Wright, a Mexia, Texas, native, completed Baylor and Tulane before joining the Navy Medical Corps. Two years at the Armed Forces Institute of Pathology and Episcopal EENT Hospital at Washington, D.C., led to a fellowship in 1947 to study eye at the Gulf State Eye Surgery Foundation in New Orleans, after which he completed an EENT residency at the Charity Hospital there. Back in Texas after naval service in World War II, he established an ophthalmology practice at Corpus Christi while maintaining his military ties as a civilian consultant to the USN Hospital, Naval Air Station. Finally, in 1949 he began to practice at the Thomas-Spann Clinic and Hospital, where he later became a partner.

The Driscoll Foundation Children's Hospital built in 1953 had specially equipped rooms for eye, ear, nose, and throat treatment.

Dr. Fred Cooper interview;
Nueces County Medical Society records;
Nueces County Historical Society, 137-8;
Texas Medical Association records

Cuero continued to attract specialists such as Dr. Corinne Westphal, who had been born at Yorktown, Texas, and graduated from Southwestern University at Georgetown and Vanderbilt before deciding to specialize in ophthalmology. After receiving her medical degree from George Washington University at St. Louis in 1934, Dr. Westphal was the first resident in ophthalmology at Jefferson Davis Hospital in Houston. She later served in Wichita Falls and with the Columbus Eye Associates, and in 1943 was listed as an ophthalmologist at Yorktown, where the only other specialist in town was EENT specialist Dr. George W. Cross. Later she moved to Cuero, where she practiced at the Burns Hospital and retired in 1976. Dr. Vernon A. Black attended Texas A&M and the University of Texas Medical Branch at Galveston, interned at John Sealy Hospital and completed a residency at Cook Memorial Hospital in Fort Worth by 1939. By 1942, he also had completed an EENT residency at Henry Fort Hospital in Detroit and returned to Wharton, Texas, to practice ophthalmology. Active in the field, he later published an article on the Marcus-Gunn Phenomenon in the Texas State Journal of Medicine.

Texas Medical Association records

Perhaps the most well known of those outside San Antonio, however, was Dr. George E. Penny, a graduate of Baylor in 1935 who practiced ophthalmology in Laredo, along with Dr. Joshua T. Ward. By 1943 EENT specialist Dr. Newell W. Atkinson practiced at Alice and Dr. Clay C. Berry, a University of Louisville graduate who limited his practice to the eye, worked at Beeville. Eye, ear nose and throat specialists Drs. Walton E. Douthit and Guilford M. Duckworth practiced in Cuero, Drs. Robert M. Scott, Emile C. Schulze, and Elizabeth Donaldson at Del Rio, and Dr. William J. Bussey in Eagle Pass. In Harlingen, patients visited Drs. Thomas T. LaMotte, Frank D. Walsworth, and Charles S. Amidon, and, at Hebbronville, Dr. Vela-Vasquez, a graduate of the Institute Literario in Mexico. Drs. Axel J. Black and Clarence L. McClellan served the Kerrville community and Dr. Houston Brown worked in Kingsville, while Dr. Charles Langer, a graduate of Johns Hopkins, practiced in Knippa. At McAllen, there were four EENT specialists, including Drs. Frank W. Bennett, John B. Casey, James C. Ellis, and Loyal H. Moore. At Mercedes, Dr. Newton H. Bowman served the community, and at Mission, Dr. Norman T. North. Dr. Edward Ehlert, Jr. graduated from the University of Texas in 1934 and practiced EENT at Victoria. Drs. Robert E. Mann and Richard C. Youngblood offered specialized services at Pleasanton, Dr. Charles C. Conley at Raymondville, Dr. Charles L. Kopecky at Yoakum, and Dr. Oscar V. Lawrence at Brownsville. Dr. James C.B. Douthett, a University of Pittsburgh graduate, was at Seguin, Dr. Norman I. Wood at Uvalde, and Drs. Edwin Lanoier McCalip and James E. Montgomery at Weslaco. Dr. Russell A. DeVol, who trained in Nebraska and at King's Daughter's Hospital in Temple, Texas, went to Gregg County in 1948.

County medical society records;
Texas Medical Association records

## THE TEXAS OPHTHALMOLOGICAL ASSOCIATION

In one sense, the professional strength of the new configuration of specialists had its greatest impact in the creation of the first society dedicated entirely to ophthalmology in the region. The San Antonio

Ophthalmo-Otolaryngological Society simplified its name and became the San Antonio Society of Ophthalmology and Otolaryngology in 1947, but it took nearly another decade for further change in the profession to occur. Society minutes up to that time, however, clearly show a new level of sophistication in the science and indicate that San Antonio was becoming a dynamic medical community.

Society Minutes, 1947

At various O&O Society meetings, Dr. John Matthews discussed the absorption of ultraviolet, infrared, and visual light rays and lenses to protect against radiation and glare, and Dr. Edwin Sykes reported on "*Two Cases of Detached Retina*" that reflected advances in retinal specialization. When the members visited Randolph Air Force Base, Dr. Heinz Haber presented his work on a new theory of color vision, and Dr. Heinrich Rose demonstrated visual acuity at high angular speeds and new kinds of depth perception tests. Dr. Paul Cibis demonstrated spatial distortion caused by differences in retinal illumination, and Dr. Gerathewohl a supersonic radar trainer combined with an ophthalmograph for photographing eye movements during radar scope operation and a reaction test to investigate steady and flashing light signals. Lieutenant Gulley showed members new sunglasses, goggles, night flying glasses and a visor helmet developed by the School of Aviation Medicine, and Dr. Bahn demonstrated a Risley rotary prism attachment orthorater used to study prism divergence and test slides for use in the new Armed Forces visual acuity tester. Dr. Wilson showed the Rodenstock refractometer, Dr. Grunwell described a perimeter to study flicker fusion, and Dr. Ingeborg Schmidt talk on a rotator and illuminator for the automatic presentation of pseudoisochromatic color vision plates and a collection of aids for color defectives.

Society Minutes

Other programs dealt with advances in community ophthalmology. At a meeting at the Fort Sam Houston Officer's Club, members discussed treatment of the recurring Southwest problem known as pterygium, and, at another meeting, Dr. Boen Swinny requested referrals of patients with mesquite thorn injuries to determine whether their reactions were allergic or toxic. Dr. Jack Lee spoke on visual testing of preschoolers, and Dr. Henry Hilgartner of Austin spoke on civil suits brought by the United States against the American Optical Company, Bausch and Lomb Optical, and certain ophthalmologists, that charged violation of the Sherman Anti-Trust Law in owning interests in or obtaining revenue from optical firms. Dr. James A. Bethea, now Assistant Dean of the University of Texas Post-Graduate School of Medicine at the R.B. Green, spoke on the training program there. Dr. John Burleson, who remained active in the Society, spoke against the creation of a medical "*welfare state*" involving prepaid medical coverage. In this way, the San Antonio O&O Society created a platform from which new efforts to strengthen ophthalmology in Texas could spring.

Society Minutes

Although the strength of the two specialties--ophthalmology and otolaryngology--had grown considerably, the San Antonio membership of only thirty-four physicians in 1950 was not large enough to permit separation of the two specialties. Six years later, however, Texas specialists succeeded in creating the first state-level society geared strictly to ophthalmology. Facing social, political and economic problems that the Section of Ophthalmology of the Texas Medical Association and the Texas Society of Ophthalmology and Otolaryngology could not adequately address (such as whether optometrists should be allowed to dispense eye drops), ophthalmologists determined to create a permanent institution for the purpose of filling "*several voids*" in their professional lives. According to one physician, "the scientific program at the TMA meetings was "*very scanty and scattered as to ophthalmological subjects*" and there was a "*desire to increase ophthalmologic post-graduate education.*" Neither the San Antonio O&O nor the Texas O&O Society served as a spokesman for Texas ophthalmologists in the State Department of Health, the Texas Educational Agency, or other social programs where the health and function of the eyes required medical attention. Before Medicare or Medicaid existed, physicians faced many uncertainties.

Letter, Otto Lippmann to Dr. Jack Lee, June 10, 1981;
TOA brochure

After the Annual Scientific Session on Ophthalmology at the Texas Medical Association meeting in Galveston in April 1956, therefore, a group of ophthalmologists set up a temporary body to discuss the possibility of a new organization that could take an active role in representing the interests of Texas ophthalmologists. The result was the founding of the Texas Ophthalmological Association in 1956. Sixty ophthalmologists joined, including Drs. Ed Dumas, Jack Lee, John Matthews, A. Belvin Pritchett, Dan Russell, Sr., and Francis X. Weixel from San Antonio, Dor Brown from Fredericksburg, J. Gordon Bryson, Jr. of Corpus Christi, and Henry Hilgartner, Otto Lippmann, Robert Rothen, and Carey Legett, Jr. of Austin. One of the organization's first six councilors was Dr. Jack B. Lee; Dr. John Matthews and Dr. Henry Hilgartner became members of the nominating committee for the first set of officers; and Dr. John Kuppinger of Harlingen became an active member and officer.

Vanzant, Thomas J., "Texas Ophthalmological Association," Texas Medicine, 63 (March, 1967), 85;
Sandy Hirsch, Letter to Sue McDonald;
Alan C. Baum, Letter to Dr. Jack B. Lee;
Texas Ophthalmological Association, "By-Laws" and "Minutes";
"Organizational Meeting of the Texas Ophthalmological Association, April 23, 1956, 5:20 p.m., Terrace Dining Room, Hotel Galvez"

The Texas Ophthalmological Association quickly gained added strength by inviting military ophthalmologists to join and cooperating and affiliating with other institutions. With the Texas Branch of the National Society for Prevention of Blindness, which Dr. John Matthews helped to found, the new association developed statewide programs through the public schools for education on and detection of glaucoma and a program for visual screening of schoolchildren's eyes in consultation with the Public Health Department. The Association also affiliated with the National Medical Foundation for Eye Care, later the American Association of Ophthalmology, to create closer ties between ophthalmologists in Texas and the other states. TOA representatives helped reduce the intrusion of non-medical practitioners into ophthalmology and led an active and expanding program of continuing education in conjunction with Texas Medical Association annual sessions by sponsoring two-day programs, setting up links with Texas medical schools, and sponsoring two to three days meetings organized by medical school eye departments. More importantly, the Texas Ophthalmological Association developed vital connections with insurance carriers and retained legal counsel to update practitioners across the state regarding eye care legislation, judicial opinions, and other legal matters that indirectly helped to strengthen the profession, rounding out the impressive list of accomplishments resulting from World War II.

"Chronology of the Texas Society to Prevent Blindness";
Texas Ophthalmological Association brochure;
"TOA Honors Past Officers," Perspectives of the Texas Ophthalmological Association, 1;
Interview with Andy Weir, Texas State Commission for the Blind.

# CHAPTER 10

## THE SPECIALTY MATURES: RESIDENCY PROGRAMS AND EYE BANKS, 1950-1965

*Life is a residency.*

James L. Mims, Jr., M.D.

*Education is the chief agent of perfectability as of progress.*

A. A. Ross, M.D., Stepping Stones

At the end of World War II "*eye training was still recognized on an individual basis*," and was often haphazard and undisciplined. South Texas medical students continued to arrange preceptorships or to seek specialized training outside of Texas, and the quality of their training varied widely. Elder physicians reluctant to relinquish the reins of their practices often gave junior men little hands-on experience or simply exploited their labor by using the apprenticeship system for their own benefit. As long as standardized training--an essential in most professional fields--had not been established, one final step remained for the specialty to achieve maturity. By now, the complex treatment and techniques demanded by the new science of ophthalmology required more advanced knowledge and practice that eventually led to residency requirements. Across the nation, residency programs had emerged as the best way to train specialists, yet until 1950 not a single ophthalmology residency program existed in all of South Texas.

Important regional progress was made, therefore, when oph-

thalmologists replaced the outdated preceptorship system and successfully organized three approved ophthalmology residency programs in San Antonio in a single decade. As the city came of age, the local ophthalmological profession followed suit. The roots of residency training programs were commonly military and urban, and the three San Antonio programs--two military and one civilian--all developed in South Texas' principal military and urban center in the 1950s. The Brooke Army Medical Center program at Fort Sam Houston was founded in 1950. A second program was established at the city's R.B. Green Community Hospital in 1952 and was approved in 1958. The third program, located at Wilford Hall Hospital at Lackland Air Force Base, began in 1959. Seven military ophthalmology residency programs existed at the end of World War II, but today only six remain--two Navy, one Air Force, and three Army--making San Antonio's two programs an important component of modern military medicine. Three ophthalmology residency programs in a single city may seem unusual, yet was a logical outcome. By the 1950s, the Alamo City had become both a center for military operations and a major city.
By the late 1960s, Galveston also had a three-year residency in ophthalmology, with two residents each year for a total of six.

Hunt, Harold E., "Ophthalmology in Texas," 70, 72;
Dr. Jack Lee, Dr. William C. Lloyd, III interviews.

In 1949, two-thirds of U.S. physicians were general practitioners, but one third were already specialists. By 1977, the reverse was true as residency programs developed and the importance of specialization grew. Residencies were partly a byproduct of the military organization of medical forces and the concentration of medical resources in major cities that occurred in World War II and the Korean War. War transformed American medicine into a centralized system and established relationships between institutions that previously functioned in regional isolation. As returning ophthalmologists integrated information, techniques, technologies, and research questions generated by battlefield and ward experience into their profession, they developed a common approach that tended to make ophthalmological treatment uniform nationwide. Shared perspectives also made establishing common standards for basic professional training--such as using hands-on experience as a teaching tool--more widely acceptable.

Military interest in residency programs heightened at the end of World War II when the U.S. Army recognized that specialists would continue to be needed overseas and that an offer of specialty training would help the armed forces to retain specialists. Walter Reed Hospital had already initiated several residency programs successful enough to convince the U.S. Surgeon General of the importance of the new form of training. Not only were preceptorships being phased out at home, but it was clear that residencies could supply the kind of experience that had led to important discoveries during the war, something few preceptorships could promise. The outlines of a model for residency training also emerged from the realization that rotating personnel in the top echelons of any organization--a common military practice--strengthened its capacity, an idea that medical leaders employed as they combined basic scientific education with hospital duties. As residency programs developed, the mutual benefit of staffing hospitals with those in training became apparent. Higher standards for medical students kept older doctors on their toes and provided valuable assistance in dealing with cases, while students received vital hands-on experience.

Dammin, 1462;
Lloyd, Col. William C., III, "Founding of the BAMC Ophthalmology Residency Program," video.

The urban roots of medical residencies grew from the growing complexity of specialized medicine. Physicians returning from World War II frequently found themselves unable to afford the equipment required to practice their specialty and forced to affiliate with a big city hospital. Both practicing physicians and medical students were drawn to urban settings where specialists were needed to handle the large number and variety of injuries and diseases that flowed into city hospitals. Major cities also generally offered the best chance, under the watchful eye of an affiliated expert, for learners to observe cases and gain clinical experience. Residency programs, as a consequence, tended to start up in the nation's urban places, a pattern followed by the three South Texas residencies. By the 1950s, San Antonio had a population large enough to support resident staff at both its central community hospital and two large military sites.

Hunt, 72

As the supply of residency programs increased, demand swelled. Although the practice of eye, ear, nose and throat persisted, interns and practicing physicians alike, realizing a need to prepare adequately for specialized practice, sought specialization in ophthalmology. Returning physicians found that the climate for medicine in their local communities had improved significantly in their absence and that the American Medical Association and many hospitals now had higher standards and new training requirements. By 1950, for example, emphasis on an ophthalmologist's ability to operate translated into a requirement that doctors sitting for board certification needed sufficient skill to perform a cataract operation on a cat. As general medicine branched into the specialties, moreover, each branch established a separate board, a reflection of increasingly sophisticated medical techniques developed in treating wartime casualties and of growing professionalization. As a result, many of those who served in World War II sought residency training when they returned to the United States.

In founding three residency programs, San Antonio military and community ophthalmologists continued the custom of sharing resources and equipment begun during World War II and enjoyed a lively scientific exchange characterized by "*mutual active support, cooperation, and friendship*." Each residency program eventually filled a separate niche such that no single institution dominated local medicine as it did in many other places. In all, the three residency programs aimed to "*represent the combined achievements of separate institutions with shared goals,*" making a richer regional climate for medicine without harmful competition. The cooperative spirit fostered at the three training sites and the new level of sophistication among local practitioners also laid the groundwork for sub-specialization, encouraged the development of new technologies, and enriched the environment for ophthalmic research. Until the 1950s, Dr. Everett L. Goar of Houston could be considered perhaps the only ophthalmologist of national stature in South Texas, but this distinction would soon be shared with others.

Dr. Richard Ruiz interview;
Dammin, 1464.

Once in place, the three residency programs exerted pressure on the profession that amounted to a systematic effort to improve its quality. Eventually, the introduction of residency training not only ended the custom of relying on specialists brought in from outside South Texas, but also reinvigorated efforts that had failed in 1949 to create a medical school outside of Galveston, stimulated interests that led to the creation of the Baptist and Wilford Hall Eye Banks, and motivated ophthalmologists to create the Texas Ophthalmological Association. Creation of the University of Texas Health Science Center a decade later made it a formidable era of medical progress, indeed. A generation after World War II ended, America trained the majority of its ophthalmologists at home, ophthalmologists trained in San Antonio filtered out across Texas to the nation and beyond, and American medicine led the world.

Dammin, 1462

## THE FIRST OPHTHALMOLOGY RESIDENCY PROGRAM: BROOKE ARMY MEDICAL CENTER, FORT SAM HOUSTON

The first approved ophthalmology residency program in South Texas was organized in direct response to the Korean War that began in 1950. In the interim between World War II and Korea, Brooke General Hospital at San Antonio's Fort Sam Houston staffed its eye surgery service with civilian ophthalmologists serving as visiting consultants. With the onset of fighting in Korea, however, Brooke replaced the Army Eye Center at Valley Forge, Pennsylvania, in handling the majority of Army eye casualties and, henceforth, evacuees were sent to San Antonio.

Dr. William Sichi interview, Lloyd, William C., III, "Brief History of the BAMC Ophthalmology Service," typescript, AIRMED Museum Collections, Fort Sam Houston, San Antonio

Beginning on June 25, 1950, the Korean War transformed Brooke General Hospital into a bustling center of activity with a shortage of medical personnel. Seven barracks, whose first floors initially had been used by the cavalry as stables, were rapidly converted into hospital space, while up to 2,000 patients were hospitalized in Beach Pavilion, known as Annex 4. As "*air evacs*," or men who had made the long airplane trip from overseas battlefields, began to arrive, the eye surgery operating room ran five days a week and clinic began after the surgical cases were completed. Major George Lathrop, who was trained at Detroit's Henry Ford Hospital, could be seen leaving the hospital in his surgical gown and returning the next morning wearing the same gown to the operating room. For the trip to the United

States, Korean casualties were given atropine and had their eyes covered to allow for rest. At Brooke enucleations of the eye were the most common procedure performed, followed by retrievals of intraocular foreign bodies. Globe trauma was common, and orbital prostheses frequently prescribed; others suffered burnt lids that often resulted in loss of an eye. The new Army Eye Center also drew patients from across the Southwest. Eventually, Brooke treated local active duty and retired servicemen, their dependents, and referrals from as far away as Panama and Canada, and served as the regional VA hospital before new facilities could be built at Kerrville and San Antonio. Roughly ten per cent of casualties flown in from the West Coast and Hawaii were eye-related, hence the Brooke ophthalmology residency program was "born of necessity."

Later, Lathrop was replaced by Dr. Robert Kennedy, who was trained at Johns Hopkins.

Lloyd, Col. William C., III, "Brief History of BAMC Ophthalmology Service: The Second Decade," typescript.;
Lloyd, Col. William C., "Founding of the BAMC Ophthalmology Residency," video;
Dr. William Sichi interview.

## DR. WILLIAM T. SICHI

The choice of Dr. William T. Sichi to head up the Brooke ophthalmology department and establish the new residency program was a wise one. Colonel Sichi was an outstanding ophthalmologist who, before coming to Texas, had helped to organize the nation's medical response in World War II and gained valuable experience as a medical administrator. With a distinguished background and extensive training, he represented a significant addition to the military medical community and to San Antonio.

Sichi came from Valley Forge, bringing the heart of operations there with him. Ordered to Fort Sam Houston as chief of the Brooke eye section at the beginning of the Korean War, he arrived in San Antonio in 1950 accompanied by members of his staff, including his operating room nurse, Major Dentfip, and an ocularist and former dentist named Lt. Col. Smolczynski, who had developed a device known as the Valley Forge socket implant. The Germans used glass eyes, but Americans developed plastic ones. These ingenious products were fitted with stainless steel mesh that could be sutured to surrounding eye muscles. Sichi set up centers for Plastic Surgery and Ophthalmology with Smolcznski as chief of the plastic eye section, and transferred "*a sufficient inventory of equipment and supplies from Valley Forge to open an eye service*." His personal tasks included examining pilots before facilities were established at Lackland Air Force Base.

Lloyd, William C., III, "A Brief History of the BAMC Ophthalmology Service," typescript, Ft. Sam Houston Archives; Dr. William Sichi interview.

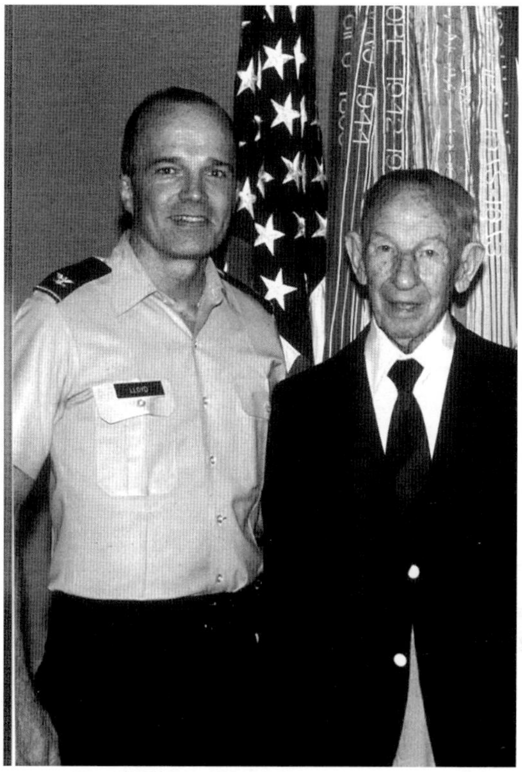

Dr. William T. Sichi (r ), first Chief of Ophthalmology at Brook Army Hospital. On his right is Col. William C. Lloyd, III, M.D., who taught eye pathology to the military and civilian residents and, in 1989, became the Director of the Lions Eye Pathology Laboratory at The University of Texas Medical School.

Sichi gained his awareness of national medical issues from his early military assignments in the nation's capital. Born the son of Italian immigrants in New York City on August 18, 1906, he had grown up in Kutztown, Pennsylvania, and moved to Washington when his father, a sculptor, was hired to make stone carvings for the Lincoln Memorial, Washington Cathedral, Supreme Court, and other government buildings. Although he first majored in engineering at the University of Maryland hoping to become a mechanical engineer in the auto industry like a cousin who found opportunity there, Sichi revised his plan when his cousin lost his job. He then acceded to his family's wish that he become a doctor. By the time he received his medical degree from George Washington University in 1931, moreover, he had benefited from contact with several distinguished professors who had trained in Germany.

Dr. William Sichi interview

Although he left Washington to intern at Garfield Memorial Hospital in Utah and completed a six-month pediatrics residency at the Children's Hospital there, Sichi returned to Washington after he applied for a reserve commission and joined the Army in 1934. His first assignment took him to the center of military medical operations at Walter Reed Hospital, where he crossed paths briefly with Dr. Frederic H. Thorne before being sent to the Medical Field Service School at Carlisle Barracks, Pennsylvania. Whether Thorne influenced him is not known, but he did find mentors who sparked his interest in ophthalmology at Fort Meade, Maryland, where he subsequently served as a general practitioner. Colonel Daniel P. Card and General Dwight D. Eisenhower's physician, Lt. Thomas Mattingly, in particular encouraged him to specialize in ophthalmology rather than pediatrics, convincing him that pediatrics had little use at a time when the military discouraged enlisted men from marrying. Ophthalmologists, Sichi also learned, generally had few emergencies and night calls, another attractive feature of the specialty.

Dr. William Sichi interview

World War II gave Sichi's professional development, as it did that of many others, a new dimension when he returned to Walter Reed once more in 1938 to work with doctors responsible for orchestrating the nation's response to World War II. The Surgeon General's Office had sent him to study eye, ear, nose, and throat, but, with the added encouragement of Colonel John R. Simmons, Sichi decided to specialize in ophthalmology. Assigned to Panama's Gorgas Hospital in 1941, he observed individuals with the temporary blindness that results from malaria and learned to administer intravenous quinine. He also served at a medical training center at Abilene, Texas, and at Camp Ellis in Illinois helping to form the 37th Field Hospital. The greatest medical innovations of the war, according to Sichi, were penicillin and the use of fresh blood that was more highly effective than artificial plasma. He also remembered using cortisone in eye drops to settle inflammations in only a week whereas iritis had formerly required a month for recovery with the application of atropine. After 1944, Sichi went to the jungles of New Guinea (an environment so threatening that nurses were not allowed to serve there), and last served in the Philippines.

Medical battalions collected casualties, brought them to aid stations, and ultimately moved them to field or evacuation hospitals made up of 200 enlisted men plus doctors and nurses, a vital part of a complex medical chain capable of supporting divisions of up to 25,000 enlisted men. Hand-held magnets were used at these facilities to remove foreign bodies.

Dr. William C. Lloyd interview with Drs. Matthews et al;
Dr. William Sichi interview

In 1946 Sichi returned for a third time to Walter Reed, this time to increase his skills in military administration. He also completed his postgraduate training at the University of Pennsylvania, passed his boards in 1947, and then went to Valley Forge, where he worked for a time with one of the nation's outstanding leaders in ophthalmology, Dr. Harold Scheie. With this remarkable combination of military experience and specialty training, therefore, Dr. Sichi brought distinction and dimension to ophthalmology when he arrived in Texas at the start of the Korean War.

Before Dr. Sichi was reassigned as chief eye consultant to the 97th General Hospital Frankfurt in 1953, he also developed a blind rehabilitation program. He later retired to San Antonio and practiced as a civilian until 1983 in the Olmos Medical Center and the Metropolitan Professional Building. In 1980 he was designated Consultant Emeritus by the Brooke Commanding General for his many contributions to ophthalmology.

Dr. William C. Lloyd interview with Dr. John Matthews et al;
Dr. William Sichi interview

## THE BROOKE OPHTHALMOLOGY RESIDENCY PROGRAM

Dr. Sichi set up what would eventually become a three-year ophthalmology residency program serving both Army and Air Force physicians. In creating the program, he drew upon the diagnostic and surgical skills of civilian consultants who staffed the Brooke eye surgery service to head up the residency program. Dr. John Matthews, who retired in 1944 to civilian practice but returned to Brooke in 1946 as a civilian consultant, now took charge of the three-year residency program. Dr. Alfred Nisbet also joined the effort, and together the two local physicians provided sufficient expertise to satisfy both the patients and the accreditation teams. Drs. Richard Stern and Herbert Olsten graduated in 1951, and more residents followed. The first Air Force resident in the Brooke program was Dr. Harold Lewis, and the Army and Air Force were equally represented among the new residents who subsequently arrived every July. Colonel Rex House, who had entered the U.S. Army Medical Corps in 1934 and, beginning in 1946, ran the ophthalmology service before Dr. Sichi arrived, also enlisted the support of another outstanding San Antonio specialist, Dr. W.E. Muldoon.

Lloyd, Col. William C., interview with Dr. Matthews et al;
Lloyd, Col. William C., "Brief History of the BAMC Ophthalmology Service," typescript, AIRMED Museum Collections, Fort Sam Houston;
Dr. John Matthews interview.

During the Korean War, the first Brooke residents faced an average daily inpatient census reaching up to 180 individuals and, with a few lectures, received training consisting primarily of "hands-on" experience. Early residents were responsible for separating arriving casualties into groups according to need for treatment and performing all visual fields. Drs. Matthews, Nisbet, and Muldoon, who had completed residencies at such premier institutions as the Mayo Clinic and Johns Hopkins, oversaw the training activities. "*Our main responsibility*," they explained, "*was to examine patients there so as to instruct the residents who were in training*." The idea was to "*enable the residents to get a little bit different perspective on the practice of ophthalmology than they were getting from the military people*" and "*broaden their horizons*." "*They would have cases lined up, and we would examine these cases. Then we would discuss them and present to the residents interesting cases that we ourselves had had in our office*." Residents also enjoyed a weekly literature review. Despite the hectic schedule, the fact that graduates were obligated to three years additional service, and occasional sparks thrown by the giant magnet in the eye surgery operating room threatened annihilation, only a single resident quit the program. Some observers attributed this to the fact that the only two air-conditioned facilities then at Fort Sam were the operating rooms and the Eye Clinic.

Lloyd, Col. William C., "Founding of the BAMC Ophthalmology Residency Program," video;
Dr. John Matthews interview;
Dr. Lloyd interview with Dr. Matthews et al.

By the time the Korean armistice was signed, it was clear that postgraduate medical education had become "integral to Brooke's mission." In the late 1950s, when Drs. Frank Weixel and Dan Russell served as co-chiefs of the ophthalmology service, residencies were done at six-month intervals and included a rotation through the Robert B. Green Hospital. Later, as Brooke Army Medical Center's mission expanded beyond education, training, and hospitalization to research, the program introduced residents to the latest in treatment, technique, and technology, drawing on such outstanding ophthalmologists as Walter Reed graduate and former Letterman chief, Dr. John Shock, a pioneer in the techniques of phacoemulsification used to perform cataract surgery.

Dr. Lloyd interview with Dr. Matthews et al

Brooke ophthalmology residents in the 1960s focused on equipment innovations and new treatment techniques, doing troop sick call using Schiotz tonometry for screening exams and providing eye care for Job Corps volunteers. Each completed the Lancaster course in Maine plus the Armed Forces Institute of Pathology course in ocular pathology. Residents used two slit lamps that replaced older Posner Universal apparatus, although operating microscopes were not yet in use. They were also introduced to phoropters and the gonio prism, and shared a room for indirect ophthalmoscopy. Electrodiagnostic studies and fundus photography were done at the visual physiology lab at the nearby School of Aviation Medicine. A laser was installed in 1965, but surgery continued to be conducted with surgical loupes for corneal grafts or by the naked eye since black silk thread for suturing was easily visible.

Medical students took the 12-week Lancaster course in Waterville, Maine, after their first year of training. First given in the 1940s, it covered academic and clinical ophthalmology, including clinical examination methods and discussion of optics, inflammation disorders, pathology, and other subjects. Though the American Board of Ophthalmology required it at one time, courses developed by Stanford and others eventually competed with it, and it was later largely replaced by residency training.

See Albert, Survey of Ophthalmology, 1993, for details.
Lee, Lloyd, Weixel interviews;
Lloyd, Col. William C., III, "Brief History of the BAMC Ophthalmology Service," typescript;
Barksdale, 1.

After its inception, 135 residents comprising forty-five classes graduated from the three-year Brooke Army Medical Center ophthalmology residency program by 1995, including a significant number who settled in San Antonio. New equipment and technology brought refinements to the program, residents treated a new influx of casualties in the Vietnam War, and BAMC patients in time included both President and Mrs. Johnson and a prince from Saudi Arabia, but its importance for the city lay not only in the communication it stimulated between military and civilian practitioners, but the addition of trained ophthalmologists and improved ophthalmological services to the community.

Lloyd, Col. William C., III, "Founding of the BAMC Ophthalmology Residency Program," video.

## THE R. B. GREEN MEMORIAL HOSPITAL OPHTHALMOLOGY RESIDENCY PROGRAM, 1952

The community counterpart of the Brooke Army Medical Center residency, the R.B. Green Memorial Hospital ophthalmology residency program, followed the paradigm of residencies that began in major urban settings. Local ophthalmologists established the Green residency to meet the needs of a community that had become the fastest-growing urban center in Texas. The San Antonio population of 400,000 in the 1950s represented an increase of 60% in only a decade. The city now boasted a new airport that linked the community to the rest of Texas and beyond and two television stations that broadcast regularly to the surrounding hinterland. It had also become a major urban center for medical care. When the program began, the city had five general hospitals--the Santa Rosa, Medical Arts, Nix, P&S, and the Medical-Surgical. It was also home to a uniquely large population of Hispanic-Americans/Latinos and poor people for whom little access to eye care had previously existed. Dr. Francis X. Weixel recalled that a common remedy for eye inflammation among these groups had been to place a cut potato over it.

Drs. Dan Russell, Frank Weixel, John Matthews, James Mims interviews

The R.B. Green Hospital took its name from the colorful county judge who first called for a charity hospital in Bexar County, where San Antonio is located. So loved by the public that he was called the "*Abraham Lincoln of Texas*," Green endeared himself to his constituents by reducing his own salary until the county was out of debt. He was also the youngest Court Judge in the United States at the age of twenty-eight and later served as a state senator, but died eight years before the hospital named for him was finished. Green would have been proud of the institution that bore his name since the new center of San Antonio community medicine was operated as a joint city and county project, employed tax funds allotted for medical care to the "*medically indigent*," and served large numbers of the needy. The hospital was intended to serve primarily as a Bexar County hospital, but eventually served patients from the Texas hinterland with its emergency room services and outpatient dispensary and became the campus for the community's first postgraduate medical training efforts.

R.B. Green Archives clipping file: "History-Robert B. Green Memorial Hospital," "Robert B. Green" bio, "Fact Sheet;" and "History of the Robert B. Green--once neglected, now proud and strong;" Dr. Dan Russell interview.

When it opened in 1917 "*the Green*," as the hospital came to be known, was considered one of the finest, most modern institutions in the nation. Local physicians staffed the hospital on a volunteer basis, and it had an intern training program and school of nursing from the start. Dr. Edward Dumas was one of three interns in training in 1921 along with Dr. Reuss of Cuero and Dr. Scott, who later helped to found the Scott and White Hospital in East Texas. At the time, diphtheria was rampant and the hospital handled cases of typhoid, leprosy, and consumption, requiring the young interns to do emergency treatments in the Great Flood of that year when fifty people drowned.

Dr. Jack Lee interview

Technically, ophthalmology residency training began at the Green in 1933 when Dr. Marion Wallace McCurdy, who also completed a traditional preceptorship under Dr. John Burleson, began a yearlong EENT residency after his internship in general medicine there. In 1939, however, the city terminated its portion of the hospital's funding, and by July of 1946 or 1947 financial difficulties forced the Green to close for lack of support. Residency training ceased. The polio ward and the Eye Clinic were the only outpatient clinics that remained open until 1949. At that time an agreement was reached between San Antonio and Bexar County providing a levy of ten cents on every one hundred dollars for hospital maintenance. Under this arrangement, most of the Green's patients continued to come from the city, but some taxpayers paid both city and county taxes.

Support for the program, however, came from other sources as officials recognized the need to expand the region's medical resources. Specialization fragmented medical school programs into separate branches, making the addition of residencies a natural extension of fundamental training. When the Texas Legislature in 1949 decided to locate a new University of Texas Medical Branch in Dallas rather than San Antonio, the Bexar County Medical Society formed a committee to support the idea of a postgraduate school and formal residency training programs rather than an undergraduate medical school to the University of Texas Board of Regents and the Legislature. According to committee member Dr. Charles Venable, more than 100,000 persons were coming to San Antonio for treatment every year, and each spent an average of seven days and was accompanied by two persons. He also indicated that, "*Texas doctors have always had a heck of a time getting to New York, Boston, Philadelphia, Baltimore or the Mayo Clinic in Minnesota for post-graduate training.*" San Antonio newspapers reported that the greatest benefit from such a program would be "*to the people of the small cities and towns of South Texas, since the intent of the postgraduate school is to give general practitioners training in various specialties, making them better qualified in diagnosis and treatment in their home towns.*" In cases where there wasn't time to "*bring the patient to a large city*" such as Dallas, the presence of a specialist could mean the difference between longevity and fatality for the "*rancher, farmer, or traveling man.*" Unfortunately, Texas legislators declined to appropriate money for the project. In response, the San Antonio Medical Foundation shifted its interest from the medical school and instead provided funds of $12,000 a year to initiate a postgraduate program, leaving the creation of a medical school for the next generation to complete the region's medical infrastructure.

Engelke, Louis B., "*The Doctors Study Over Time,*" San Antonio Express Magazine, February 17, 1952, n.p.

Until a formal residency program could be established, interim measures were taken. Credit for founding the R.B. Green Ophthalmology Residency program that began in 1952 goes to a handful of community practitioners led by Drs. John Matthews and Alfred Nisbet. With the help of the San Antonio Medical Foundation, Drs. John Matthews and Al Nisbet oversaw the "*pilot operation*" that enabled Dr. David McClure from Louisville, Kentucky, to complete a one-year residency in 1949. By this time, the medical staff had been reorganized with one hundred and fifty local doctors donating time for charity patients as attending staff at the Green's free clinic. In addition, thirty-five physicians, "*half from the city and about half from the country,*" were enrolled at the R.B. Green "*campus*" from different specialties, including doctors from Cuero, Crystal City, Goliad, Junction, Del Rio and Austin, allowing the institution to function informally, yet successfully. By now, the Green averaged 5,000 inpatients, 50,000 outpatients, 1,400 obstetric cases, and 17,000 emergencies in a typical year. Dr. Charles Venable explained the resulting residency program by linking it with training programs in Europe. "*The system in effect here today has been used in Europe, especially Vienna, for many years, but Texas was the first to adopt it this side of the ocean. In recent months, Michigan and Virginia followed suit.*" Although the claim to being first may be disputed, residency training did develop at a relatively early point in South Texas history when one considers how recently the region's first specialists had arrived.

San Antonio Medical Foundation leaders included Col. W.B. Tuttle, Melrose Holmgreen, John M. Bennett, Jr., Albert Steves III, Mrs. Edgar Tobin, a UT regent, and A.J. Lewis. From 1950 to 1953, Medical Foundation funds were used as a salary supplement for residents.

Weixel interview and Matthews interview with Dr. Lloyd;
Louis B. Engelke, The Doctors Study Overtime, San Antonio Express Magazine, February 17, 1952, n.p.;
Dr. Weixel interview.

According to Dr. Frank Weixel, "*when I came out of the service and went into private practice, it was customary at that time for every new physician (in San Antonio) to put in his time working at the Green, and it was completely donated time.*" Each physician did surgery and made rounds, often bringing someone from their own office to help them go through the clinics and spending at least one afternoon a week there. When a new doctor came to town, the oldest doctors left or, as Weixel described it, "*dropped off like billiard balls.*" Local specialists taught at the Green, but enjoyed no special status; their title as "*Lecturers of the University of Texas Post Graduate School of Medicine*," according to one local physician, didn't mean anything. While the R.B. Green Hospital awaited re-accreditation in 1950, Dr. Dan Russell, Jr. externed there between his junior and senior years of medical school. American Medical Association re-accreditation of the intern training program was soon secured, and by 1951 there were seventeen interns in service, most of whom went on to become board-certified. By this time also, consulting physicians at the Green enjoyed an affiliation with Baylor University in Waco that gave them the status of associate professors.

Dr. Frank Weixel, Dr. Dan Russell interviews

The second resident to complete his training at the Green after Dr. McClure, Dr. Joseph De Gasperi, did so as a direct result of seeking help from Dr. John Matthews. Faced with few local training opportunities and unable to afford to leave the state, De Gasperi contacted Dr. Matthews who responded by setting up a program that allowed De

Gasperi as a resident to successfully tap into both the R.B. Green and Brooke Army Medical Center programs and the mentorship of an outstanding community practitioner. Between 1951 and 1952, De Gasperi completed a residency that included attending lectures and seeing problem cases with Matthews in his role as consultant to the Brooke residency program, assisting his mentor in surgery at the R.B. Green, and learning to handle private patients in Matthews' office.

Dr. Joseph De Gasperi interview

As De Gasperi and other ophthalmologists approached him, Dr. Matthews realized the acute need for a locally-based approved residency program with accompanying research capabilities. By this time, the distinguished ophthalmologist had what could be described as a "*high society*" clientele including members of important local families such as the Kennedy ranching clan, and was prepared to assume a leadership role in the community. Matthews had already established an Eye Clinic in the Green's basement and outfitted it with some of the latest Bausch & Lomb equipment, including a slit lamp and lensometer. To acquire the equipment, he applied the rebates optical companies gave out each time a prescription was sent in to the purchase of equipment for the Eye Clinic. Now Matthews gathered local ophthalmologists Drs. Jack Lee, Graham Milburn, James L. Mims, Jr., and Russell Snip to organize the teaching and experiential components of a residency program. Credit for supporting the Green residency program also goes to pathologist Dr. Herman Wigodsky, who ceased his medical practice when he inherited a local store, the Pincus Store, and Tulane's Chairman of Ophthalmology, James Allen, M.D., who helped to obtain certification for the new program.

Dr. Joseph De Gasperi, Dr. Jack Lee interviews

The R.B. Green Ophthalmology Residency Program officially began when the Texas legislature passed a state constitutional amendment authorizing the creation of countywide hospital districts with taxing power. Initially turned down by voters across the state, the law passed in 1955 with a maximum tax rate of seventy-five cents per $100 evaluation. Weeks later, Bexar County voters approved their county hospital district, approved a budget for the R.B. Green, and began to call for other additions to the region's medical infrastructure. Dr. James Mims, Jr., one of San Antonio's first ophthalmologists to complete residency training and an individual highly interested in developing a local residency program, now came on board to help supervise the clinics and establish the program's monthly lecture series. Mims also gained permission for Green residents to visit the State Hospital eye clinic where community ophthalmologists provided care once or

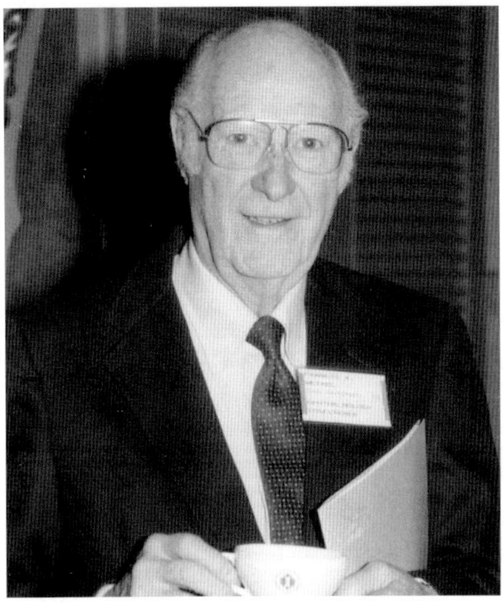

Dr. Francis X. Weixel, first Chief of Ophthalmology at Wilford Hall Medical Center, and first co-Chief of the Ophthalmology Department at the Robert B. Greene Hospital, as well as the UT Medical School in San Antonio. In 1995, the following tribute was paid to Dr. Weixel for major contributions to ophthalmology in South Texas.

"During your lifetime, which has spanned most of this century, you have experienced some of the greater challenges to our civilization, especially the Second World War and the Korean War. Through those and other challenges, you have, nurtured by your religion and your family, continued to adapt yourself to the changes of your times by being selflessly available for duty whenever needed, while never losing sight of your goals.

Your success as a family man is evidenced by a highly supportive spouse, five children and six grandchildren, who already demonstrate the benefits from your touch and your genes.

As a military man, you helped forged the eye departments at Brook Army Hospital and especially at Wilford Hall Medical Center, where you helped design the eye clinic and became its first Chief.

As a physician, your excellence, early recognized when you were appointed Chief of Ophthalmology at Letterman Army Hospital even before you had completed your residency, has resulted in an exemplary career as a highly capable, caring and ethical ophthalmologist.

As a teacher, after initiating the ophthalmology training program at Wilford Hall, you became an early Chief of Ophthalmology at the Brady Green, at that time called the Robert B. Green Hospital, where you began a residency training program even before the U. T> Medical School existed. Since 1968, without cessation, you have voluntarily and without pay, taught residents and medical students the science and art of ophthalmology. As evidenced by your students' written evaluations, you are a favorite because, and I quote, 'You are interested in the student, kind, patient, nurturing, well informed, experienced, up to date, and all-in-all outstanding.'

We, the Ophthalmology students and teachers at Brooke Army Medical Center, Wilford Hall Medical Center, and the University of Texas Health Science Center in San Antonio, honor you today as an outstanding teacher and role model by giving you the Alamo City Ophthalmological Residents Association Award."

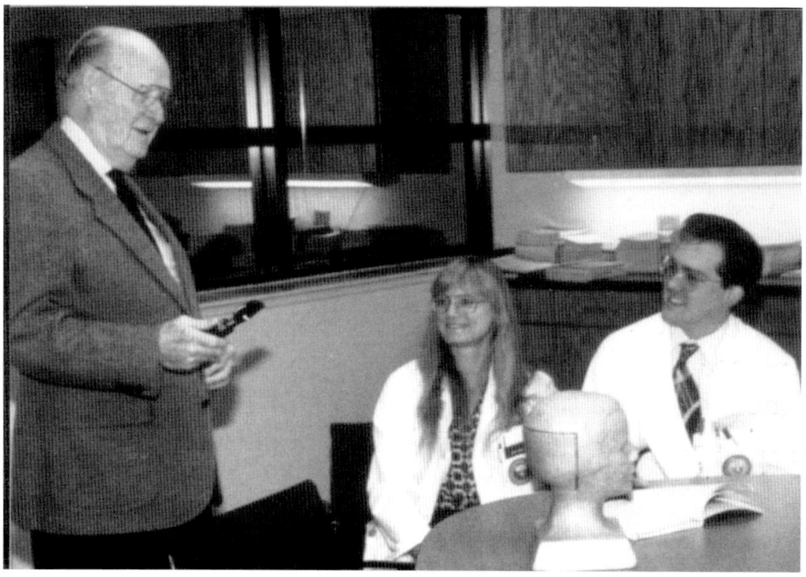

Dr. Weixel continued to teach residents and especially medical students until his retirement.

twice a month to widen their clinical experience and they continued to attend the Lancaster course at Waterville, Maine, organized by the Massachusetts Eye and Ear Infirmary through which many outstanding regional specialists were recruited to serve on its faculty. Later, as Dr. Harold Scheie and Stanford University developed competitive courses, residents went to Maine for three to six months to complete the didactic, or pure science as opposed to clinical, aspects of the program. Back in San Antonio, Dr. Rex House ran the ophthalmology service and oversaw the residents' work at the Green and Santa Rosa Hospitals where they helped with cataract operations at a time when patients spent up to two weeks in the hospital. Dr. Jack Lee served as Chief of Ophthalmology at the R.B. Green in 1954, followed by Dr. James Mims, Jr. from 1955 to 1957. Drs. Frank Weixel and Daniel Russell served as co-chiefs each for a six-month period in 1958. Other early associate chiefs of the Green's EENT service were Drs. Wesley Dallas Hicks and J. K. Beck.

See Dr. Albert, Survey of Ophthalmology, 1993 on the history of the Lancaster course.

As the program developed, a San Antonio news reporter noted its positive impact with satisfaction, claiming the benefits outweighed even the absence of a medical school or were "*more direct to the people of South Texas than they might have been if the school had been put here in the first place*." In time the program also began to attract ophthalmology residents from beyond the boundaries of the state of Texas.

The first residents to complete the residency after it became a three-year program in 1949 were Dr. Dilip Kumar Patel, who had trained in India and later became a retinal surgeon in Rochester, New York, and Drs. Richard Stern and Herbert Olsten in 1951. Dr. Matthews recalled that during Dr. Stern's training, before steroids were available to treat uveitis or iridocyclitis, foreign proteins were used to stimulate febrile response. Stern had developed a potent strain of boiled milk known as sternolac that once infected, produced a powerful febrile response. The first woman to complete the three-year residency was Dr. Joan B. Nickol, who finished in 1962. Residents were proud to work at the Green despite the fact that a first-year single resident made only $275 monthly, and from 1950 to 1953 medical foundation funds supplemented resident salaries. The American Medical Association Joint Commission on Accreditation re-approved all the hospital's residency programs in 1958, before the ophthalmology program relocated to the University of Texas Health Science Center medical school. Eventually, the R.B. Green program also accepted military residents from Brooke Army Medical Center and Lackland Air Force Base when the program had no senior resident, affiliated with the Santa Rosa Hospital as well as Brooke, and became part of the new University of Texas Health Science Center known as the Post-Graduate Medical Training School of the University of Texas, San Antonio Division, headquartered at the Robert B. Green Hospital.

Col. William C. Lloyd interview with Dr. Matthews et al.

In time, a close alliance developed between the R. B. Green residency program and Dr. James A. Bethea's administration at the Brooke Army Medical Center. Dr. Bruce Bowers was the first BAMC resident to participate in the Green program, and after 1962 the Green regularly had first, second and third-year residents and one from Brooke Army Medical Center rotating through on a regular basis. Each program made its facilities available to the other; residents from the Brooke program provided free service at the Green on a rotation basis and Green residents attended Brooke lectures. When there were two senior residents at Brooke, there was so much to do at the Green that a senior resident was allowed to spend six months of his last year there, receiving valuable experience in cataract surgery. Populations treated at the two facilities differed significantly. According to one resident, one in ten patients at Brooke had something serious while one in ten at the Green didn't. When the Green program began to take a resident every other year, Brooke rotated one of its senior residents through the Green every three or four months in years when the Green had no senior resident of its own. Later, Air Force residents from Wilford Hall Hospital participated in a similar fashion. In general, cooperation between the residency programs translated into a wider experience for all with each program offering a place for scientific exchange between local physicians and military doctors.

Weixel interview;
Lloyd, William C., M.D., "History of the BAMC Ophthalmology Service," archives typescript.

It may be of interest to note that the development of the three San Antonio ophthalmology residency programs preceded the provision of basic medical training in South Texas. Roots of the medical school and the University of Texas Health Science Center Ophthalmology Residency Program, however, both lay in the successful advances in professional training that began at the Green. With the announcement of authorization for the medical school, efforts began to organize a clinical faculty in the city, and before a single medical school building had been constructed, residents at the R.B. Green considered themselves part of the new Health Science Center program. The first official ophthalmology resident at the Medical School was Dr. Dudley Harris, and the first non-military resident Dr. Al Burden after 1965 when the Green program affiliated with the UT School of Postgraduate Education, forerunner of the University of Texas Health Science Center (UTHSC) Department of Ophthalmology.

Drs. Frank Weixel, Wilbur Matthews, James Mims interviews.

The R.B. Green residency program had fitful beginnings between 1949 and 1953 and ceased to function several years before the University of Texas Medical School residency received formal approval in 1957, but nonetheless had a major impact on South Texas through ophthalmologists who went on to practice in the region. Among those who did so, Dr. Barney Williams came to San Antonio from New Orleans' Smith-Clark Eye Clinic and a year at the Hurst Clinic in East Texas in 1956 and went on to practice in Kerrville. Williams was invited to join the program by Dr. Dan Russell, Sr., whom he met at a social program at the Pearl Brewery following a medical meeting. Russell convinced him that the program would be approved so he that could take his boards, and Williams became the first full-time certified resident at the R.B. Green, assisting in surgery, going to Maine for his basic science course, and helping to build up the eye clinics. He was followed by Dr. Joseph Badone and a host of others that included Drs.

Joseph Neigut and Roger Hernandez, the last resident in the program. Subsequent Green residents who entered practice in the community included Dr. Thomas Folbre, Dr. Joe Frey--who worked at the State Hospital after his residency--and Dr. Doyle Leslie of Austin. Kirbyville native Dr. Bernard Gene Hewitt graduated from the Galveston Medical Branch in 1959 and went to Lackland, but completed part of his training at the R.B. Green.

Dr. James Mims interview

By 1968 when the R.B. Green residency was reaccredited and transferred to the new University of Texas medical school facilities at Oak Hills, the local newspaper reported that Green interns and residents were "*gaining diversified experience envied by many colleagues in private hospitals*," including a volume of patients and "as wide a variety of medical problems as any hospital's likely to have." At the new facility, Drs. Weixel and Russell served as co-chiefs of the service until Dr. Weinstein came to head the Division of Ophthalmology in 1970. With at least 100,000 indigent residents in Bexar County, the majority of whom qualified for "*free*" medical treatment at the Green, the "*multitude of unusual medical maladies*" in this population made the residency experience one that was profitable and sought after. It was also noted that strong intern and residency programs "*allowed staff specialists to concentrate on teaching and research*."

"*24 Green Hospital Interns Live Fast Pace*," San Antonio Express, March 9, 1964, 4D;
Col. William C. Lloyd, III interview

## THE WILFORD HALL OPHTHALMOLOGY RESIDENCY PROGRAM, LACKLAND AIR FORCE BASE: 1958

Although the Army Medical Services were no longer responsible for the medical care of Air Force personnel after the United States Air Force joined the Armed Services in July 1949, the old Lackland Air Force Base hospital at San Antonio was all but dismantled, its patients shipped to the Army's Brooke Army Hospital at Fort Sam Houston, and its equipment transferred to other facilities. The Air Force, responding to flight surgeons' wishes, planned instead to create dispensary facilities at air bases and allow the hospitalization and training of Air Force personnel to continue at Army hospitals. When the

Korean War started, however, these plans changed and activity at both Brooke and Lackland ballooned. Lackland's military population quickly exploded to 60,000 trainees and 70,000 military personnel and dependents. Construction began on a new 1,000-bed hospital known as Wilford Hall, while in the meantime doctors converted existing structures to respond to the crisis. As case numbers escalated, the old hospital formerly used for rehabilitation of patients evacuated from overseas was connected to a double cantonment or wooden barracks by ramps to create a 1,200 bed facility. Once again war stimulated medical advances as Lackland doctors realized that residents could provide valuable assistance while receiving advanced professional training in their specialties. This activity gave rise ten years later in 1958 to the Wilford Hall Hospital ophthalmology residency program.

Historical Files, Department of Ophthalmology, Wilford Hall Hospital;
Dr. Francis X. Weixel, Dr. Stephen G. Waller interviews;
Alcott, Edward, Aerospace Medical Division, 70-72

Dr. Francis X. Weixel, the first Chief of Ophthalmology at Wilford Hall and the creator of the only ophthalmology department in the Air Force in 1951, offered apprenticeship-type training for general medical officers before the residency program began. Another of the generation shaped by World War II, Weixel had extensive experience in the field and the kind of military background that gave a medical community depth. Born during World War I in New York City, Weixel was inspired to become a doctor by stories of his grandfather, a New York general practitioner named Patrick Byrne. Another ancestor had been a vice president of the Southern Pacific Railroad, who surveyed railroad routes in West Texas. Entering college during the Depression, Weixel majored in engineering for one tuition-free year at the Cooper Union on a state scholarship, but abandoned the idea and graduated instead from Manhattan College in 1941 before setting out for Creighton University Medical School in Omaha, Nebraska. Like his contemporary, Dr. William Sichi, Weixel finished a nine-month internship (in his case, at St. Francis Hospital in New York) before he joined the Army just prior to the start of World War II.

Col. William C. Lloyd, III, Dr. Stephen F. Waller, Dr. Francis X. Weixel interviews

For the next two years, Weixel traveled on hospital ships conveying injured soldiers and their dependents to and from Europe and the Caribbean. These floating hospitals held as many as 1,500 beds compared with an average hospital that had only 500 beds, visiting ports at Cherbourg, Le Havre, and Bremerhafen before making the five-day trip back to New York. Adapting to the needs of his situation, he was enlisted briefly to serve in the absence of superiors as Chief Medical Officer for the Port of New Orleans and the Port of New York where as many as 800 ships were anchored. During the war, Weixel simply found himself "*drafted*" into ophthalmology to satisfy a shortage of doctors. The experience was a positive one, however, and led to his decision to become an ophthalmologist.

Dr. Francis X. Weixel interview

When the war ended, Weixel went to San Francisco's Letterman Army Hospital for residency training and also completed a preceptorship under Letterman's outstanding chief of service, Colonel Earl Maxwell. Maxwell was an inspiration, and the young doctor chose to become a charter member of the Air Force because Maxwell had chosen to join. Because of his timing in beginning his residency in 1948 just as the Air Force became a separate service, Weixel was the Air Force's first ophthalmological resident at a time when it had only 369 regular medical officers. He was also in a position to become involved in the Korean War. When Maxwell left in 1950 for Washington, D.C., to become Chief of Professional Services, Weixel was a senior resident and Maxwell's logical successor as Letterman's Chief of Ophthalmology.

Dr. Francis X. Weixel and Col. William C. Lloyd, III interviews; Joseph S. Weisman, Major, USAF, MC, Chief, Neuro-Ophth Service, Residency Program Director, Report, 1992

In the thick of the Korean crisis, Weixel's next assignment brought him to San Antonio. As the first ophthalmologist assigned to the 3700th Air Base Wing and Lackland's only ophthalmologist in 1951, his initial task was to treat casualties evacuated from overseas. His schedule required seeing 100 to 120 patients daily and, in the absence of an optometrist, teaching a corpsman to do refractions. Because most Air Force members were young, Weixel treated more retinal detachments than cataracts, did almost no glaucoma surgery, and concentrated largely on squint operations and plastic surgery for land mine injuries, using what he had learned from an expert in ocular plastic surgery at Letterman, Dr. Crowell Beard. He also served as a preceptor for a Lackland resident in 1951, an activity that called to his attention the need for a residency program. After a discussion with his mentor, Col. Maxwell, Weixel decided to wait until three ophthalmologists were on staff before offering residency training. Although he left Lackland in 1954 to join Dr. Matthews in private practice,

Weixel continued to support the idea of creating a residency program. At the time, he recalled there were roughly a dozen ophthalmologists in San Antonio, a city he described as "*a large village*." Among his patients were a number of physicians from Mexico.

Dr. Francis X. Weixel, Col. William C. Lloyd, III interviews

Although Lackland closed for a time after the Korean War, its medical facilities were designated as an Air Force hospital with a continuing role in delivering eye care to active duty servicemen, dependents, and retirees, including surgical and medical diagnosis and treatment of ophthalmic disease, making them a logical place to locate the Air Force ophthalmology residency program. Weixel's effort bore fruit in 1958, when San Antonio's second military and third ophthalmology residency program began. At that time, Alfonso C. Tenney, Lieutenant Colonel, USAF, MC and Lackland's Chief of Ophthalmology, applied to the American College of Surgeons on the first day of the New Year to establish the program. Not only did this event enrich the mixture of local medical institutions but, as the Air Force's only ophthalmology residency, soon attracted "premier ophthalmic academicians in the Air Force" from around the world.

Wilford Hall Ophthalmology Residency Program Directors have included Dr. Alfonzo C. Tenney, 1959-61; Dr. James L. Curtis, 1961-65; Dr. Glen P. Johnston, 1965-1968; Dr. Jerry V. (Virgil) Shepherd, 1968-1972; Dr. Lydell C. Kiplin, 1972-1977; Dr. David L. Shacklett, 1977-1982; Dr. Jack O. Sipperley, 1982-1983; Dr. John W. Shore, 1983-1987; Dr. H. Michael Lambert, 1987-1990; Dr. Raul J. Moreno/Dr. Robert Ward, 1990-1991; Dr. Joseph S. Weisman, 1991-1994; and Dr. Christopher T. Westfall, 1994-,

Historical File, Department of Ophthalmology, Wilford Hall Hospital;
Col. William C. Lloyd interview with Dr. Francis X. Weixel

The original three-year residency program consisted of "*a nine-month basic science course at an approved civilian institution followed by a two-year, four month program of didactic and clinical teaching leading to eligibility for certification by the American Board of Ophthalmology*." To obtain valuable clinical experience, Lackland residents--whose numbers increased to a total of 12 beginning in 1991--participated in citywide training opportunities, regularly completing their programs at Brooke General Hospital as well as spending time at the R.B. Green and the Colby College Basic Science Course and a one-week course on ophthalmic pathology at the AFIP. Dr. James Raspberry and Dr. Herschel Phelps, the first to complete the program, graduated in 1961. Residents also commonly rotated to the Santa Rosa Clinic beginning in 1957, thereby extending the links between the Air Force and civilian medicine. Since its beginning, Wilford Hall Hospital has trained over eighty residents, and nearly all have become board-certified.

Dr. Russell interview with Dr. Lloyd;
"Milestones" and "USAF Hospital, Lackland, San Antonio, Texas," typescripts,
Ophthalmology Department, Wilford Hall Hospital

In 1962 the Wilford Hall Ophthalmology Department reported 24,332 annual visits, handled by the chief and only two full-time staff ophthalmologists. Rapid advances gave residents a high-quality experience. By continually upgrading and modernizing its equipment, the program remained in the forefront of ophthalmology training programs and constantly improved the quality of patient care. In 1964 San Antonio's second eye bank opened at Wilford Hall to collect eyes for teaching purposes and the study of eye pathology. Residents also were encouraged to participate in clinical research. In 1970, when the program affiliated with the University of Texas Health Science Center, Dr. David M. Hunter performed the first fluorescein angiography there, and a year later the facility acquired its first argon laser capability. By 1975 modern extracapsular cataract surgery was done, and Wilford Hall staff ophthalmologists implanted their first intraocular lenses. Only a year later B-scan ultrasound and ERG/EOG units had been set up in the clinic, anterior chamber lenses were commonly employed, phacoemulsification and intraocular lens training established and vitrectomy capability acquired. Around 1977 staff gained the capability for Ocutome posterior vitreous surgery, and two years later began a vitreo retinal surgery service. Corneal transplant surgery and surgery to implant posterior chamber intraocular lenses began after 1980. The hospital acquired an argon/krypton laser in 1982 for treatment of macular disease. For some years, Wilford Hall ophthalmologists also regularly provided ophthalmic care for Oklahoma Indian reservations. This program ceased in 1977, however, as the need for military readiness for possible deployment to third world countries increased in priority. More recently, residents have gone to Central Mexico, Honduras, and the Dominican Republic as part of readiness training.

"Milestones," typescript, Historical Files, Ophthalmology Department, Wilford Hall;
Dr. Stephen G. Waller interview.

Against this backdrop were corresponding changes in the residency program. Residents acquired clinical knowledge of glaucoma, motility, retinal, and refraction cases, discussed problems related to flying and ophthalmology, did microscopic work, completed research projects in their last years, and participated extensively in surgical procedures. By 1976 all regularly completed an animal surgery program for phacoemulsification. A year later team teaching began, with teams led by senior residents and supervised by staff physicians. In 1979 senior residents began attending extracapsular cataract extraction intraocular lens cases to advance the department's capability. The program began to accept three residents instead of two in 1980, and a senior resident implanted his first posterior chamber intraocular lens. In 1981 senior residents began attending the Knolle extracapsular cataract surgery and intraocular lens course earlier to allow for a greater volume of intraocular lens cases and permit earlier training of the junior residents. Sub-specialty rotations for second-year residents were formalized and residents began rotations into civilian facilities in pediatric ophthalmology and oculoplastics.

"USAF Hospital, Lackland, San Antonio, Texas," typescript, Ophthalmology Department, Wilford Hall Hospital.

According to BAMC Staff Ophthalmologist William Lloyd, from their beginnings, "*the three independent eye surgery programs were united by mutual friendship and cooperation.*" Dr. Matthews recalled that, "*there was a 'very fine rapport' at the time through the San Antonio Society of Ophthalmology and Otolaryngology.*" Residents at Wilford Hall, like those at BAMC, were encouraged to participate in all citywide training opportunities, and regularly rotated to BAMC and the University of Texas Health Science Center to complete their residency programs. To maximize its offerings or capitalize on the possibilities of joint information exchange, Wilford Hall affiliated with UTHSC as early as 1970. In 1984 the first tri-service Cataract and Intraocular Lens Course was established at USUHS, and in 1985 residents participated in tri-service ocular trauma courses at Letterman in San Francisco. By the 1990s, the program boasted that its residents scored in the 97.5th percentile on the Ophthalmic Knowledge Assessment Program board examination, placing it fourth among the nation's 156 programs.

Col. William C. Lloyd, III interview

Wilford Hall ophthalmologists also did significant research. In the 1970s and 1980s, the Department participated in an FDA investigational protocol for intraocular lenses, a Vitrectomy/Chronic Aphakic CME Study, an Ocular Melanoma Study, and the National Eye Trauma Registry. Senior residents were actively involved in an intraocular lens study. Other Wilford Hall studies have investigated drug effects on intra-ocular pressure in cataract surgery and the effects of hyperbaric oxygen therapy on ophthalmic disorders.

"USAF Hospital, Lackland, San Antonio, Texas," typescript, Ophthalmology Department, Wilford Hall Hospital.

Like their counterparts at BAMC, some Wilford Hall ophthalmologists eventually moved into the community. Among them, Drs. David Shacklett and Patrick O'Connor entered the civilian sector by joining the faculty of the University of Texas Health Science Center in 1981. Distinguished Air Force practitioners arrived continuously, bringing with them knowledge and techniques in new subspecialties such as kerato-refractive surgery, while others moved into private practice or service at some of the nation's most prestigious hospitals and universities.

Today, the Alamo City Ophthalmology Clinical Conference sponsored by the UT Health Science Center Medical School enriches the lives of residents from all three area programs. In each case, residency programs combined the forces of local and military practitioners, such that ties between the institutions remained strong and each was strengthened by the other's presence.

## RESIDENTS WHO BECAME SAN ANTONIO SPECIALISTS: DRS. JAMES MIMS JR., BLAND SCHWARTING, AND JOSEPH DE GASPERI

The careers of three early residents demonstrate the importance of San Antonio's three ophthalmology residency training programs to the community. That of Dr. James Mims, Jr., one of the last in the pioneer tradition of those who specialized in ophthalmology before professional residencies had entirely replaced the preceptorship, illustrates how residency training changed the field. A transitional figure in ophthalmology, Mims created the prototype for a new type of Texas physician, the modern specialist whose background combined old-fashioned and residency training. One of Mims' English forbearers created the equivalent of the *Physician's Desk Reference*, an index of medical specialties, for that country in 1900. He also was related to the pioneer Texans who established the frontier Texas

Republic through his maternal grandfather, Reuben Hornsby, who had served as a surveyor for Stephen F. Austin, the man who set up the first Anglo colony in the region. Mims' father was well educated and his mother attended both the University of Texas and Miss Whiting's Finishing School in Austin.

Col. William C. Lloyd, III, M.D. interview with Drs. Matthews, Russell, Weixel, Mims et al.

Mims' own colorful history began in 1920 when he was delivered into the world by a second cousin employed as a veterinarian. Born in Austin and raised in Ft. Worth and Dallas, his family traveled around the state while his father worked as a State Insurance Department actuary. Accustomed to living in hotels, Mims recalled throwing rocks at the alligators in San Antonio's Menger Hotel pool and frequenting the magnificent Galvez Hotel at Galveston. Despite his family's itinerancy, however, he finished Paschal High School in Fort Worth and enrolled at the North Texas Agricultural College, now known as Arlington State. Without his experience in World War II, Mims' medical career would likely have taken a different direction. As Europe headed toward the brink of war, he began pre-med courses at the University of Texas in Austin, and then entered the Galveston Medical Branch when the medical school course was only a year old. He graduated in 1943 in the midst of World War II just as the school's surgical hospital became the 30th Evacuation Hospital destined to be sent to New Guinea. The 12th General Military Hospital Unit at Galveston was also activated in 1943, and wound up in eastern Brittany some time after D-Day.

Dr. James Mims interview with Col. William C. Lloyd, III, M.D.

From this point on, experience became Mims' teacher and military medicine began to shape his career. After receiving a medical administrative corps commission from the Galveston Medical Branch, he took a position in general medicine at a charity hospital in Wichita Falls, Texas, where he treated few patients because the defense boom had given almost everyone in the community enough money for private care. From there he went to the Medical Field Service School at Carlisle Barracks, Pennsylvania, and briefly in Colorado Springs before boarding a troop ship for the Philippines.

Like many in his generation, James Mims was something of an autodidact. While serving as a junior officer for a psychiatric service at a field hospital in the Philippines, he began to read May's *Diseases of the Eyes*, to do photography, and study optics on his own time. Among the problems in the Philippine population were cases of eye disease, especially the optic atrophy common to starvation and vitamin B-12 deficiencies. This condition often produced the epidemic blindness that was the scourge of countries with poor nutrition, much as trachoma was common among people living in arid countries. Slowly Mims' interest turned to ophthalmology and the precision science of optics. Although he later spent a year at Galveston's state psychiatric hospital and worked at Brentwood Hospital in Long Island, New York, with psychiatrist Milton Heptmacek (who later headed Psychiatry at the Galveston Medical Branch), Mims' military experience convinced him to pursue ophthalmology when the war ended. He returned to the United States weakened by tropical disease, however, and first went to San Antonio to recover his health.

San Antonio's senior ophthalmologists, including Dr. Daniel Russell, Sr., Jack Matthews, William Gill, and Ed Dumas, soon "*adopted*" Mims. In order to qualify him as a specialist, they recommended that he sign up for training with Dr. Scott Bronson, an elderly local eye, ear, nose, and throat specialist. He recalled the preceptorship experience as a mixture of learning and labor that required him to boil up fifty eyedroppers each morning and prepare eye drops of sterile saline and a drop of methiolate. For clinical experience, he was also allowed to assist Drs. Gill, Matthews and Dumas with their patients. In what remained still a largely informal medical world, Mims remembered his colleagues as "*extremely friendly and helpful.*" They "*just treated me like a son*," he claimed, while he was "*trying to make a living until I could get into a residency*" and completing a home study course in ophthalmology. Clearly, however, this experience did not suffice to qualify him as a professional.

Lacking access to residency training in San Antonio, Mims now went to a major city where the urban setting had created a rich medical environment. Accepted into the residency program at Tulane University in New Orleans, Mims found himself in a regional medical center for much of the Southwest and the place where many of the region's early ophthalmology professors got their training. At the New Orleans Eye, Ear, Nose, and Throat Hospital, the young resident found powerful mentors in Dr. William Clark and department chairman, Dr. James (Jimmy) Allen. The residency increased his level of expertise and introduced him to the ophthalmic subspecialties when he attended part of the seven-year medical meeting cycle focused on a different sub-specialty each year that Allen had established.

When Mims returned to San Antonio, he did so as a highly trained ophthalmologist and a force in the still old-fashioned community for more sophisticated medical practice. Patients continued to schedule cataract surgery after August until 1952 when air-conditioning became available and society functioned much as it had for generations. Mims not only brought expertise and state-of-the-art technique into the community, but familiarity with medical issues and ideas that helped to end the provincial isolation of the region. On the negative side, others like him had also joined the community and he now faced an increasingly crowded medical environment. The Baptist Memorial Hospital had taken over the old Physicians' and Surgeon's and Medical and Surgical Hospitals in 1948, and the Nix, Medical Arts, and two floors of the old Medical and Surgical Building offered the only office space available. He later recalled that, "*someone had to die in the Medical Arts for an office to open.*" His community connections, however, now served him well. Mims opened an office in the Medical Arts Building in the space occupied by the now-deceased Scott Bronson and soon operated a small eye service at the R.B. Green Hospital. He was fortunate to begin his practice just as the city's population soared and patients began to arrive from the surrounding countryside, Northern Mexico, Beeville, Cotulla, Carrizo Springs, and New Braunfels.

Mims' subsequent contributions to the field of ophthalmology, therefore, reflect to a considerable degree the impact of his training. Not only is he credited with the first cataract, glaucoma and eye muscle operations at the Methodist Hospital, but with early operations on detached retinas, developing an erisophake suction device to remove the cataract and lens, and improving a manipulator created by Dr. Daniel Kendrick. Mims' colleagues recalled his enthusiasm for technology at an American Academy of Ophthalmology meeting in Dallas where he exhibited the model of an eyeball that turned on a lathe to simulate movement. Set in an orbit made of wood, the contraption was a masterpiece of ball bearings, fishing weights, strings, pulleys and indicators. It was also an appropriate symbol for the kind of technology soon to be replaced by the innovations resulting from the latest ophthalmic research. Mims went on to do research, but was recalled for being so thorough he was accused of "*seeing his patients too much.*"

By the 1960s, he maintained a highly successful practice and had founded a dynasty beginning with his son, James Mims III, who later became one of a new generation of San Antonio ophthalmologists. Those who followed Mims, however, would find their way to a career in ophthalmology via a more direct route.

During Mims' career, American Academy of Ophthalmology meetings brought the most people to Dallas of any kind of event held there and they were responsible for the design of that city's vast Convention Center. His wife, Mary Charline McGehee, was the daughter of a doctor with a degree in microbiology. The Gilbert family on his grandmother's side who came to Texas as early as 1836 included several physicians. The rest of the Southern family entered the state in 1870 to escape Alabama carpetbaggers, and settled on the Robinson grant.

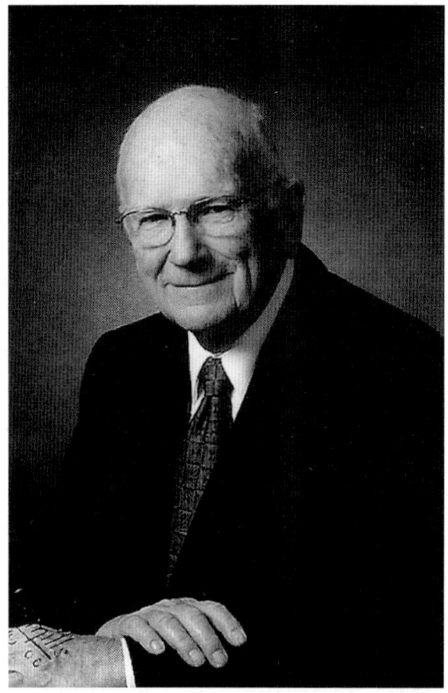

Dr.Bland Schwarting

## DR. BLAND SCHWARTING

The first graduate to affiliate with the Brooke residency program as a consultant, Dr. Bland Schwarting graduated from the military residency program but spent the bulk of his career as a San Antonio community ophthalmologist. His military career developed out of his youthful fascination with airplanes. The native Texan fell in love with flying after a ten-minute ride for a dollar in a Ford trimotor plane that circled Waco's tallest building and returned to the airfield. Between his college and Baylor medical school years, Schwarting became a World War II pilot. After medical school, faced with low-paying internships at civilian hospitals, he reentered the military and completed an internship at Honolulu's Tripler Army Hospital and a residency at Walter Reed in Washington, D.C. with the service branch that became the U.S. Air Force Medical Corps.

Dr. Bland Schwarting interview

Schwarting's early interest in ophthalmology began when a younger brother lost an eye to a BB gun, but grew primarily out of a fondness for physics and the inspiration of his chief at Tripler. In 1953, Schwarting volunteered to fill a vacancy opened for a senior ophthalmology resident at Brooke Army Hospital, and soon he found himself tending Korean casualties and their dependents arriving at Beach Pavilion, the hospital component where eye cases were treated. As a resident, he treated shrapnel injuries from hand grenades, removed intraocular foreign bodies, and handled traumatic cataracts and inflammations at the same time Hazel Colombe ran the prosthetics laboratory that provided many of the injured with artificial eyes. Among soldiers' families, he recalled numerous cases of strabismus, and also victims of the Bataan Death March who came to Texas suffering from optic atrophy, a degenerative condition of the eye resulting from malnutrition.

Dr. Bland Schwarting interview

After three years paying back the cost of his education as Chief of Ophthalmology at Wright-Patterson in Dayton, Ohio, Schwarting returned to San Antonio to fill the space left by the recent death of James Aderhold in the private practice of Dr. Alfred Nisbet, a friend of his chief at Brooke. Schwarting's memories of Nisbet's barbecue and fried corn bread picnics at his Sisterdale ranch capture the informal and collegial tone of the medical community in the period. In 1958 Schwarting opened a San Antonio practice in the office where he was still at work in 1998 after a distinguished career of service, including research projects on visual acuity in infants and eye muscle imbalance.

Dr. Bland Schwarting interview

## DR. JOSEPH De GASPERI

Among early R.B. Green residency program graduates who provided medical care for generations of South Texas residents, Dr. Joseph De Gasperi enjoyed a transitional career much like that of James Mims. In this case, the Green residency did not fully qualify the young man as an ophthalmologist, but provided key contacts that launched his career. The son of an Italian father and Spanish mother who came from Barcelona, Spain, De Gasperi was born in San Antonio and received his medical degree from Baylor University in 1945 but deferred his education to serve in the Navy during World War II. Home after the war, he completed a one-year rotating internship at the Santa Rosa Hospital and then set out for Maine in 1948 to complete the didactic part of his training. The twelve-week Lancaster course drew prospective specialists from around the country and maintained an excellent reputation, fulfilling board requirements with components in academic and clinical ophthalmology, optics, clinical examination, study of inflammation disorders, pathology and other subdivisions. De Gasperi then returned to enter the residency program at Fort Sam Houston.

Dr. Joseph De Gasperi interview

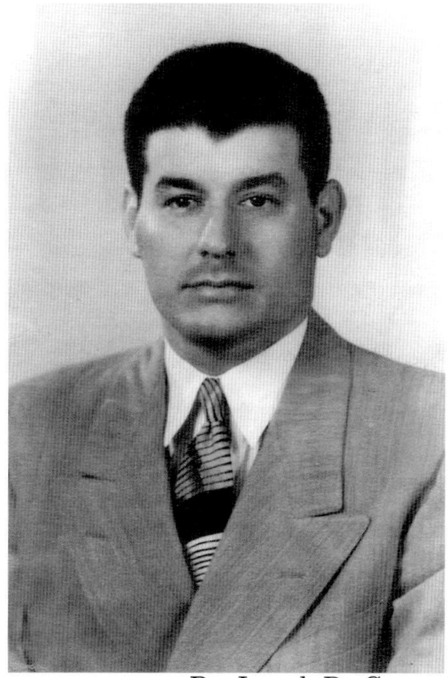

Dr. Joseph De Gasperi

In order to complete his training, the young doctor contacted Dr. John Matthews, and subsequently spent a year-and-a-half with Matthews who agreed to a preceptorship. Here De Gasperi learned how to handle private patients, take histories, and conduct preliminary examinations. In addition to Dr. Matthews' professional blessing, however, De Gasperi also received a recommendation to Dr. Donald Atkinson, the contemporary of Dr. John Burleson who belonged to San Antonio's first generation of ophthalmologists. Atkinson had prospered during World War II and developed an outstanding reputation as ophthalmology gained prominence after the war, drawing patients from all over South Texas. Now winding down his career, the older ophthalmologist used his influence to make his young partner highly successful and, in return, the young man introduced his mentor to equipment such as the streak retinoscope he had learned about in Chicago. The process was successful, and De Gasperi practiced for the rest of his career in San Antonio.

Dr. Joseph De Gasperi interview

## THE FIRST SOUTH TEXAS EYE BANK, 1965

With a growing professional community of specialists, San Antonio next acquired its first eye bank. In 1965, community ophthalmologists Dr. Jack B. Lee and James L. Mims, Jr. along with Dr. Dan Kendrick, helped Baptist Hospital administrator David A. Garrett to create the first "eye-banking service" for the residents of Central and Southwest Texas, the Baptist Memorial Hospital Eye Bank or Eye Bank at Baptist Medical Center, to supply eye tissue for corneal transplants. Dr. Mims's mentor, Dr. William Clark of Tulane, a former Secretary of the national Eye Bank Association, provided information and assistance for the effort. The new facility represented the combined efforts of the entire community, however, including volunteers and ophthalmologists from both civilian and military sectors of the city. Together, these individuals formed a committee and succeeded in obtaining approval for a San Antonio Eye Bank from the national Eye Bank Association. Among local ophthalmologists who served as board members were Dr. Charles Leone, Dr. Lydell Kiplin, Dr. Robert Snip. Initially, the South Texas Lions did publicity to develop support for the Eye Bank.

David Garrett interview, 1-31-91;
"The Eye," Encyclopedia of Medicine, 574;
"Eye Bank Gets First Donations," BMH Newsletter, June 1965 in Baptist Eye Bank Historical Information brochure, compiled February 1991.

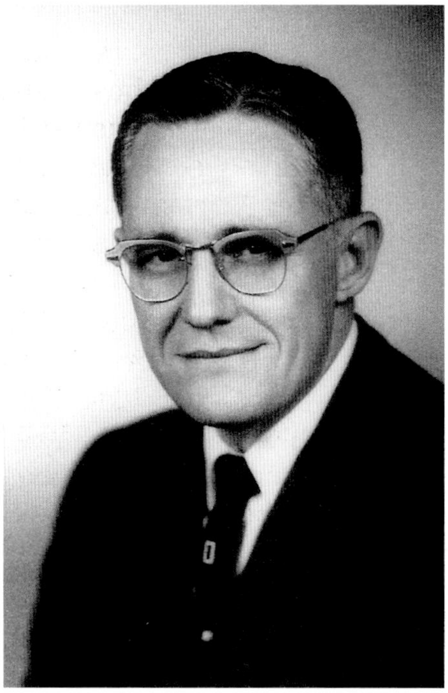

Dr. James Mims, jr., who together with Drs. Kendrick and Lee, helped create the first South Texas Eye Bank. Dr. Mims son, James Mimms III, followed his father's footsteps and became a pediatric ophthalmologist.

Blood banks had established a precedent for the idea of collecting and distributing materials from the human body some time earlier and organ transplants would begin roughly a decade later, but the nation's first eye bank was a product of the 1940s. The first effort to gather fresh eye tissue for use in sight-restoring corneal implant surgery began when Dr. R. Townley Paton, a corneal surgeon, obtained eye tissue from Sing Sing Penitentiary to help his patients with corneal blindness. Soon thereafter Paton founded the nation's first eye bank at the Manhattan Eye, Ear, and Throat Hospital. By the 1950s, most eye banks were located in university centers and efforts were being made to coordinate, accredit, and standardize eye banking practices. While eye banks are widely accepted today, early institutions met with public resistance. Success in creating an eye bank for South Texas required overcoming opposition to eye banking from the area's Hispanic and largely Catholic population, who resisted the practice based on religious beliefs. The Baptist Memorial Hospital Eye-Bank was the first institution of its kind in South Texas. As a service of the hospital laboratory, it also constituted the first effort in developing what by 1978 had become a more extensive facility known as the Eye Treatment Center for testing and treatment. One of every twenty blind persons in Texas was capable of regaining vision after a corneal transplant, but until this time the nearest eye bank was over 300 miles away.

Farge, 260-263;
"Eye Bank Anniversary," BMH Newsletter, May 1969;
"Ophthalmology Seminar Newsletter, September 1978.

Ophthalmologists did corneal surgery at public and private hospitals including teaching, federal, state and county hospitals. According to Baptist Eye Bank procedure, individuals who wished to donate tissue at the time of their deaths were matched with recipients in need of surgery anywhere in the United States. A nationwide network of amateur radio operators working with the American Association of Eye Banks worked to relay information about donors and recipients, and eyes were shipped in sterile cold containers by commercial airlines. Doctors later organized procurement centers at rural substations and the Department of Public Safety enlisted to transport tissue to the eye banks. Initially only whole globe donations were accepted and tissue had to be transplanted within twenty-four hours. Unlike other types of transplants, corneal replacements tended to be successful and could be repeated in cases of initial rejection.

David Garrett interview;
"Growth of a Service," typescript, Eye Bank Archives reprinted in the Eye Report, December 1984, 1-2

The Baptist Eye Bank helped old and young alike to receive the gift of sight, including mental patients at the Texas State Hospital and charity cases sponsored by Texas Commission for the Blind. By 1975 the number of donations had increased to fifty per year. Legislation in 1977 allowed corneal tissue to be retrieved from the Medical Examiner's Office, and eventually state legislation approved "*Routine Inquiry*" for donations at hospitals. Although ophthalmologists initially required only the transparent covering of the front part of the eye to replace the clouded tissue of the blind, they later acquired tissue for retinal detachment surgery and other operations. A close relationship developed with the South Texas Organ Bank and tissue was ultimately procured for research, pathological study, and teaching purposes. Diseased tissue sent to the medical center also was used for research purposes, and after 1988 all research tissue was distributed to the University of Texas Health Science Center ophthalmology department for their studies.

"Visions of Sight at BMH," BMH Newsletter, June 1967;
"Eye Bank at Baptist Hospital Celebrates Sixth Year," BMH Newsletter, May 1971.

Ultimately, the Eye Bank gave San Antonio the capacity to provide much-needed total eye care. As new technology became available for diagnosis and treatment, the Eye Treatment Center acquired instruments ranging from an ophthalmoscan for diagnosis to lasers for treatment. By 1969 the facility had a Zeiss Light Coagulator to prevent or repair retinal detachments, a SITE Unit to cut and remove part of the lens while keeping the eye inflated, an operating-room microscope and a tool for phaco-emulsification that enabled ophthalmologists to treat diseased lenses by disintegrating and removing them without damage to surrounding tissue. Ultrasound equipment diagnosed tumors, trauma, retinal detachments, vitreous hemorrhage and foreign bodies by producing an image of the eye on an oscilloscope recorded with a Polaroid camera. Dr. Stuart Terry was the first to use therapeutic ultrasound for treatment in Texas and lasers were used here before anywhere else in Bexar County. An Argon laser to treat diabetic retinopathy, YAG lasers and an intraocular argon laser were made available, and cryopexy instruments sealed retinal tears with intense cold. In 1976 Dr. Sheldon P. Braverman and Dr. John Y. Harper, Jr. donated the first automated vitrectomy unit in a San Antonio hospital for replacing the vitreous fluid filling the eyeball. A digital biometric ruler for mapping irregularities in the eye came a year later to help treat cataract patients, and a Micro-Vit unit for vitreous surgery. Use of advanced techniques and improved instruments furthered sub-specialization in cornea, retina, glaucoma, pediatrics and plastic surgery.

"Ocular Tonometer Installed," BMH Newsletter, March 1966;
"Equipped for Excellence," Tres, August 1986;
"Eye Care Combats Eye Disease," BMH Newsletter, February 1975

By 1980 the Baptist Eye Bank was one of seventy-five eye banks nationwide, had processed 155 corneas used by doctors throughout South Texas, received 165 donations, and performed 55 corneal transplants. Its services expanded into Mexico in the 1980s when doctors established a program with the Pan American Eye Bank Association to provide care in Monterrey, Mexico, and a satellite eye bank was established at Laredo's Mercy Hospital. Outreach eventually extended as far as an affiliated eye bank in Venezuela. By 1988 there were thirteen eye banks in Texas, including the one at Wilford Hall Hospital founded in 1970. It was estimated that over 280,000 persons had regained their sight as a result of this activity in the United States and Canada.

Karen May, "Sight Center," Tres, August 1986.

The definition and standardization of medical training to assure continuity in ophthalmological practice had been essential to the growth of the profession. The post-World War II realization that more uniform standards of training were needed, the Korean War, and simply an increasing cosmopolitanism in medicine increased the demand for better preparation and mobilized individuals to create residency programs. Ophthalmology residencies in South Texas developed in a unique way as military and community ophthalmologists worked together in close cooperation to produce not one, but three, programs before a medical school was established. The combination of military and community residencies at San Antonio, in particular, increased its influence as a regional medical center, hastened the acceptance of specialized medicine in rural areas, and helped routinize growth in ophthalmology in a way that enabled the profession to adapt more readily to change. The products of the three efforts, a generation of new ophthalmologists, added a new dimension to medical excellence in the region, and led to the development of resources such as the Baptist Memorial Hospital Eye Bank at San Antonio, and new federal support for medicine and the beginnings of Medicare in 1965 further emphasized the importance of specialists. With multiple hospitals, well-trained physicians, and growing resources, San Antonio was the logical place to locate other military and community medical institutions, and these would come in the years to follow.

Dr. Richard Ruiz interview, February 6, 1996;
David Garrett, "Growth of a Service," Eye Report, December 1984, 1-2.

# CHAPTER 11

## THE BEGINNINGS OF AEROSPACE MEDICINE AT SAN ANTONIO, 1950-66

*As man sought to fly like an eagle, he needed to see with an eagle's eyes.*

Thomas Tredici, M.D.

Before America sent its first astronauts into space, the strong relationships that developed between ophthalmology and aviation in two World Wars deepened in the 1950s and early 1960s. Reflecting on this history, Dr. Thomas Tredici, Senior Scientist, Aerospace Ophthalmology Branch, Brooks Air Force Base, Texas, and Clinical Professor, Department of Ophthalmology at the University of Texas Health Science Center in San Antonio, who spent over thirty years conducting visual experiments at San Antonio's School of Aerospace Medicine, said, "*As man sought to fly like an eagle, he needed to see with an eagle's eyes.*" Ultimately, efforts to achieve this goal also fueled the formation of new branches on the tree of ophthalmology. The added professional expertise that was required to facilitate adequate visual and other physical performance under extreme conditions above the earth's surface had made aviation medicine a separate field. Now, further progress in aviation science coupled with growing national concern about problems relating to thermonuclear warfare and new discoveries about how the eye functions in space fostered the development of a new sub-specialty field in ophthalmology. In part, at least, sub-specialization in ophthalmology may be viewed as an unintended consequence of the progress of military research at the School of Aviation Medicine.

A generation earlier, Dr. Donald Atkinson predicted that the future of medicine would see both a return to the family doctor and movement toward "ultraspecialization." At the time, the latter possibility so puzzled observers that one jokingly wondered if the zeal to specialize would eventually produce ophthalmologists who limited their services to treatment of the "*right or left eye*." What Atkinson could not foresee was that the demands of aviation and space flight would necessitate the further specialization he had predicted. The School of Aviation Medicine played a central role both in the emerging space program and in the history of ophthalmology. In the process of finding ways to improve human performance, ophthalmological research teams expanded vision science to meet the challenge of space flight by actually creating new ways of seeing.

Nineteenth-century practitioners succeeded in curing eye diseases and helping those who suffered eye injuries in the course of everyday living, but aviation demanded uses of natural vision that the ophthalmic pioneers scarcely could have imagined. Good depth perception and the ability to judge altitude helped in any takeoff and landing and good visual acuity and night vision were essential in wartime, but pilots had new needs as well. While airmen were regularly selected for the excellent quality of their vision and many pilots possessed the almost-perfect sight necessary to navigate the skies, coping with flash blindness, radiation, and the visual experience of space travel necessitated even greater visual capacity. Among those responsible for adding new dimensions to eye science were such experienced military ophthalmologists as Drs. Victor Byrnes, James F. Culver, and Thomas J. Tredici. Much as Ferdinand Herff advanced medicine on the Texas frontier, these individuals pioneered the development of the complex role that San Antonio ophthalmology played in the growth of the American space program.

Dr. Thomas Tredici interview;
Dammin, 1454-1471;
Peyton, Green, San Antonio, City in the Sun, 97-118.

## THE BEGINNINGS OF SPACE MEDICINE

If most Americans associate the U.S. National Aeronautics and Space Administration's (NASA) Houston Manned Spacecraft Center or Florida's Kennedy Space Center with the U.S. space program, fewer people are able to recognize the links that exist between South Texas and events leading up to the 1957 Russian Sputnik launch that began the Space Race. Long before NASA was founded in 1958 or completed its Houston headquarters, the School of Aviation Medicine in San Antonio served as the backbone of the nation's medical endeavors relating to preparations for the first manned space flight.

Alcott, Edward, Aerospace Medical Division, 19

Long before the drama of the Cold War space race began to unfold, the American Aeronautical Society set out in 1911 to obtain federal support for a national laboratory dedicated to space flight, resulting in the government's creation in 1915 of the National Advisory Committee for Aeronautics (NACA). While public feeling remained ambivalent about airplanes due to the high number of fatalities in World War I, NACA oversaw experiments in the 1920s to test airfoils and explore engine and other aviation design. Within a decade, however, the agency left safety and operations issues behind and began to consider questions of maneuverability, jet propulsion, high altitude function, and breaking the sound barrier. In medicine, corresponding activities to prepare for sending human beings into space began in 1917 when the War Department established a Medical Research Board to deal with issues of pilot fitness, and created the School of Aviation Medicine, which in 1925 adopted as its motto the phrase "Volanti Subvenimus," or "We support the flyer."
Bilstein, 1-15;

Air Training Command, Aerospace Medical Center, ii;
Ashcroft, Bruce A., "A Brief History of the School of Aviation Medicine with an Emphasis on the Randolph AFB years, 1931-59"

By the end of World War II, however, a new agenda had developed, and officials acknowledged that Texas, with its history of aviation research dating back to the time Ocker and Crane conducted local eye-related research in Texas when they informally consulted ophthalmologists following World War I, was the logical place to conduct the nation's aerospace enterprise. The classic motion picture Giant recalls the impact of airplanes on the lifestyles of Texas ranchers

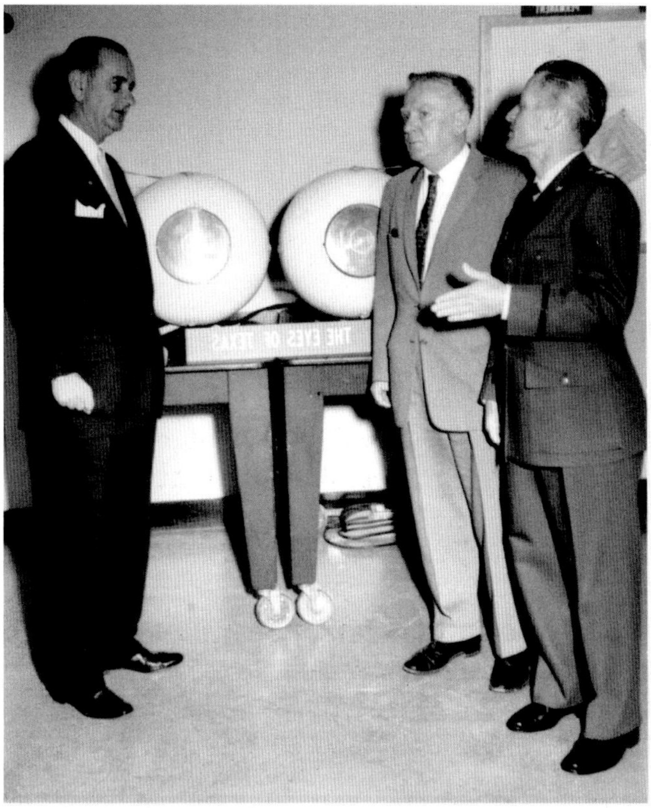

President Lyndon B. Johnson (L) visits the School of Aviation Medicine to meet Dr. Humburtus Strughold (C), and Major General Otis Benson (R), Commander. Dr. Strughold became known as the "father of space medicine."

and oilmen after World War II when personal aircraft replaced the railroads as a basic means of transportation. Bic Benedict and his family in that film went from horseback to airplane in a single generation. Businessmen quickly learned to fly to cover the state's vast territory and reach its financial centers in Houston and Dallas. Texans started a host of airlines, and the coming of aviation "ushered in a new saga of manufacturing in Texas." World War II made the state a cradle for the birth of the nation's aerospace industry by concentrating resources and operations at Texas military posts, and by the time it was over Texas had leaders capable of winning in the political competition for national resources. In the 1950s, Texas politicians succeeded for the first time since Reconstruction in winning national office and bringing federal support back to the region. Lyndon Baines Johnson's presence in Congress was instrumental in making the School of Aviation Medicine at Randolph Air Force Base the nation's sole training center for flight surgeons and a major player in the space program. Two years after the Air Force became an autonomous branch of the armed services in 1947, the task of developing aptitude tests for pilots was assigned to the Human Resources Research Center at San Antonio's Lackland Air Force Base. It is no mere coincidence that in 1958, when Airman Donald R. Farrell emerged after seven days of testing human reactions to space conditions in SAM's tiny "*space cabin simulator*," the man who greeted him was Lyndon Johnson. The

National Aeronautics and Space Administration (NASA) found its home in Texas partly because of Johnson's zeal and interest. At every stage in these advances, moreover, ophthalmologists had served as essential, if silent, medical partners.

Barksdale, 1; Bilstein, 1-15

## PROJECT PAPERCLIP

In 1941, the School of Aviation Medicine created an independent Research Division with an ophthalmology department, and in 1943 a new Medical Research Laboratory was established that became a natural gathering place for the nation's aerospace scientists. In particular, the U.S. government effort known as "Project Paperclip"--the "*brain drain*" project that brought some of the finest European researchers to the United States--sent a number of German scientists to the Eye Department in the 1950s. Echoing nineteenth-century immigration patterns that had brought large numbers of Europeans to South Texas, twenty-five scientific experts from Germany were split between the nation's primary military medical research facilities, including School of Aviation Medicine, the Aero-Medical Laboratory at Wright-Patterson in Ohio, and the Navy School of Aviation Medicine. Among those who joined the ophthalmology department at San Antonio and later became United States citizens were color-vision expert, Dr. Ingeborg Schmidt, and Dr. Heinrich Rose, the man who had been in charge of the eye department for the Luftwaffe at SAM's German equivalent during World War II. Dr. Paul Cibis, later a retinal specialist at Washington University in St. Louis, was also among them. This outstanding group participated in a wide range of studies that grew out of war-related interests, but also enjoyed a common interest in vision outside the boundaries of normal physiology. Soon, they were busily engaged in research on human adaptation to new environments, including those in space.

Cibis' son, Gerhart, and his daughter, Andrea, also became ophthalmologists. Dr. Schmidt later moved to the University of Indiana and Dr. Rose to Stanford.

Dr. Hubertus Strughold interview with Ingrid Kokinda, April 5, 1982;
Ashcroft, Bruce, "A Brief History of the School of Aviation Medicine," 5-6;
von Braun, Werner and Frederick I. Ordway, III, 163-4

Another Project Paperclip scientist, Dr. Hubertus Strughold, had come to the United States before World War II at the invitation of the Rockefeller Foundation to study the effects of oxygen deficiency on the heart, but returned to Germany's Aero Medical Research Institute sometime between 1935 and 1942. After becoming an American prisoner of war, Strughold was subsequently relocated to the School of Aviation Medicine and assigned to the Department of Ophthalmology, a decision that reflected his interests in vision studies. Like both Helmholtz and William Ocker, who made major contributions to ophthalmology but were not ophthalmologists, Strughold was a physiologist and an M.D. While he lectured on flight physiology and experimented on alternative pressures for use in airplane cabins, sensory perceptions, and nerve reactions to flight conditions, Strughold also studied the effects of airplane environments on the eyes. Because he had received a retinal burn when he looked through smoked glasses at the solar eclipse of 1910, he volunteered as a guinea pig in the first experiment that televised a picture of the retina, a technique that became known as "*intraocular television*."

Strughold, Dr. Hubertus interview with Ingrid Kokinda, April 5, 1982;
Dr. Thomas Tredici interview

Years before the historic Sputnik flight of 1957, Dr. Strughold wrote an important article entitled "Where Does Space Begin" that delineated the relationship between the earth's atmosphere and space. In addition, the article "*set forth a clear and comprehensive sequence of human problems in space flight to be resolved by medical science*." Space flight was defined as travel within the atmosphere between twelve and 120 miles up; until 1956, no human being had flown above twenty-four miles. Strughold also wrote one of the first theoretical works on space medicine, entitled <u>The Principles of Aviation Medicine</u>, in which he established paradigms that dictated a new focus for ophthalmological research. On February 9, 1949, roughly three months after a scientific meeting on the "*Aero Medical Problems of Space Medicine*" at Randolph Air Force Base, School of Aviation Medicine officials founded the world's first "*Department of Space Medicine*" and appointed Strughold the first Chief of the new department. In this position, he swiftly redirected the research agenda, began to lay the foundations for the man-in-space program and, in time, came to be known as the "*Father of Space Medicine*."

The scientific meeting on aeromedical problems of space medicine was held

November 10, 1948. The meeting was co-sponsored by the Lovelace Foundation of Medical Education and Research, founded by Dr. W. Randolph Lovelace II, who also had connections with South Texas. Lovelace, a flight surgeon and pilot, had graduated from SAM, worked as part of a Mayo Clinic research team, and then created the Lovelace Foundation for Medical Education and Research in Albuquerque, New Mexico, to conduct research on the medical problems of flight.

Air Training Command, Aerospace Medical Center, 1;
Peyton, Green, San Antonio, City in the Sun, 97-118;
Peyton, Green, 50 Years of Aerospace Medicine, 1968, 151;
Ashcroft, 59)

Given the strength of operations in San Antonio, the first plans formulated for NASA envisioned an engineering facility for which the School of Aerospace Medicine at San Antonio would provide all necessary medical assistance. Just as the U.S. Army recognized that it had "*an excellent source for research in aviation medicine*" where medicine might move from a clinical to a laboratory setting and researchers gain access to a patient population with the highest visual potential, not sick patients but healthy individuals who could demonstrate optimal levels of human performance-- planners realized that aeromedical research had been conducted in San Antonio for some time already and a distinguished team of doctors and scientists had been assembled there. The public became aware that important things were happening when the School of Aviation Medicine co-sponsored a Symposium on the Physics and Medicine of the Upper Atmosphere that brought four hundred scientists, engineers, and international authorities in the physical and biological sciences to the Alamo City to discuss space flight. In November 1951, the event was opened to the press, allowing public attention to focus for the first time on the possibilities of flight outside earth's atmosphere.

Peyton, Green, 50 Years, 155-56;
Benford, Robert J., 258;
Alcott, Edward, Aerospace Medical Division, 30-31;
Alcott, Edward, "Brief History of Brooks Air Force Base"

Among scientists who attended the program at downtown San Antonio's Plaza Hotel were rocketry expert Wernher von Braun; James A. Van Allen, the discoverer of radiation belts in the earth's magnetic field and later a professor at the University of Iowa; Fred L. Whipple of Harvard University's Department of Astronomy; radiation expert Titus Carr Evans; and Brussels solar physics authority Dr. Marcel

Nicolet. Their counterparts from the School of Aviation Medicine included German scientists Konrad J.K. Buettner, ophthalmologist Paul Cibis, and ENT specialist Paul Campbell, then serving as the School of Aviation Medicine's Director of Research. Among other scientific celebrities, the 250 Air Force, Navy, Army and civilian specialists who came included test pilot Major Charles E. Yeager, the first American to break the sound barrier in 1947. Journalists from *Collier*'s magazine, the *Reader's Digest*, *The Saturday Evening Post*, and a number of metropolitan dailies assured that news of the event reached the public beyond San Antonio. Discussion topics ranged from cosmic rays to the design of space ships and everything from pumpkins as the logical crop to cultivate in space gardens to questions about visual responses in space. The importance of the meeting, however, lay in the public recognition it generated for the School of Aviation Medicine as the national institution most closely linked with the excitement, mystery and romantic promise of space flight until the completion of NASA facilities almost a decade later. Henceforth, the School would be associated less with defense-related efforts than space flight and medical activity conducted there would be less concerned with warfare than humanitarian purposes.

Peyton, Green, 50 Years, 154-7;
San Antonio Express coverage, November 6-9, 1951

By 1959, when the Aerospace Medical Center moved back to Brooks Air Force Base, a foundation for space flight had been established. Center Commander Major General Otis O. Benson, Jr. could say "*If we were asked right now to provide a livable cabin for a craft built to operate in outer space, we could write specifications which the engineers would be able to meet.*" Quoting Dr. Strughold, who claimed that an American ship could land on the Moon in five years, an observer wrote that the idea rested on "*a solid bulwark of scientific fact, most of which was established through research carried on for more than ten years at the School of Aviation Medicine.*" The same observer also noted that the School provided "*specialized medical practice*" to treat flying personnel with difficult, obscure, or borderline diagnostic problems that affected their flying status, a reference in part to ophthalmology as one of six sections making up the School's Clinical Medicine Department. Coupled with the objectives of space flight, SAM ophthalmologists were in an ideal position to widen the base of the science, open new avenues of research, and, ultimately, to develop levels of knowledge that would constitute the basis for sub-specialties in the

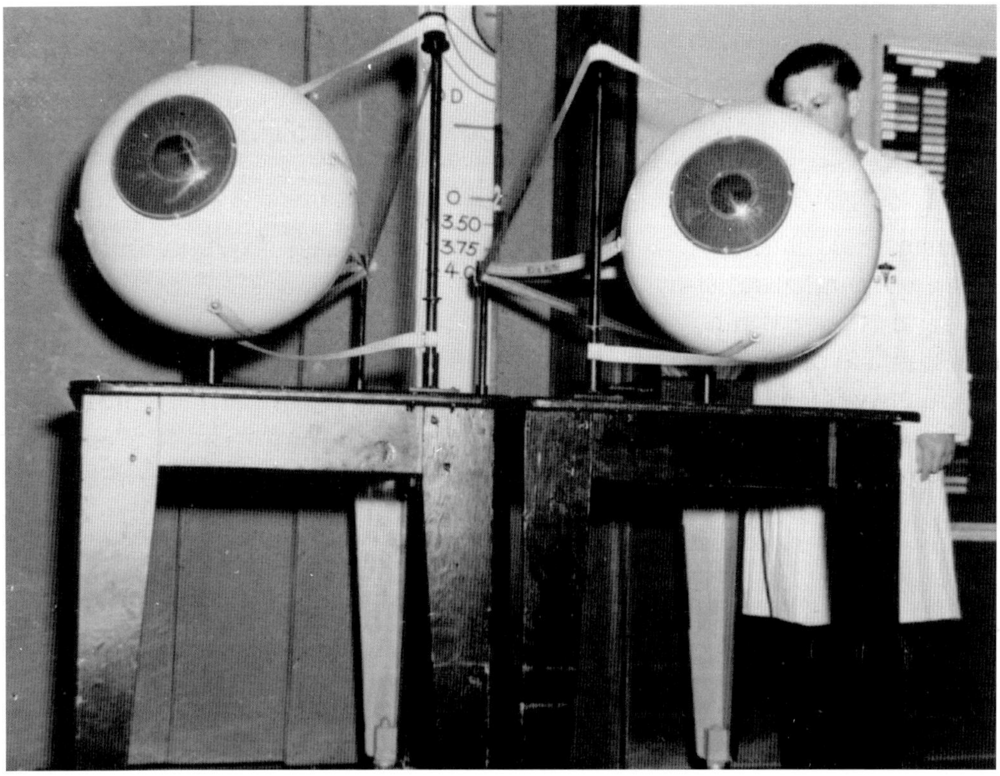

The School of Aviation Medicine model to study and teach about the muscle disorders during flight.

field. The School moved into 36 existing buildings and hangars at the Brooks site, and a research institute, academic building with 16 classrooms, altitude laboratory to house pressure chambers and a human centrifuge, flight medicine laboratory, and various research components, television studios, and support services were constructed as well. Soon thereafter, the School also established links with the hospital at Lackland AFB for use as a teaching facility.

Air Training Command, Aerospace Medical Center, 1, 5;
Ashcroft, Bruce, 8;
Alcott, Edward, Aerospace Medical Division, 19

## SAM RESEARCH PROJECTS IN THE 1950s

School of Aviation Medicine researchers initially focused on the problems of World War II pilots reported by flight surgeons and sought applications of this research in domestic contexts. After 1950, attention shifted to the threat of thermonuclear war and investigations relating to space travel that raised the possibility of enhancing normal visual capacity. Dr. Victor Byrnes, who oversaw the work of up to fifty people and dozens of research projects, laid the foundation for research on muscle disorders, the relationship between psychological factors and vision, training to perceive objects more rapidly, reaction time, color vision, and innovations with implications for transportation, traffic signals, airplanes and other vehicles. Byrnes also shared information with the wider medical community by participating in early efforts at international scientific cooperation, being active in numerous ophthalmological organizations at home, and lecturing to ophthalmologists in Europe.

Dr. Thomas Tredici interview

As School of Aerospace Medicine researchers and their Project Paperclip counterparts began to consider the requirements for space flight, ophthalmology researchers adopted a new mission not only to maintain pilots' visual performance and keep highly trained fliers in the air, but to compensate for their vision defects, improve their capacity to perform at supersonic speeds and high altitudes, and help them adapt to new environments. Pursuit of these objectives led to the development of a motion-parallax tester that measured candidates' potential for flight training and answers to a key challenge to ophthalmology in the atomic age, the need to know more about the visual effects of thermonuclear explosion and the use of rocketry.

Byrnes biographical records;
"Research, Development Keep Brooks AFB Busy, 84-P

The National Institutes of Health at Bethesda, Maryland, already had test-fired biological experiments in V-2 rockets at the White Sands Proving Ground near Alamogordo, New Mexico, and the Aero Medical Laboratory at Wright-Patterson Air Force Base in Ohio had sent mice and Rhesus monkeys aloft there. Now SAM conducted experiments at White Sands to study the visual aspects of everything from ultraviolet light and G forces to instruments for movement detection. Air Force officials needed to know how much efficiency pilots might lose should an atom bomb be unexpectedly detonated within their field of vision, producing a fireball. Assuming that an aircrew could not be adequately shielded without some exposure to radiation, it was agreed that pilots should not be expected to fly this type of aircraft except in cases of extreme national emergency. Nonetheless, knowledge was essential since conditions might arise in which such flights would be needed. Observations made from these experiments gave rise to new discoveries with implications not only for space travel, military aviation, and all the armed forces, but for the ophthalmic profession as well.

Peyton, Green, 50 Years of Aerospace Medicine, 147-50

Within a few short years, SAM researchers produced nearly fifty publications on experimental and clinical ophthalmology dealing with the ocular effects of radiation, retinal burns, flash blindness, glaucoma and other concepts in aerospace medicine. The effort also produced several conferences on the subject of "*radiation cataracts*" and a tribute to Dr. Byrnes in the form of a certificate from his co-workers for membership in the "*Royal Order of Radiated Desert Rats*." Byrnes summarized what was known about the results of such effects on humans in a paper entitled "*Human Chorioretinal Burns from Atomic Fireballs*," while another paper on "*Chorioretinal Burns Produced by Atomic Flash*," recorded the results of animal studies in Project Upshot-Knothole, an experiment used to test the response of 700 pigmented rabbits to six atomic detonations at the Nevada Proving Grounds in 1953.

Byrnes biographical records

Scientists learned that the human eye sustained its greatest injury from retinal burns by gathering energy at great distances from a thermonuclear explosion. This type of injury could occur up to 300 miles from ground zero. Pilots would need protection against intense light within extremely minute periods of time, much shorter than the blink reflex. The intensity of radiant energy released at detonation of an atomic bomb in the form of infrared and visible light is extremely high. It is a physical agent with which ophthalmologists are familiar because it produces the well-known eclipse burn of the retina. It is this infrared and visible light which produces the atomic chorioretinal burns. The pigment of the retinal epithelium and choroid was the principal site of absorption of the energy from atomic flash which produced intraocular lesions. In the atomic burn most of the energy is delivered so rapidly as to be almost instantaneous, thus giving no opportunity for vascular dissipation and very little for dissipation by conduction. In addition, it may well be delivered through the widely dilated pupil occurring at night that admits roughly 50 times the energy passed by the small pupil in the same period of time.

Byrnes, Col. Victor A. et al., 1-8

To solve the problem, the School of Aviation Medicine Ophthalmology Department, in cooperation with the Department of Radiobiology, designed an experiment that was known as Operation Snapper to simulate what would happen if a bomb were detonated during daylight hours. Teams of physicians made photo stress tests to determine how long it would take to recover from the intense light that produced flash blindness and began to explore the hazards of radiation in space. Other researchers conducted tests and evaluated protective filters. In Project Upshot-Knothole and other experiments, animal subjects were placed in a light-tight trailer where different types of shutters and protective lenses could be placed over their eyes, some transmitting less that a fraction of the light passing through them. Red-lighted aircraft instruments called nyctometers along with scotometric devices and other types of examiners installed in the vehicle measured the animal's responses.

Air Training Command, 27;
Byrnes biographical records

Aware that exposure to radiation produced cataracts, Dr. Heinrich Rose conducted experiments to measure the thresholds at which cataracts would be produced and the doses necessary to induce them and others that simulated the retinal lesions caused by atomic explosions using a heliostat to focus rays of the sun. These data were then compared with others compiled by researchers at Stanford University. Researchers at SAM used Strughold's description to set up a Los Alamos project with the help of William Ham, Col. John E. Pickering, David V.L. Brown, and G.C. Bahn there to study the cataractogenic effects of fast neutrons on monkey eyes in an effort to develop possible defenses. Other ophthalmological studies "rode piggyback" on thermonuclear explosions at Christmas Island in the Pacific, allowing researchers to test equipment and gather data from other animal experiments.

Byrnes, 351-364

One result of this testing was a remarkable observation, published in 1955, worthy of being expressed in the researchers' own words, foreshadowing an important windfall for the public:

*The clinical observation of a sharply circumscribed coagulated area in the fundus, together with the pathological finding of solid fusion of the retina, choroid, and sclera, immediately suggested the use of visible and infrared radiations as potential agents in the therapy of such intraocular diseases as retinal detachments, small malignant growths, retinal cysts, and the like. Such small areas within the eye could be coagulated by the focusing of large amounts of radiant energy. Technically the procedure is entirely feasible. Radiation from a carbon arc concentrated by means of lenses will give sufficient energy per unit area. The direction of the beam could be controlled under direct vision by means of partially transmitting mirrors. This method offers the advantage of making unnecessary such surgical procedures as the opening of Tenon's capsule, tenotomy, and perforation of the globe.*

Byrnes, 10

A USAF arc lamp was given to researchers Drs. William Hamm and Dupont Guery at the Medical College of Virginia for such experimental work. Other researchers, focusing on the problems of radiation and space travel, developed experiments requiring extended time in space. Some of their experiments fired monkeys downrange to determine the effects of space flight and consider the impact similar experiences might have on human subjects. Projects conducted in close communication with military flying units to investigate eye problems caused by flight at supersonic speeds and under G forces led to the discovery of a hazard in the lag in visual perception that occurs between the time an event takes place and the time it registers mentally. The results of these experiments resulted in a paper by Dr. Victor Byrnes entitled "*Visual Problems of Supersonic Speeds*," along with several technological applications for general vision. In 1953, Byrnes' connection with SAM ended for a time when he left to become Deputy Surgeon of the United States Air Forces in Europe and Consultant to the Eye Service at the principal American hospital in Europe at Wiesbaden, but his connection with San Antonio was not yet finished.

Dr. Victor Byrnes, Richard Fixott interviews

In Byrnes absence, ophthalmic researchers devised equipment to protect pilots from flash blindness and radiation and methods to measure the impact of a nuclear blast on pilots' ability to fly. In 1958, the year NASA was created, the Zeiss Corporation began production of a device to coagulate light for the treatment of retinal disease known as the Zeiss photocoagulator under the guidance of Dr. Meyer-Schwickerath of Essen, West Germany. Related research produced improved aviator sunglasses and these, in turn, led to the manufacture of better civilian sunglasses. Meyer-Schwickerath later served as a professor of ophthalmology at Essen.

Byrnes biographical records

Impressed by advances in Texas, the U.S. government acknowledged the School of Aviation Medicine's achievement by adding to its resources. To increase its capacity to conduct advanced research, construction began in 1957 on a complex of laboratories and offices that eventually housed research, teaching, and clinical treatment operations just as Randolph became the world's largest training system and the Air Training Command Center. Until the creation of NASA, "*the laboratories at Randolph entertained a constant stream of visiting newsmen, feature writers, film and television producers, and authors of books and magazine articles, often from abroad, in search of material on the technical and human aspects of flight beyond the atmosphere.*" SAM now became the only Air Force unit to provide medical care and clinical evaluation of flyers, a group soon to include astronauts when NASA founded its headquarters in South Texas.

"Randolph AFB celebrates 60th Anniversary This Year," San Antonio Express News, June 24, 1990, 25-R;
Alcott, Edward, Aerospace Medical Division, 25-30

## NATIONAL AERONAUTIC AND SPACE ADMINISTRATION (NASA)

After President Dwight D. Eisenhower signed the bill that launched NASA in 1958, the national space program officially "got off the ground" when space scientists targeted a lunar landing as their goal. A year later NASA began its first aeronautics and space flight operations, and the School of Aviation Medicine moved to its original location at Brooks Air Force Base to concentrate on the medical aspects of space flight under a new name as the School of Aerospace Medicine. As the 1960s began, a new Aerospace Medical Division emerged from the combination of the Aerospace Medical Center and a group of other laboratories. With the help of now Senate Majority Leader Lyndon B. Johnson and Texas Congressman Paul Kilday, SAM underwent a series of reorganizations that created the United States Air Force Aeromedical Center at Brooks Air Force Base with jurisdiction over a number of subordinate institutions around the country including Lackland Hospital (later Wilford Hall Medical Center) and the Air Force Epidemiology Laboratory as well as the Medical Service School at Gunter AFB, Alabama, plus the arctic laboratory in Alaska. At the new site, the five buildings making up the School included a research institute, an academic building with classrooms and an auditorium, an altitude laboratory with pressure chambers, a flight medicine laboratory, and other support services and research areas. After flying activities on the base ceased in 1960, thirty-six of the existing buildings and hangars at Brooks housed offices, labs, and equipment. With the 1,000-bed hospital at Lackland AFB nearby serving as its teaching facility, the School was ready to begin training astronauts and attendant medical personnel. Here it would continue its "*transition from a flight-training base to a center for medical research, development, and education*" with an expanded staff of physicists, psychologists and other scientists.

Ashcroft, Bruce, 8-9;
Alcott, Edward, Aerospace Medical Division, 19-30

In 1959 research adviser Dr. Hubertus Strughold moved to Brooks, where he developed a new terminology for life in space including the terms "*spatiography*" to refer to the geography of space, "*bioastronautics*" to contemplate the effects of space travel on man, and "*gravisphere*" to connote the places influenced by the gravitational field of a body. Physical plant improvements allowed SAM researchers to study ergonomics, or human reactions in extreme conditions, and attracted an increasingly high level of research staff. In 1959 the Space Medicine Department comprised three sections dealing respectively with weightlessness, effects on the body, and instruments. The physiology building had acquired a centrifuge that simulated conditions above 15,000 feet where temporary blindness resulted from G forces and, for pilots to survive, oxygen and pressurization were necessary, while altitude chambers and hypo and hyperbaric chambers allowed scientists to study human reaction to conditions from 400 feet under the sea to outer space. A separate laboratory dedicated to the study of night vision and a program known as "*Dyna-soar*" to plan and develop an aerodynamic spacecraft that could be fired into space aboard a Titan missile, much like today's space shuttle, also came to San Antonio.

Alcott, Edward, Aerospace Medical Division, 34; Pisano, 8T

From the beginning, NASA relied on the School of Aerospace Medicine for medical advice and personnel. Officials transferred the job of "*conducting medical examinations and developing medical standards for the first Air Force astronauts*" from Wright Patterson to San Antonio. The choice of the first seven astronauts was based on visual evaluations of 162 original candidates by SAM ophthalmologists. Some personnel, however, went to Houston, including a lieutenant colonel trained at SAM: Dr. Charles Berry. After resigning his Air Force commission to go to NASA, Berry became one of the first physicians to care for the astronauts. Because NASA initially intended to "*manage the American space effort as a civilian agency*" and was "*interested in creating a civilian atmosphere*," personnel like Berry at first wore business clothes rather than uniforms to create a more "*civilian atmosphere*." According to those at SAM, these individuals "*took off their blue Air Force uniform and went downtown and bought a blue blazer*."

Dr. Thomas Tredici interview;
"Aviation in Texas"; "Aerospace Medicine," "Air Force," "Brooks AFB,"
New Handbook of Texas

Dr. James F. Culver, an ophthalmologist who returned to the Air Force at the invitation of General Otis Benson to take the aviation medicine course, became the School of Aerospace Medicine's Chief of Ophthalmology and senior instructor just as activity at NASA commenced. Later he was named Assistant Director of Research and Development and Deputy Surgeon General for Operations and Commander of the Air Force Medical Service Center/Aerospace Medical Division. At Brooks until 1966, Culver found himself in what he described as "*the most exciting time in my life*," dealing with the medical problems of flyers and training flight surgeons and nurses.

Working in conjunction with Project Paperclip scientists, Culver helped to develop everything from dark glasses to windscreens, closure techniques using a "*picket fence*" effect, and photochromic dyes.

Drs. James F. Culver, Richard Fixott interviews

Under Dr. Culver's leadership, the School of Aerospace Medicine designed contact lens fitting and fabricating components initially to solve the problems of pilots, but that eventually led to a new technology for public use. While Dr. Heinrich Rose developed a type of contact lenses suitable for use in full pressure suits, Dr. Hubertus Strughold published a paper entitled "*Investigations on the Usefulness of Contact Lenses in Flight*" and in 1961 Culver wrote another on "*Contact Lenses for Flying Personnel*" that was printed in the Aeromedical Digest. This research benefited not only America's newest pioneers, the astronauts, but the

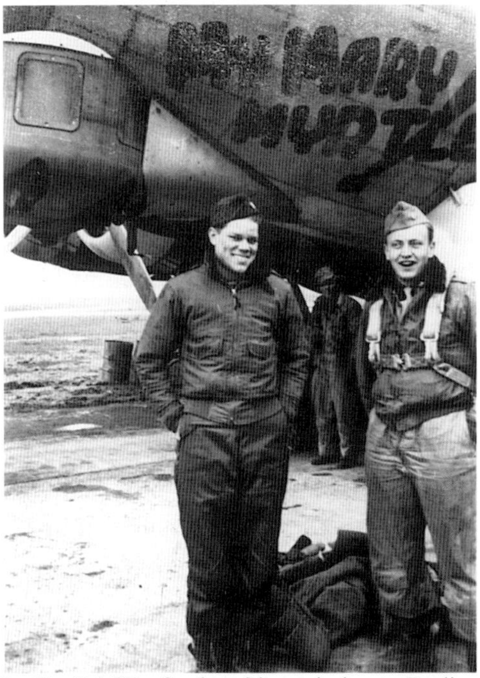

Lt. Tredici (R) after bombing mission to Berlin in 1945 in his "My Mary Myrtle" with 2nd Lt. John Seef (L).

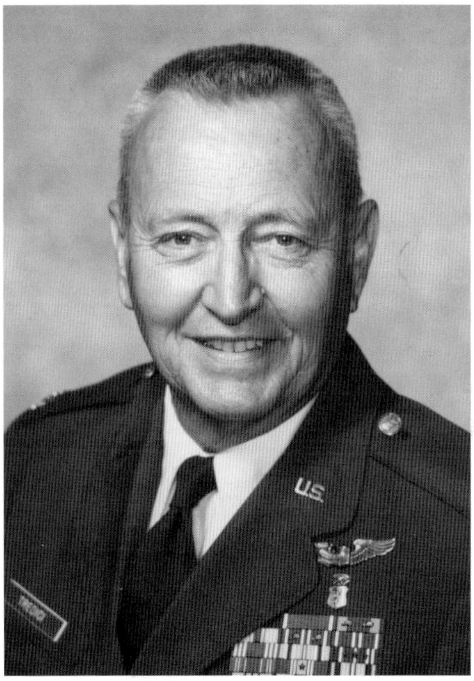

Colonel Thomas J. Tredici, M.D.

surrounding community as well when physicians at SAM communicated their discoveries to their counterparts in local practice.

Bexar County Medical Society records;
Culver, Brigadier General (Dr.) James F., USAF Biographical Sketch, 1980;
Culver, James F., "Contact Lenses for Flying Personnel, "Aeromedical Digest 12 (7 July 1961.

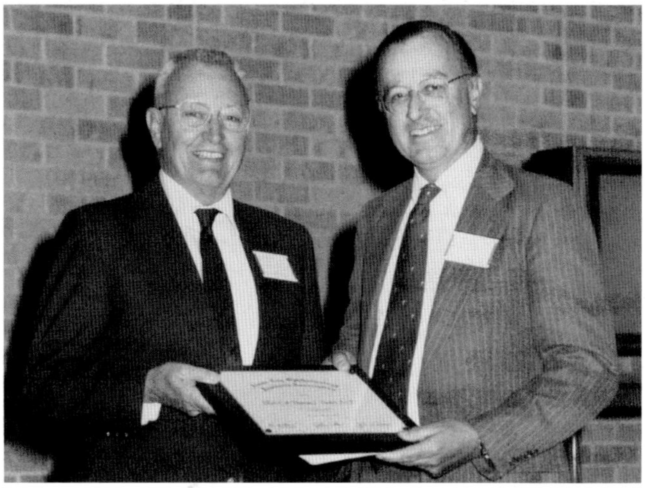

Dr. van Heuven honors Col. Tredici with the A.C.O.R.A. Award.
The citation reads:

*Dr. and USAF Colonel (Ret.) Thomas J. Tredici, the members of the Alamo City Ophthalmology Residents Association honor you today as a person who has contributed greatly to Texas ophthalmology in all its aspects.*

*As a soldier and pilot during World War II, you were where the action was, taking the ultimate risk to save America and its educational institutions, which are the backbone of our democracy. As a teacher, your enthusiasm continues to inspire many, including ophthalmic technicians, flight surgeons, residents, fellows and your peers. As a researcher, you were the first to apply ophthalmic science to military needs, now even affecting civilian eye care and safety. As a doctor, you made excellence in patient care a priority while sacrificing personal monetary gain. As an adviser, your honesty and quick appraisal of complex situations, using common sense, has given you a reputation which our government has recognized.*

*As a success story, you represent the immigrant's dream of success in America where, as the son of Italian born parents, speaking only Italian in early childhood, you helped America win the war which threatened Western civilization. You then reached the highest honors in advanced education, became an innovator in research, a teacher of teachers and finally an adviser to government. We, the San Antonio students and teachers of ophthalmology, your chosen profession, honor you with the ACORA Award.*

For the Bexar County Medical Society, Colonel Culver also reported on "*Common Errors in Ophthalmologue Examinations of Candidates for Flight Training*".

Efforts to create lenses capable of protecting pilots against thermal flash led scientists to the discovery of photochromic dyes that changed color in milliseconds when exposed to light. Initially, efforts to paint the dyes on lenses proved unsuccessful, as did an electronic device that increased the density of the lens, but a later process that melted the substance and made it integral to the lens proved more effective. Polocoat, Inc. of Cincinnati, Ohio, held the patent for the process until Bausch and Lomb purchased it. This discovery eventually enabled the public to enjoy the benefits of light-sensitive sunglasses and also facilitated the design and manufacture of light-sensitive windows and related technologies.

Dr. Thomas Tredici interview

In addition to pursuing specific research problems, personnel of the Aerospace Medical Division also worked closely with NASA to develop the Gemini, Apollo, and other space programs. By this time, the School of Aerospace Medicine had acquired a host of elaborate facilities, including a Bioastronautics/Biodynamics Laboratory, Bionucleonics Laboratory, and more. NASA officials selected Dr. James Culver to become a member of its Bioastronautics Task Force in support of the Mercury and Gemini projects, and in this position he performed preflight and postflight ophthalmological exams on astronauts beginning with the first suborbital flight of Alan Shepard in 1961. As part of the surgical team that flew to Grand Bahama Island, Culver helped to set up the quonset hut where the astronaut underwent a post-flight exam after being picked up from his spectacular landing in the ocean.

"NASA Manned Space Center," Handbook of Texas;
Dr. Culver biographical sketch

At the dedication of Brooks Air Force Base in 1963, President John F. Kennedy acknowledged the importance of ophthalmology to America's space efforts before a crowd of 10,000:

*. . . medical space research may revolutionize the technology and the techniques of modern medicine. Whatever new devices are created to monitor our astronauts--to measure their heart activity, their breathing, their brain waves, and their eye motions at great distances and under difficult conditions- will also represent a major advance in general medical instrumentation.*

John F. Kennedy, Address at Dedication Ceremony,
Brooks Air Force Base, November 21, 1963;
"JFK's Visit to Brooks Recalled," San Antonio Express-News, November 1, 1987

San Antonio supported NASA's efforts again in 1962 when John Glenn prepared for his flight at Lackland Air Force Base and was examined there on his return. In that year, however, a new agreement transferred control of nearly all manned space flight and aerospace medical research from the jurisdiction of the Air Force to NASA. Thereafter, SAM joined other businesses conducting testing and research projects under contract with NASA and continued its vision research projects already underway. Technology firms soon ringed San Antonio military installations, but the School of Aerospace Medicine's importance to the American space program was still of sufficient magnitude that the Manned Orbiting Laboratory was transferred there in 1964. Among new local firms, a branch of Technology, Inc., originally founded in Dayton, Ohio, worked on blind flight problems and tested eyewear and lasers. Later renamed Krug Life Sciences, Inc., this enterprise developed a more permanent role by providing increasing scientific, administrative and maintenance support for NASA operations. By the 1970s, Krug had become part of TASC, a Boston company that took over local Air Force contracts and moved its headquarters to Houston.

Alcott, Edward, Aerospace Medical Division, 21, 34;
Ralph Allen, Ph.D., Technology, Inc. interview

## DR. THOMAS J. TREDICI

When Russia broke the moratorium on nuclear testing in 1962, the "*big project on flash blindness*" once again became a priority, causing Colonel James Culver to take two important steps. Returning to the project to initiate a new generation of research discoveries, he also invited Dr. Thomas J. Tredici to join the project in 1964, thereby beginning a long and fruitful association with the School of Aerospace Medicine. As clinical professor of ophthalmology responsible for eye pathology on the project, Dr. Tredici brought new expertise to the endeavor. At the same time, in the context of the region's history, Tredici was simply the latest in the long tradition established by Ferdinand Herff and other nineteenth-century immigrant physicians who brought new skills and knowledge to the region.

Like many a typical Texan, Thomas Tredici was the son of immigrants. His father and mother, Marino Tredici and Maria Pizzanelli, were Italians who had come to the United States from an area near Florence known as Pistoia and from a place near the marble centers of Tuscany. After settling in western Pennsylvania at a steel town called Monessen, the Tredicis welcomed their new son to the family in 1922. Tom went on to become the first member of his family to complete a college degree.

By the time Tredici arrived in Texas, he already possessed an outstanding medical reputation. In World War II he passed the entry examination despite his lack of a college education and joined the Army Air Corps Aviation Cadet Program in 1942. During the war, he flew 18 combat missions in B-17s, serving with the 457th Bomb Group of the Eighth Air Force. Inspired by watching the precision of the science practiced by flight surgeons, Tredici was attracted to medicine and decided to become an ophthalmologist. When the war was over, he not only took his chemistry degree *magna cum laude* at Washington and Jefferson College in Pennsylvania, but also was selected as a member of Phi Beta Kappa and in 1952 graduated from the University of Pittsburgh School of Medicine.

Dr. Thomas Tredici interview

Tredici came to Texas as one of seven or eight out-of-state members of a group of thirty-three interns at Fort Sam Houston's Brooke Army Hospital. He chose to return to the service because of his prior association with the military as a pilot, arriving when Brooke Army Hospital was filled with Korean War casualties. Beds filled with orthopedic patients in Annex 3 and 4 touched each other, while some unfortunates were confined to the porch. For the young man, however, these conditions offered a unique opportunity to work with difficult cases. Brooke Hospital and the Southwest, meanwhile, remained a world without air conditioning, dominated by ceiling fans and high ceilings. Living in hot second floor quarters at Fort Sam Houston, Tredici's wife Margaret (De Santis) Tredici, a former industrial nurse back in Pennsylvania, took their newly born son in the family's 1948 Chevy to downtown San Antonio and occasionally spent the afternoon staying cool at Joske's, the first air-conditioned building of its kind in the region.

Dr. Thomas Tredici interview

His internship completed, Tredici set off for a three-year residency at the University of Pittsburgh Eye and Ear Hospital and two years of service as Chief of Ophthalmology at Scott AFB, Illinois. He also served overseas as Chief of Ophthalmology at Clark AFB in the Philippines, where he handled patients from Southeast Asia, the 7th Fleet, Okinawa, and Saigon. He was still at Clark in 1961 when cases began to arrive from Vietnam after President John F. Kennedy sent advisors there. By now a seasoned practitioner with extensive experience, Tredici was selected in 1961 to attend the Air Force Command and Staff College at Maxwell AFB in Montgomery, Alabama, and then to complete a fellowship in ophthalmic pathology under Dr. Lorenz Zimmerman at the Armed Forces Institute of Pathology at Walter Reed Hospital (AFIP). This program was "*better*," he claimed, "*than anything in civilian education*," and he remained on the Walter Reed staff until 1964 when his expertise in ophthalmic pathology attracted Colonel Culver's attention and produced the invitation to return to the Southwest.

Dr. Thomas Tredici interview

When Dr. Tredici returned to San Antonio after the long hiatus, the "*age of air-conditioning*" had begun. By that time over 11,000 airplanes were registered in the state of Texas, of which only 141 were commercial aircraft. The scale of the Texas aviation interest was also measured by the fact that 31,373 Texans with flying skills held pilot's licenses that year, and active airports across the state numbered 812. The School of Aerospace Medicine, which had come to enjoy a certain celebrity among the public at large, now occupied a place in the vanguard of American space science as a formal program of space exploration got underway. In effect, the School of Aerospace Medicine had been "*elevated to the status of a national institution*."

Peyton, Green, Fifty Years, 157

In 1965 Dr. Tredici left for a tour of duty to Clark Air Force Base and Vietnam as the Air Force's only ophthalmologist in Southeast Asia; in 1966 he returned to SAM to continue his career as Chief of the Ophthalmology Branch at the USAF School of Aerospace Medicine when Dr. Culver left in that year. Working as a clinician and researcher, he was "*instrumental in establishing and implementing U.S. Air Force policy on glaucoma for aviators*." Other research work with the glaucoma group developed techniques and drugs that ultimately returned over 500 medically grounded aircrew members to the cockpit, including a method for detecting "*preglaucoma*" and selection of drugs to treat the disease better.

"Louis H. Bauer Founders Award," 759

As Tredici joined the flash blindness project, researchers began a series of experiments known as Operation Dominick that gathered a joint task force of eight scientists to study the retinal burns caused by thermonuclear explosion, but this time to test the use of a new technology associated with laser light. Using ten aircraft for altitude comparisons, researchers developed a model to predict the amounts of retinal burn experienced by pilots in different atmospheric conditions. Culver, Tredici, and the SAM research team established standards for the use of lasers, developed aiming devices, and defined necessary precautions for military operations in places where lasers might be used. Responding to the importance of the new technology, the School established a laser hazards laboratory at Building 803 in 1969, the first in the Department of Defense, and published the first laser health hazard handbook in the United States. Tredici helped to establish the laser laboratory, and aided in developing filters and other materials to protect the eyes from various wavelengths of intense laser light. In the area of radiation hazards, he also helped to develop a model to predict the effect of laser-induced flash-blindness on battlefield performance, and to write Air Force safety standards for individuals working with lasers in both military and domestic contexts.

Alcott, Edward, Aerospace Medical Division, 64, 139;
Dr. Thomas Tredici interview;
"Research, Development Keep Brooks AFB Busy," 84-P.

During this period, other SAM researchers tested visual problems that appeared at altitudes over 10,000 feet, including everything from the effects of sunlight on the eye to conditions that bleached eye pigments. Teams explored the experience of blackout under intense G forces that caused blood to drain away from the retina, resulting in loss of vision and a lag in visual perception when traveling at high speeds. The same Barany chair that led William Ocker to his discoveries about blind flying was used to test the flight disorientation and a phenomenon known as nystagmus in which the eyes move rapidly back and forth when middle ear cells are activated. Other efforts clarified the limitations presented by ocular disease in qualifying pilots for flying and aerospace duties.

Dr. Thomas Tredici interviews;
"Research, Development Keep Brooks AFB Busy," 84-P.

Under Tredici's direction, SAM researchers supplied data used to make visors capable of protecting astronauts from the ultraviolet energy present in space that were also made available to manufacturers of ultraviolet protective spectacle lenses. Another research group explored the use of hard contact lenses by aviators and their use in the treatment of corneal disease, returning an additional 225 aviators to service and making Dr. Tredici one of the nation's leading authorities on the use of contact lenses. In 1969 the first USAF aviator returned to the cockpit after cataract surgery, using contact lenses prescribed at Brooks. Dr. Tredici also explored the implantation of intra-ocular lenses in primates, a technique that eventually helped aviators and one astronaut to return to full flight status using these devices.

Culver, Tredici interviews;
"Louis H. Bauer Founders Award," 759

Construction of a clinical electrophysiology laboratory at the School of Aerospace Medicine in 1970, the first complete laboratory of its kind in the military, allowed ophthalmologists to make more definitive clinical diagnoses and resulted in the development of microminiaturized electronics to protect and monitor the health of astronauts during space flight. This knowledge generated hundreds of medical devices and techniques for saving lives and improving health care. Meanwhile, teams of space technicians, ophthalmologists, and other medical researchers produced heart pacers, patient monitoring systems, sensors to test for change in temperature, heartbeat, and blood pressure, simulators, and an aspirin-sized transmitter pill that could radio back information from deep within a subject's body.

Bilstein, 66-7;
Alcott, Edward, Aerospace Medical Division, 64, 89;
Dr. Thomas Tredici interview

When a new reorganization transferred SAM's flash blindness research and related projects to the Radiation Division in 1972, Dr. Tredici became involved with studies in the windscreen evaluation laboratory on visual distortions, made recommendations to aircraft windscreen manufacturers, and developed optical standards for bird-proof windscreens and polycarbonate spectacle lenses. LexanTM glass, transparent but capable of withstanding considerable physical force, was a byproduct of this research used to make multi-layered aircraft windscreens. Tredici also oversaw a 1970s study in conjunction with the U.S. Air Force Academy on orthokeratology, proving that this contact lens technique could not permanently alter a subject's refractive status. Dr. Tredici's discovery of the principal reason for failure of stereopsis in aviators, the phenomenon known as microstrabismus, led to the development of an ocular prism test to facilitate diagnosis. Other researchers worked on the minimum dosage of microwave energy an aircrew could receive safely and other effects of microwave technology. By 1976, research resulted in changing the 20/20 minimum vision standard without glasses for pilots to 20/50 visual acuity--correctible with a -1.25 diopter prescription--and also produced the design for a "trifocal" for pilots and other flying personnel that represented a further advance on more familiar bifocal vision enhancements.

Tredici, Thomas, "Aerospace Ophthalmology," 1-6

Among his numerous responsibilities, Dr. Tredici taught the ophthalmology component of the Primary Course in Aerospace Medicine, that was attended until 1996 by all NASA trainees. He also trained numerous servicemen who went to Wilford Hall for ophthalmology residencies and prepared ophthalmic technicians in the first military courses of their kind in the United States. Although he officially retired in 1987, the year in which the Aerospace Medicine Division changed its name to the Human System Division, Dr. Tredici was still training young ophthalmologists in 2000 and was part of a laboratory that provided clinical consultation for an average of 1,000 aviators a year to salvage the military investment in pilots trained at the cost of approximately one million dollars each. In addition, Tredici instituted a pre-clinical fellowship for flight surgeon trainees that staffed his department with ophthalmologists.

By 2000, after teaching 10,000 flight surgeons and lecturing classes of Residents in Aerospace Medicine and Advanced Aerospace Medicine International medical officer classes, Tredici rounded out his career as a contributor to a project dealing with refractive surgery in the aviator. Among other activities, he also initiated a project to train Branch Fight Surgeons in Aerospace Ophthalmology.

Dr. Thomas Tredici interview

In the 1980s, ophthalmic researchers at SAM also directed their attention to the field of chemical defense, and in 1982 cooperated with the AMD on a Military Space Biotechnology program using the space shuttle to conduct medical experiments. Early experiments tested visual function in response to astronauts' comments about both their increased and reduced ability to see in space, with the goal of predicting vision changes and developing methods to minimize them. In 1984 Dr. Tredici oversaw the creation of a night vision laboratory under the direction of Lt. Col. Bob Miller to study the medical and physiologic aspects of scotopic (night or rod vision as opposed to photopic or day vision) and mesopic vision that resulted in a publication of major importance, the first night vision manual for flight surgeons. Devices to permit night vision, Tredici indicated, were among the "*newest, most significant innovations used in flying during the last decade.*" Development of instruments relating to this project gave rise to a host of civilian applications.

Alcott, Edward, Aerospace Medical Division, 61;
Dr. Thomas Tredici interview; Tredici, Thomas, "Aerospace Ophthalmology," 1-6;
"Louis H. Bauers Founders Award, 759

When pilots complained that their lenses dried out in an aviation environment, researchers conducted new studies of soft contact lenses. Hypoxia, or insufficient oxygen to the cornea, was a problem, along with low humidity environments that made contact lenses uncomfortable, G forces that caused temporary loss of vision, and the physical effects produced by long term missions. Scientists developed new tools to simulate flight conditions, made statistical evaluations, and ultimately developed a biodynamics branch at SAM to study pilot responses and develop ways to compensate for temporary vision loss. Through systematic research, scientists explored all of the "parameters important in aviation," including humidity, long periods in space, types of lenses, size of lenses, cleaning systems, and more. By introducing flying personnel to the use of intraocular lenses, ophthalmologists returned numbers of aviators to flight duty after cataract surgery who would otherwise have been permanently grounded with loss of binocular vision, and in 1990 SAM published a book dealing with the medical management of combat laser eye injuries. Laser light, depending on the type of laser involved, clouded the cornea or permanently damaged the retina. Dr. Donald N. Farrer, a psychologist who specialized in vision and human perception, lab tested a specially tinted, laser-screening visor to protect pilots' eyes and worked to develop more effective cockpit canopies. In another vision-related area, Dr. Patrick O'Connor studied acephalgic migraine, a condition in which pilots suffered from the perception of auras and scintillations.

Tredici, Thomas J., Aerospace Ophthalmology, 1-6;
Pisano, Marina, 8-T

In the 1980s and after, the approximately 6,600 people of the AMD moved beyond abstract research and testing to develop a constant stream of new and innovative products. While work on laser protective devices continued at the Armstrong Aerospace Medical Research Laboratory, researchers developed a Visually Coupled System (VCS) technology that produced a Helmet Mounted Sight and Display to improve the aiming accuracy of weapons, shorten reaction times, and allow head tracking. This invention worked by projecting a sight reticle on the pilot's visor, measuring the line of sight of the reticule and transmitting the line of sight to aircraft subsystems. The display received video signals from the subsystems that allowed for the generation of an image on a small cathode ray tube and projection of the image to the pilot's eye. According to Dr. Tredici, future objectives for San Antonio's AMD research facilities in 2000 included the production of technologies required for manned systems in space, including space station design, improvements in human-machine performance, simulation, robotics, and remotely piloted vehicle control.

Dr. Thomas Tredici interview;
Alcott, Edward, Aerospace Medical Division, 96-9, 109

Over its long history, the School of Aviation and Aerospace Medicine trained nearly 20,000 physicians, including flight surgeons, residents in aerospace medicine, and allied medical officers in ophthalmology and the visual aspects of aerospace medicine. The proximity to unique cases and problems, the opportunity to concentrate on research, and the stimulus of national interest in developing applications at this institution reproduced the conditions that enabled the first doctors to specialize and produced new levels of professional expertise. General Otis Benson's creation of an Air Force aviation medicine residency program contributed to the growth of ophthalmology as a whole, and to the San Antonio community. Finally, the civilian impact of SAM research can be measured in the use of fluorescein angiography, photochromic lenses, color vision testers and other visual screening devices, new visual standards, sunglasses and contact lenses.

While research in and of itself was significant, however, the impact of San Antonio military medical research had been more far-reaching. If research had created new technologies and innovations, training programs in aerospace medicine fostered the growth of a new level of specialization in ophthalmology and produced the first ophthalmic sub-specialists. The next generation of ophthalmologists would specialize in fields including retina, vitreous, pediatrics, cataract surgery, motility, and more to bring new benefit to society as a whole. Among Tredici's students who entered sub-specialty fields were Dr. James Mims, III, who later specialized in pediatric ophthalmology at San Antonio, and Dr. David Epstein, who became a Harvard professor and glaucoma specialist at the Massachusetts Eye and Ear

Infirmary in Boston and later chairman at Duke. The School of Aerospace Medicine also trained numbers of sub-specialists who became area practitioners, including Drs. David Shacklett, Gene Kirby, David Tasker, Ward Heinrich, George Lowry, Jed Howard, Douglass Ivan, Lee Arnold, and Jack Muckleroy. By 1983, roughly twenty-five per cent of San Antonio's population was military. In addition to advances from military research, therefore, South Texas military medical facilities contributed numbers of community ophthalmologists to the field.

Benford, Robert J., 283; Bexar County Medical Society records.

## CHAPTER 12

# FROM WESTERN FRONTIER TO THE FRONTIER OF MEDICINE: THE UNIVERSITY OF TEXAS HEALTH SCIENCE CENTER DEPARTMENT OF OPHTHALMOLOGY AND THE SEARCH FOR NEW KNOWLEDGE, 1960-1990

*Thoroughly equipped laboratories, in charge of men thoroughly equipped as teachers and investigators, is the most pressing want to-day in the medical schools of this country.*

Sir William Osler, Aequanimitas

Between 1960 and 1990, the idea of creating The University of Texas Health Science Center at San Antonio (UTHSCSA) led to the construction of an institutional setting in which the integration of academic and clinical ophthalmology could be achieved and the first ophthalmic subspecialty training programs in South Texas begun. This chapter focuses on the roles played by outstanding eye specialists in these advances and the accomplishments of those who followed once the new regional educational and professional medical infrastructure was in place, including the beginnings of South Texas-based eye research, the growth and acceptance of sub-specialization, and the definition of new horizons for ophthalmology in the region.

Construction of The University of Texas Health Science Center at San Antonio (UTHSCSA), a thirty-year project that is still ongoing, created an impressive medical establishment that today includes the University of Texas Medical School with its Department of Ophthalmology and eighteen related medical institutions including a Dental School, Nursing School, six major hospitals, and, under Medical School supervision, the Robert B. Green Hospital in downtown San Antonio, now the Brady Green clinics. Built at a cost of over $560 million dollars, the Health Science Center complex in the 1980s had over 16,000 employees and housed 3,500 patient beds plus office space for physicians. In 1990, the UTHSCSA service area encompassed Bexar County and the surrounding counties of Kendall, Comal, Guadalupe, Wilson, Atascosa, Medina, Bandera and Kerr, extended as far as Val Verde, Edwards, Real, Kinney, Maverick, Dimmit, Zavala, Uvalde, Gillespie, Frio, La Salle, and Karnes counties, and provided treatment to a clientele of international patients as well. When Dr. David Hunter began YAG laser surgery at the Nix Hospital in the mid-1980s, South Texas ophthalmology no longer followed paradigms for medical practice that had originated elsewhere and, henceforth, knowledge propagated in the region as fast as it did in other places.

Matthews, Wilbur L., 27; John Matthews interview. The context in which the Health Science Center developed included Alcon Laboratories, Inc. of Fort Worth, the oldest U.S. eye preparation firm (established in 1947) which made 61 ophthalmic products by the late 1960s, and Professional Pharmacal Co., Inc. of San Antonio, that also produced eye-related pharmaceuticals.

Two special features characterized San Antonio and South Texas ophthalmology during this period. The first was a high density of skilled clinicians in local practice, including, late in the period, numbers of sub-specialists. According to Texas Medical Association statistics, San Antonio was one of four places in Texas with the highest concentration of eye specialists in 1966. Of approximately 400 ophthalmologists or eye, ear, nose, and throat specialists statewide, there were 19 ophthalmologists in San Antonio, 50 in Houston, 33 in Dallas, and 13 in Fort Worth. Professional organizations in the region included the Nueces County Eye, Ear, Nose and Throat Society; the Houston Ophthalmological Society; an Eye, Ear, Nose and Throat society in Fort Worth; the Academy of Ophthalmology and Otolaryngology in Dallas; and the Texas Society of Ophthalmology and Otolaryngology, a social and scientific organization made up of eye, ear, nose, and throat specialists. In South Texas, physicians created the Bexar County

Medical Society and the San Antonio Ophthalmological and Otolaryngological Society. Because this community would play a key role in the growth of the Department of Ophthalmology at the Health Science Center, a profile of some of its members may help the reader to better understand the professional forces that shaped it, including such "*representative men*" as:

*Dr. Thomas F. Hogan, Jr., a San Antonio native who established a practice at the Nix Building in 1956 and formed a partnership ten years later with Dr. Joe R. McFarlane. Following in the footsteps of his predecessors who had taken active roles in the community, Hogan became a member of the German Club, the Town Club, the Order of the Alamo, the Texas Cavaliers, and the Argyle Club. In 1970, with Dr. McFarlane and Dr. David M. Hunter, he opened a group practice known as Ophthalmology Associates of San Antonio. After traveling to Bern, Switzerland, to study the use of lasers for treating retinal diseases and glaucoma, Hogan and Hunter became the first South Texas physicians to use the YAG laser in the 1980s. In 1984, with John A. Evans and Aureliano "Bud" Urrutia, a general surgeon, Drs. Hogan, McFarlane, and Hunter formed the Physicians Group and acquired the Nix Hospital.

*Dr. Alfredo Trevino, Jr. attended Laredo Junior College, graduated from the Galveston Medical Branch, completed his training at Wilford Hall, and practiced in San Antonio for a time before moving back to Laredo in 1978.

*Dr. Ruben F. Salinas-Garcia was born in Nuevo Leon, Monterrey, attended the Colegio Justo Sierra there, and received his medical degree from the University of Nuevo Leon. After an internship at the Memorial Medical Center in Corpus Christi, he completed his residency at Vanderbilt University and postgraduate work at the Bascom Palmer Eye Institute before opening a South Texas practice at McAllen.

*Dr. David Dean Pfaffenbach, a neuro-ophthalmologist typical of area sub-specialists, had graduated from the University of Wisconsin, interned at Boston City Hospital, completed his residency at Johns Hopkins, and finished his postgraduate work at the Mayo Clinic.

Hunt, Harold E., "Ophthalmology in Texas," 67;
San Antonio Medical Society records.

Military ophthalmologists further enriched South Texas ophthalmology. As they had throughout the region's history, such men as the following added a dimension of expertise, experience, and wider perspective to the community:

*Dr. Daniel Lee Kendrick was born and educated in Virginia, interned at William Beaumont Army Hospital at El Paso and completed his residency at the Medical College of Virginia in Richmond, doing research at A.H. Robins, Inc. during the summers between his residency years. As earlier military doctors who served as vehicles for the transfer of medical expertise to the region, he subsequently joined the U.S. Army Medical Corps and spent the next five years in Japan and at DeWitt Army Hospital in Fort Belvoir, Virginia. He opened a San Antonio ophthalmology practice in 1965, and later entered into a partnership with Dr. James Mims, Jr.

*Dr. Robert William Wolters, a University of Texas at Austin graduate, earned a UT Dallas-Southwestern medical degree, interned at Galveston, and specialized in ophthalmology at the UT Health Science Center. After serving at an Air Force Dispensary and as a flight surgeon in Danang, Thailand, he returned as an instructor at the Bexar County Hospital and studied corneal disease before eventually moving to Colorado.

*Oklahoma native Dr. Doyle C. Leslie spent four years with the U.S. Marine Corps in the Pacific before enrolling at Stephen F. Austin and Southwestern and completing his internship at the VA Hospital in Dallas. In 1965 he came to San Antonio to begin an R.B. Green Hospital ophthalmology residency as preface to an Austin career.

*Dr. Emanuel Newmark, a New Jersey native and Rutgers graduate, spent three years at the University of Amsterdam in Holland tapping into international medical advances. Newmark then returned to Duke University, interned at George Washington University Hospital, and finished his ophthalmology residency at the University of Florida before coming to Brooke General Hospital in 1971.

*Dr. James Leroy Curtis arrived at Lackland Air Force Base in 1961 to study visual problems above 50,000 feet after training in the Midwest, conducting a general practice at Hill Air Force Base in Utah, and doing postgraduate work at Tulane. He also served as an ophthalmologist at Maxwell AFB in Alabama and at the USAF Hospital in Wiesbaden, Germany.

Bexar County Medical Society Membership Records

The second feature that made ophthalmology in San Antonio medically unique was the city's high number of eye residency programs. Though programs existed at The University of Texas Medical Branch in Galveston, at Baylor University College of Medicine in Houston, at Scott and White Memorial Hospital in Temple, and at the Southwestern Medical School through Hermann Hospital in Dallas, no other Texas city trained as many ophthalmology residents annually as did San Antonio. In fact, the city's three residency programs trained more ophthalmology residents per capita than any other place in the nation in this period. Each year, while only a single resident entered Scott and White's 3-year program, one San Antonio resident annually entered the R.B. Green Hospital program, two started at Wilford Hall, and two began at Brooke Army Medical Center. Typical of this group was Dr. Richard Doyle Swindle, a Pennsylvanian, who came with degrees from Princeton University and the University of Pennsylvania Medical School to complete his ophthalmology internship and residency at Brooke Army Medical Center. Coupled with the city's long tradition of successful eye specialists and active medical institutions, the eye residency programs created the kind of atmosphere associated with a major medical center.

William C. Lloyd, III, M.D. interview

Despite these conditions, however, the region continued to experience a shortage of ophthalmologists since military residency program graduates commonly left the state after their training. For South Texas ophthalmology to be fully developed, therefore, one important component of San Antonio medical infrastructure was still missing. The absence of a medical school meant that insufficient numbers of medical students could be trained to satisfy the region's need for eye specialists. Access to a basic medical education close to home, however, would not become a reality until a group of interested individuals, including such key ophthalmologists as Dr. John Matthews, developed a proposal to complete the constellation of area institutions.

William C. Lloyd, III, W.A.J. van Heuven interview

States outside of Texas commonly developed one or two medical schools, usually in major population centers along with a few others at private institutions of higher education. In all of Texas, however, only three medical schools granted medical degrees at the end of World War II. Twentieth-century North Texas, West Texas, and South Texas each defined separate regions with major cities and different identities, but only Baylor University, the University of Texas Southwestern Medical School at Dallas, and the University of Texas Medical Branch at Galveston provided a basic medical education. A South Texas medical school, in other words, was a logical outgrowth of the need for medical care in this expansive territory, and its creation marks a watershed moment not only in the history of ophthalmology but of all medicine in the region.

Brown, Clayton, 52;
William C. Lloyd, III, interview, Panill, F. Carter, 380-388

The first effort to obtain a Medical School for San Antonio was made at a Chamber of Commerce luncheon at the Plaza Hotel in 1944. Initially, attendees discussed the possibility of removing the Texas University Medical School from Galveston in order to better deal with the medical needs of all South Texans. The luncheon produced such local interest that supporters in 1947 created the San Antonio Medical Foundation and charged it with doing whatever was necessary to realize the vision of a Medical School in the city. (Coincidentally, one of the original Trustees named in the Foundation charter was Melrose Holmgreen, the President of the Alamo Iron Works Railroad who would later carry the Burns Collection from Cuero to the Medical School's new Briscoe Library). Eventually, efforts to move the Galveston school were abandoned and the decision reached not only to secure a separate University of Texas Medical Branch at San Antonio, but also to build the giant medical complex known today as the University of Texas Medical Center. The initiating moment came in 1956 at a meeting of the Foundation at the newly organized Argyle Club in Alamo Heights. There, the decision was reached to introduce a bill at the next legislative session, requesting state support of the plan.

Matthews, Wilbur L., 1-40;
Pannill, F. Carter, 381-399;
Handbook of Texas, 596-598.

In the years that followed, the San Antonio Medical Foundation enlisted the aid of the Texas State Legislature, the University of Texas

Board of Regents, hundreds of individual San Antonians, and a new generation of pioneers in ophthalmology. Chief among this group was Dr. John L. Matthews, one of the prominent physicians who attended early meetings of the Medical Foundation and went on to play a key role in establishing the new Medical School and Health Science Center. As San Antonio O&O Society President in 1950 and President of the Bexar County Medical Society in 1956, Dr. Matthews was uniquely positioned to attract other key leaders to the cause and to work "*behind the scenes*" to supply the required resources. He remained involved in efforts to carry out the plan until 1970, communicating to raise funds with the personal network of friends and patients he had built over a lifetime, negotiating with decision-makers, and gathering representatives from military and civilian medical institutions to work together for mutual benefit. In the early stages of the project, he also enlisted the support of another local ophthalmologist, Dr. W.M. McCurdy, who with John Steen and other Chamber of Commerce representatives made up the delegation that went to Austin on six separate occasions to convince the Texas legislature to support the proposal.

Matthews, Wilbur L., 15-25

Although the original objective of local leaders was to realize the possibility of a regional medical school, numbers of forces and important synergies coalesced to accomplish the much greater goal of establishing a vast new type of national medical complex, the University of Texas Health Science Center. Just as the San Antonio Medical Foundation began gathering support for the idea, federal government officials realized that more uniform access to medical education was needed and made federal support available to establish regional medical schools and research-oriented university medical centers. More specifically, in 1963 the federal government passed the Health Professions Educational Assistance Act to support the construction of new medical schools by providing matching grants. Behind the legislation lay the idea that universities had become society's principal reservoirs of research and scientific knowledge, and that medical schools and teaching hospitals should be more closely linked. Ideas about how to structure a quality medical education were suggested by an evaluation of existing medical schools and their curricula conducted by the Carnegie Commission on Higher Education.

Carnegie Commission on Higher Education, 25, 54-55.

This study, widely circulated and eventually published in 1970, highlighted the importance of regional medical training and the need to "*achieve a better geographical distribution of education facilities, particularly for the sake of central city and rural areas.*" In addition, the report introduced another powerful new idea with its recommendation that a "*university health science center*" be built in every metropolitan area with a population of 350,000 or more, for a total of nine proposed health science centers across the country. Stressing the need to "*bring more equitable distribution of the financial burden between the federal government and the states,*" the report concluded that, "*what colleges of agriculture once did for a rural society can now be done for an urban society by the health science centers--and that is to improve the quality of life for nearly all people in their areas.*" University health science centers offering care capable of reaching a network of outlying areas were an idea whose time had come.

Matthews, Wilbur L., 1-40;
Carnegie Commission on Higher Education, 25, 54-55;
Brown, Clayton, 49-52

When the Texas State Legislature met, the San Antonio delegation of medical and community leaders argued convincingly that the Alamo City was the appropriate and best location for placement of a regional medical school, based on its sizeable and growing population and the fact that it was already a major medical center. The local population had reached nearly 700,000, and the city was experiencing the start of a Sunbelt boom that in time would make it one of the country's largest metropolises. By 1970, the region's population would rise to over 1.1 million residents with fourteen hospitals in operation, including the Alamo General (45 beds); Audie Murphy VA (776 beds); Baptist Memorial (776 beds); Northeast Baptist (190 beds); Southeast Baptist (190 beds); Bexar County (425 beds); R.B. Green (57 beds); Lutheran General (204 beds); Methodist (441 beds); Metropolitan (228 beds); Nix (190 beds); Park North (102 beds); Community (216 beds); Santa Rosa (725 beds); Wilford Hall (1,000 beds); and Brooke Army Medical Center (1,000 beds).

Matthews, Wilbur L., 1-40;
Brown, Clayton, 49-52;
"Fact Sheet," Bexar County Medical Society archives

In 1959, the fifty-sixth Texas State Legislature passed an act that "*authorized and directed*" the University of Texas Board of Regents "*to establish a medical branch or department of the University*" in Bexar County. According to its original mandate, the principal responsibility of the new Medical School would be to care for all the people of South Texas. No expenditure of funds would be permitted until a teaching hospital was established to serve both indigent and private paying patients, or "*a complete cross section of society.*" The legislation also emphasized the importance of giving medical students an opportunity to "*experience all types of diseases and the effects of economic and social factors on the long-range care of the patient.*" Ultimately, this endeavor would also obtain federal funding made available for the construction of health science centers around the country.

Pannill, F.C., 381-402;
Matthews, Wilbur L., 25-35;
Brown, Clayton, 52

With the necessary state approvals obtained, the San Antonio Medical Foundation in 1960 organized a Committee of 100 to draw up plans for construction of the new Medical School. After a series of meetings to present relevant information, Foundation board members selected a 700-acre construction site on the Nix dairy farm and surrounding ranchland in the Oak Hills section of San Antonio. The wisdom of their choice to dedicate a separate sector of the community to medicine would become clear as the city expanded outward. The Medical School would occupy a parcel of land known as the "*Arsenal property*," a choice that would have pleased Major General Edward A. Noyes, a Commander at Brooke Army Medical Center, who, some years earlier, had noted that Brooke was the only Army teaching hospital not near a medical school. The new facility, first named the South Texas Medical School, later would come to be known as the University of Texas Medical School at San Antonio.

Wilbur L. Matthews interview;
Matthews, Wilbur L., 16, 23, 27;
Daughters of the Republic of Texas Library clipping file, 2-18-92;
Pannill, F. Carter, 381-402

As the Committee of 100 obtained set out to cost estimates for the proposed construction, a prominent ophthalmologist on the board of both the Medical Foundation and the Bexar County Hospital, Dr. Walter Walthall, joined the enterprise to help select the engineers and architects required to make the plan a reality. A Master Plan Committee, appointed in 1961, followed up on the work of the Committee of 100 by developing plans for the emerging center that were compiled into a document called the Ellerbe Plan, and building got underway when the public approved a bond issue that tagged over six million dollars for the project.

Mathews, Wilbur L., 20-30.
Dr. Elbert DeCoursey, another outstanding community ophthalmologist, joined the board of the Medical Foundation in this period.

As the need for a South Texas medical school became increasingly apparent, ophthalmologists recognized and acknowledged the importance of the project for their profession. In 1966, when Dr. Harold E. Hunt addressed the Texas Ophthalmological Association in Austin, he acknowledged that ophthalmology had become "*a growing and developing specialty in Texas*" and that two branches of the military service now did "*most of their main eye research within the state*," yet "*many areas of Texas*" were "*still without specialists to take care of people's eye needs*." Reiterating a problem long recognized in the region, he set out three principal objectives for the profession to move forward in coming decades: further growth of the specialty, increased research capability, and the capacity to train enough new specialists to attend to eye needs across the region. Dr. Hunt did not recognize, however, that tensions within the profession would lead to conflicts and cause delays in the process by which these goals would ultimately be achieved.

To qualify as members of the Association, specialists needed to have practiced ophthalmology for five years and/or to have received their board certifications. They also needed to be regular members of their county medical society and to have practiced in that county for three years.

For a summary of eye research and other activity in ophthalmology in Texas in the 1960s, see Hunt, Harold E., M.D., "Ophthalmology in Texas," 67.

As construction of the health science center progressed, substantial work was needed to assemble a basic administration plus the necessary personnel to staff the complex before the new institutions could officially open. Efforts to assemble clinical faculty and all other activities relating to the Medical School were conducted in the basement offices of the R. B. Green Hospital, while the first administrative offices for the complex were housed at nearby Trinity University. As the new Medical School and Health Science Center took shape, plans for an ophthalmology component grew slowly. In 1968, the Medical School opened five basic divisions that grew to include Pathology, Medicine, Surgery, Biochemistry, Microbiology, Anatomy, Obstetrics and Gynecology, and Radiology. Despite the large indigent population to be served, sufficient need for a full-fledged Department of Ophthalmology was not anticipated, given the city's large number of practicing ophthalmologists and the steady but small number of medical students interested in the specialty. Instead, early administrators made Ophthalmology a division of General Surgery in what was to be a significant decision for the future of the unit. Its first mission was to focus exclusively on teaching, to train residents, and to supervise patient care at the R. B. Green Hospital and the teaching hospital complex at Oak Hills, known successively as the Bexar County Hospital and the Medical Center Hospital. One room in the R.B. Green basement was set aside for the Department of Surgery of which Ophthalmology was a part. To start with, administrators hired four faculty members in Ophthalmology whose task would be to develop a curriculum and to collect applications for the first residencies to be offered. Plans were also made to open the search for a suitable head for the new Ophthalmology Division.

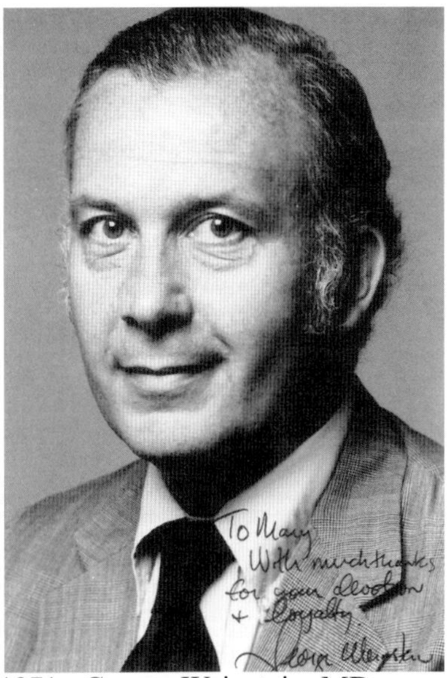

1971. George Weinstein, MD, first head of the Division of Ophthalmology at UTHSCSA.

Dr. Francis X. Weixel, Wilbur L. Matthews, Dr. W.A. van Heuven interviews; Matthews, Wilbur L., 22

Casting a nationwide net to find the best possible candidates, Dr. J. Bradley Aust, the Chairman of Surgery, selected to serve as first Chairman of the Ophthalmology Division a highly recommended ophthalmologist from the Wilmer Eye Hospital with a background in teaching, administration, and medical publication: Dr. George W. Weinstein. Weinstein had trained at the State University of New York and been a Fellow in Ophthalmology at the Wilmer Eye Hospital at Johns Hopkins and the National Institutes of Health in the Institute of Neurological Diseases and Blindness. He was an experienced researcher with a background that included testing new equipment and studying retinal adaptation and Horner's Syndrome. He also had worked with the Vision Research Training Committee for the United States Public Health Service and had taught clinical ophthalmology at the Georgetown University School of Medicine and at Johns Hopkins.

George W. Weinstein, M.D., Curriculum Vitae;
J.B. Aust, Letter to George Weinstein, November 17, 1969;
George Weinstein, Letter to J.B. Aust, November 21, 1969;
Dr. George Weinstein interview.

Both the handsome younger man who came to head the Ophthalmology Division and the jocular Chief of Surgery had charismatic personalities. Weinstein drove a foreign sports car of a type seldom seen in San Antonio, and was considered something of a visionary as well as a distinguished educator. Echoing earlier generations of eye specialists who came to the frontier, he was no doubt attracted by the freedom of an opportunity to develop an educational program "*from scratch.*" He arrived in the Southwest bringing with him much of his Wilmer research laboratory under the direction of Robert R. Hobson, a distinguished researcher whose career in Texas would last into the next century.

J.B. Aust, Letter to George Weinstein, November 17, 1969;
Mary Hicks interview;
UTHSC Department of Ophthalmology archives;
Dr. Richard Poirier interview

When Dr. Weinstein arrived, the furnishings on the second floor of the Medical School set aside for the Division of Ophthalmology consisted of kitchen chairs and minimal equipment, yet despite relatively slow beginnings these proved to be heady times. A key administrator remembered the period as one of rapid growth. In 1969, just a year after the school opened, over one hundred medical students were in training at the new University Hospital and residency programs had been established in a number of specialized fields, of which Ophthalmology was the first. The Medical School advertised quality residency training that, according to published guidelines, provided residents "*by precept and practice*" with knowledge and skills sufficient to deliver a high quality of ophthalmic care and "*to enable him to cooperate with other physicians in the care of the complete individual.*" Weinstein, working with other administrators, coordinated clinical rounds at the Medical School with those at local military institutions almost from the beginning. As first-year residents attended clinics, conferences, and courses on eye pathology and basic science, they learned to use diagnostic instruments and to perform minor surgery. Second-year residents completed the Lancaster Course, participated in clinics, deepened their experience in all areas, and performed their first cataract operation. Senior residents administered the Ophthalmology Section of the hospital, supervised younger residents, conducted ward rounds, supervised the Eye Bank, and by year's end were required to have performed 200 operations, including major intraocular surgery. They also were expected to complete up to 2,500 refractions and numerous consultations. Early animal research proj-

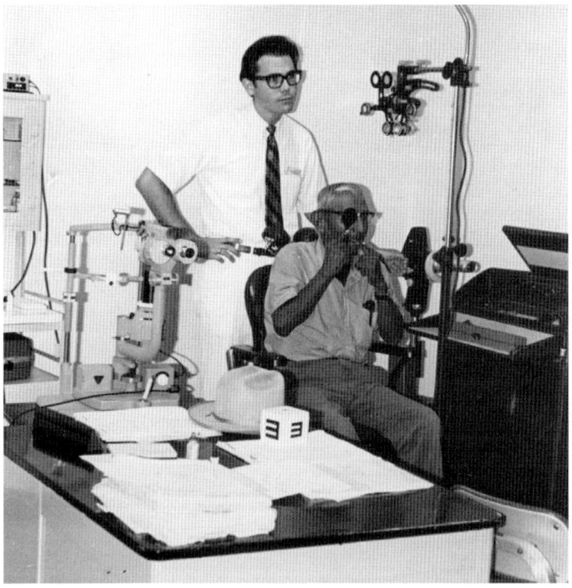

1972. Original Eye Clinic at the Brady Green Hospital in downtown San Antonio. Resident Dudley H. Harris tests patient's vision. Dr. Harris later established a thriving ophthalmic practice in San Antonio.

ects got underway to study the effects of retinal damage due to chronic light exposure in rats and monkeys, and later faculty studies focused on the effects of drugs on retina specimens from animals that could be kept alive in the laboratory for several hours.

William C. Lloyd, III, M.D. video;
UTHSC Department of Ophthalmology archives;
Dr. George Weinstein interview

When the Ophthalmology Division assumed responsibility for supervision of ophthalmology services offered at the Robert B. Green Hospital, the downtown facility had only two eye lanes and limited equipment. By the late 1970s, however, conditions improved when a local socialite known as "*Lady Brady*" bequeathed the bulk of her estate to the hospital to create the Brady Memorial Clinic. Henceforth, the facility was known as "*The Brady-Green*." Because it continued to serve as a key site for medical care of the area's Hispanic population, including ophthalmic care, the Brady-Green grew into an important service component of the emerging health science complex and an important site for faculty and students of the Ophthalmology Division.

R.B. Green Hospital archival materials

In the early years of his administration, Dr. Weinstein strengthened the curriculum and residency training programs by drawing upon the part-time services of three distinguished community ophthalmologists, Drs. John Mumma, Shelley Braverman, and Charles Leone.

He also recruited three outstanding sub-specialist faculty members from outside the state--cornea specialist Robert H. Poirier, neuro-ophthalmologist Francisco Javier M. Bajandas, and retina specialist Michael Barricks. Together, the combined background of these individuals reflected a new dimension in the field of ophthalmology and some of the richest resources in late twentieth-century specialized medicine. Dr. Bajandas had been born in San Juan, Puerto Rico, attended Notre Dame, received a University of Louisville medical degree, and completed an internship and neuroscience residency there. After an ophthalmology residency at San Antonio's Bexar County Hospital, he finished his postgraduate work at Miami's Bascom Palmer Eye Institute, and then broadened his experience with services in the Army Medical Corps before joining the Medical School faculty as an assistant professor. Dr. Poirier's background tapped the expertise of Dr. Phillips Thygeson at San Francisco, Dr. Barry Jones in London, and Dr. Richard Schulz, who later served as Chairman of Ophthalmology at the Medical College of Wisconsin.

Dr. George Weinstein, Dr. Richard Poirier, and Mary Hicks interviews;
Bexar County Medical Society Membership Records

To further broaden the scope of the Division, Dr. Weinstein laid the foundations to begin the first full-scale ophthalmology research efforts in the region. By 1971, with the help of two institutional research grants and an award through the Seeing Eye Foundation of Morristown, New Jersey, the Division acquired a substantial collection of ophthalmological equipment, including color vision, visual field and dark adaptation testers, a fluorescein angiography camera, and instruments for electro-retinography and oculography. According to one observer, the assembled array of equipment for retinal function testing offered the "*only comprehensive retinal function laboratory in the state of Texas*." In addition, Weinstein entered into a cooperative arrangement with the Baptist Hospital to use its laser photocoagulation unit. He was proud of the fact that "*patients with interesting and unusual retinal diseases have been referred here for study from all over the state*."

Memorandum, J.B. Aust to Weinstein, January 11, 1972;
Graham, Bill, "Med School to Add 'Eye Camera' Unit, San Antonio Express-News, 1971, n.p.

By 1972, Weinstein could point to numerous accomplishments. Nearly two-thirds of all students enrolled in the Medical School chose to take the Ophthalmology rotation, and participants in the residency program expanded from one person in each of three years to two persons each year. Twenty-two of twenty-eight ophthalmologists practicing privately in the community now participated actively in the teaching program by attending grand rounds, surgery, and a weekly clinical conference. A semi-annual All-Day Clinical Conference, established in 1971, drew ophthalmologists to San Antonio from all parts of Texas. The electro-physiology laboratory had become a regional resource, and Weinstein reported that colleagues from Galveston and Houston became frequent visitors, seeking advice about how to set up laboratories of their own. By 1978, there were eight faculty members and constant innovations in technique and equipment, changing requirements for training, and growing complexity in the field. Because of these advances, however, Weinstein and his staff quickly reached a watershed moment in their expanding enterprise.

Aust, J.D., Memorandum to George Weinstein, M.D., January 11, 1972;
Robert R. Hobson interview

As Dr. Weinstein became aware of the potential of the Ophthalmology Division to develop new programs and services, he also became cognizant of the limitations inherent in its identification with General Surgery. Increasingly, both he and the faculty soon realized the need to separate Ophthalmology from the organizational structure of Surgery, as had already been done at most medical schools around the country. In 1970, the faculty took the issue to their community counterparts for discussion, and the San Antonio O & O Society wrote a letter to the Dean of the Medical School recommending that Ophthalmology and Otolaryngology "*should be organized and administered as separate, distinct and autonomous departments*." No member of either specialty, they explained, was capable of administering a department encompassing both fields.

Dr. George Weinstein interview

After a lengthy debate acknowledging the expanding roles of the Division, the University responded favorably to Weinstein's request and created a new Department of Ophthalmology. In doing so, however, it also initiated efforts to recruit a new Chairman, making Weinstein himself a candidate but opening the possibility of bringing in new leadership. Among qualifications for the position, stress was placed on the idea that the future chairman would need a strong basic science background to permit participation in the early years of students' training as well as later clinical teaching. As originally outlined, the teaching program in ophthalmology for medical students had been designed to encompass basic science, specialization, and ophthalmic sub-specialization. As a further objective, the administration now emphasized research and noted the importance of making the area's indigent population of over 200,000 a unique focus of that research.

Dr. George Weinstein, Robert Hobson interviews

Weinstein's desire to create an independent department was not one he would remain in San Antonio long enough to see realized, as it finally was in 1979. Local specialty society records and accounts of eye-related activities measure the strength of the professional forces outside the Health Science Center that he confronted in his efforts to separate the original Division from the Department of Surgery. In order to understand why Dr. Weinstein's plans did not succeed, it is particularly important to understand the shared perspective of community ophthalmologists relating to the ideas he introduced. In 1960, for example, records showing that Dr. P. E. Suchs of Austin, representing Austin practitioners, filed suit against an injunction seeking to keep ophthalmologists from owning interests in or obtaining revenue from optical companies, reinforce the idea that area ophthalmologists were interested in making their profession a profitable enterprise. In 1972, other records reflect the sophistication of the community by showing that, when local ophthalmologists incorporated the San Antonio O&O Society with a membership of sixty-five, thirty-eight members were local specialists in private practice and the Society's annual symposia drew a host of distinguished practitioners from the community, the military, and other cities. At a typical meeting, participants heard Col. Thomas Tredici talk on "*Experiences with Eye and ENT Casualties from the Vietnam Conflict*," discussed "pre-paid vision care as part of new employee health plans," attended courses on subjects ranging from the "*diagnosis and treatment of surgical diseases of the anterior segment of the eye*" to sub-specialty topics such as "*neuro-ophthalmology*," and observed case presentations at the R.B. Green. Members also participated in grand rounds at the Medical School with staff representatives from Brooke Army Medical Center and Wilford Hall. Finally, awareness of ophthalmology in the local community was high due to the success of Henry Wyneken's Association for the Blind. Though the organization suffered a decline after his death in 1938, it subsequently had received new government contracts to expand its programs and gained greater visibility as the number of blind persons increased in Bexar County to roughly 1,200 in 1949. The Association's affiliation with the National

Industries for the Blind in time helped the local blind population to become more productive, and by the 1990s the Association ran a modern, diverse manufacturing operation that produced over $10 million dollars annually.

San Antonio Association for the Blind historical materials;
San Antonio O & O Society Minutes, September 13, 1960.

In time, members of the local ophthalmology community came to see as unwelcome competition the work of Medical School faculty with clinical practices at the Medical Consultants Clinic, a University of Texas faculty private clinic that served a clientele of both indigent and wealthy patients from across the state. Though cataract operations still involved a two to three day hospital stay, microsurgery using intraocular lens implants had begun to produce higher rates of success. Surveys of local ophthalmologists reveal that typical charges for an enucleation with implant were $500, phacoemulsification $800, removal of cataracts and intraocular lens implants $1,350, and vitrectomy $2,000. Improved treatments and surgical advances had begun to make the ophthalmology profession more lucrative, and community practitioners in response tended to support the status quo and to discourage change.

Mary Hicks interview;
Dr. George Weinstein interview;
"The Eye Institute, UTHSCSA brochure, n.d.

In seeking support for a separate Department of Ophthalmology, moreover, Dr. Weinstein also introduced an idea that threatened his community colleagues with the announcement of his intention to found an Eye Institute. Believing that the potential existed to create an institution where practitioners might address all types of eye and vision-related problems by working together "*under one roof*," he proposed what he intended to become "*the newest and maybe the best of this nation's growing number of Eye Institutes*." In support of his idea, Weinstein pointed to the region's growing needs for eye care. Records from 1977 show that up to an eighteen-week waiting period was needed to schedule new patient visits at the R.B. Green Hospital, and that ophthalmology staff members and residents there treated as many as 14,000 outpatients a year. As public demand for better care of HMO patients grew, the Bexar County Hospital and other area medical facilities experienced a nine-week delay and an extensive backlog in scheduling ophthalmic surgeries. The Medical Consultants Clinic, the Health Science Center ophthalmology service, treated almost 3,000 outpatients a year and numbers were increasing at the rate of over thirty per cent annually. In a general San Antonio population that reported 2,950 cases of legal blindness, 10,874 cases of severe visual impairment, and as many as 30,402 cases of partial visual impairment, analysts believed roughly fifty per cent would respond to surgical correction and projected that 3,600 corrective surgical procedures could be conducted in 1979 with current resources.

Mary Hicks interview;
Dr. George Weinstein interview;
"The Eye Institute, UTHSCSA brochure, n.d.;
"Ophthalmic Research Foundation of San Antonio, Inc." and "San Antonio Eye Institute" files, UTHSC Department of Ophthalmology Archives;
San Antonio Express News, n.d.

The first institution in Texas of the kind Weinstein hoped to create in San Antonio--Houston's Hermann Eye Institute--would not be founded for some years. He, therefore, took as a model the extensive eye facilities of what was perhaps the nation's premier institution of its time, the Wilmer Eye Institute in Baltimore. He also explored the models suggested by the Allen C. Wood Research Center, where a floor of the building was dedicated to each of several subspecialties, and the Dean A. McGee Eye Institute affiliated with the Oklahoma University Health Science Center in Oklahoma City, that suggested productive relationships to be obtained by linking an eye institute and a health science center. Combining the most attractive features of each prototype, he began to dream of an Eye Institute that could "*incorporate activities in the area of research, teaching, and patient care*," and attend to the ophthalmic needs of children and the continuing education of doctors in the region. An autonomous Eye Institute could more easily attract faculty and patients, cover students' tuition, and draw on the region's indigent population for research purposes. He also thought such a center would facilitate "*personal referral from the ophthalmological community for evaluation and diagnosis of rare, problem or difficult cases and treatment of those cases if recommended by the private practitioner.*" Funding for these endeavors would come primarily from donations and grants.

The Eye Institute," UTHSCSA brochure, n.d.

To gather support for the Eye Institute, Weinstein formed the Ophthalmic Research Foundation of San Antonio, Inc., a non-profit corporation whose purpose--according to its Articles of Incorporation, was "*to encourage, stimulate, promote, support, and engage in oph-*

*thalmic research and ophthalmic education, to extend and enrich ophthalmic effort in the San Antonio area of Texas and to foster consistently improving quality in that effort; to contribute to improved standards of eye care in South Texas*." For help in winning support, he turned to Dr. John Matthews, the "*dean of San Antonio ophthalmologists*," and Drs. James L. Mims, Jr., Col. Elbert DeCoursey, and Thomas Hogan, Jr. to assist in presenting plans for the Eye Institute to ophthalmologists in the wider community. Prominent citizens, including local ranchers Mr. and Mrs. Robert Lee Moffett and Messrs. H.B. Zachry, Ralph Winton, and Harold M. Freeman (for whom San Antonio's Freeman Coliseum was later named) also supported the cause, and in 1978 the University of Texas Board of Regents approved Weinstein's proposal for an Eye Institute. A year later, a report to the Trustees approved the Ophthalmology Research Foundation's request for a grant of land as a construction site, building costs were estimated at $5.6 million, and arrangements made to have the new facility licensed as a hospital. Elaborate plans were developed to raise funds for the project, including a rock concert with blind performers who would call attention to eye-related issues.

Minutes, Ophthalmic Research Foundation of San Antonio, Inc., Board of Directors Meeting, June 19, 1980;
Articles of Incorporation and Bylaws of Ophthalmic Research Foundation of San Antonio, Inc.;
Department of Ophthalmology Archives;
"Eye Program Strangled, Ex-Prof Says," Clint Schroeder, Jr., Express-News, n.d.
Bisno, David C., 931;
Dr. George Weinstein interview, Ophthalmic Research Foundation of San Antonio Inc., "Minutes";
Ophthalmic Research Foundation of San Antonio, Inc., "Articles";
UTHSC Department of Ophthalmology Archives; Schroeder, Clint, Jr., n.p.

Weinstein's Eye Institute met with sufficient resistance, however, that it failed to become a reality. Though its potential to make a valuable contribution was clear, the models on which the institution would be based had been developed in places where conditions in the medical community were substantially different. In order for Weinstein to succeed, he would need to marshal support outside the Health Science Center, a step requiring that he provide assurance that the Institute would benefit both Department faculty and community practitioners. As he conceived it, the Eye Institute would be housed in its own building and governed by a Board of Trustees, acting in accordance with the rules and regulations of the University of Texas Health

Science Center. Board representation would include ophthalmologists and staff members drawn from the community on a rotational basis. Given the fact that sub-specialists were already well established in the community, however, he did not realize that the Institute's objectives would be in conflict with theirs.

Dr. George Weinstein, Mary Hicks interviews;
"Ophthalmic Research Foundation of San Antonio, Inc." and
"San Antonio Eye Institute" files, UTHSC Department of Ophthalmology Archives

Support from the San Antonio O&O Society dwindled as members began to perceive the Eye Institute as potential competition in a city where competition was already growing. Many believed the Health Science Center, and especially an Eye Institute, represented a threat to their practices, and that a specialty unit outside the structure of the Medical School was not advisable. One local ophthalmologist claimed that, "*ophthalmology might be better off if it stayed part of the mainstream. This would certainly set it aside*." Given the lengthy list of requirements to make the Health Science Center fully operational, others felt that ophthalmic subspecialty training was outside the guidelines for a fundamental medical education and a costly extravagance, and saw the rest of Weinstein's agenda as unnecessary or inappropriate. Another contingent felt the facility would duplicate existing services and never provide good eye care for the medically indigent. This issue was particularly important since, late in 1979, Health Science Center officials working with the San Antonio Chamber of Commerce developed a health care program that included plans to attract Mexican citizens to the city for treatment. One observer was fearful that publicity for the Institute would "*make it seem like the only place to go*" in San Antonio for eye care. Finally, in December 1979, the O&O Society held a secret ballot and passed a motion to "*oppose the creation of an eye institute*."

Matthews, Wilbur L., 65-66;
Dr. James Mims interview;
Aust, J.B., Memorandum to George Weinstein, M.D., January 11, 1972;
Schroeder, Clint, Jr., n.d.

While to some extent the Eye Institute was simply an idea before its time, more definite reasons why Weinstein's effort did not succeed are clear. With an original mandate from the Texas State Legislature to focus primarily on quality teaching and early Ophthalmology Division hires whose primary interests lay in training medical students, his plans for research and other types of activity represented unsanctioned and inappropriate objectives. In retrospect, however, Weinstein's not-inconsiderable achievements created a sound foundation for the emerging Department of Ophthalmology and called attention to that unit's potential for further growth. Ultimately, a new stage of development required new leadership, and Weinstein was replaced as head of the Division he had established. From an institutional standpoint, the setback was temporary and progress swiftly resumed. In 1979, just ten years after the Health Science Center opened, the Division of Ophthalmology would become a full-fledged department and enter a new era of achievement in national and international medicine.

Mary Hicks Interview

When the population living in the sprawling Bexar County that surrounded San Antonio reached nearly 905-500 people in the 1980s, the Ophthalmology Division at last sent enough of its graduates to practice in local communities to answer the region's basic need for eye specialists. Statistics in 1981 show that ninety percent (90%) of all residents trained in San Antonio were practicing in Texas, and that there were 38 ophthalmologists in the city itself. Six residents trained each year at Wilford Hall, eight at Brooke Army Medical Center, and nine at the University of Texas Health Science Center.

UTHSCSA graduates who stayed to practice ophthalmology in the region were numerous. Dr. Michael David Tschoepe, a San Antonio native, completed his Bexar County Hospital internship and residency, set up his practice in the nearby town of New Braunfels, and in 1973 was joined by Dr. David Way, an ophthalmologist educated principally at Baylor and in Dallas. Among Texas natives trained entirely within the state was Dr. Marilyn Albers Kelinske of Texas City, who followed her degree at the Galveston Medical Branch in 1977 with an internship and ophthalmology residency at the Health Science Center, and then opened a practice in Austin. Other early graduates included Dr. Dudley Harris; Dr. James Ervin Lusk, who finished his residency in 1979; and Indiana native Duane Charles Flanagan, who took a medical degree in his home state and then came to Texas to intern at Baylor before completing a San Antonio ophthalmology residency. Dr. John Ronald Fish of Salt Lake City, who attended Texas Tech in Lubbock, received his medical degree at the Galveston Medical Branch in 1970, spent two years at Kelly Air Force Base, and interned at Methodist Hospital in Dallas, before his UTHSCSA ophthalmology residency. Finally, Dr. Antonio Alejandro San Martin, a San Antonio native, graduated from the University of Texas, studied optometry at the University of Houston, received his UTHSCSA medical degree, and completed his internship and residency at Brooke Army Medical Center.

"Fact Sheet," Bexar County Medical Society Archives;
Eye Report;
George Weinstein interview.

With the achievement of this goal, however, the Health Science Center faced new challenges, particularly the need to update its training program to include clinical practice in the ophthalmic sub-specialty fields and to find support for both academic medicine and research in ophthalmology. "*Sub-specialization*" in ophthalmology had developed initially as a byproduct of Dr. Charles L. Schepens' invention of the binocular indirect ophthalmoscope. Like Helmholtz's original ophthalmoscope, the new instrument constituted an innovative technology that generated corresponding new techniques that required further specialization. After refining the instrument in 1951, Schepens was considered the founder of the field of subspecialty expertise known as "*retina*." As his students became practitioners themselves and carried their knowledge forward--much like medical missionaries--to their counterparts in communities across the nation, they established a new type of credential for the profession.

(Albert, Daniel M. and Diane D. Edwards, Eds., History of Ophthalmology, Blackwell Science, 1996, 197).

In setting up sub-specialty training programs, however, different parts of the country responded at different rates, thereby creating different attitudes within the profession toward sub-specialists. In the eastern United States, sub-specialists initially were associated with medical schools and there were few sub-specialists in private practice. Community support developed for sub-specialists in this region because, with no local counterparts, they did not represent competition. Community ophthalmologists in Boston, Miami, and Chicago commonly referred cases requiring sub-specialty expertise to their local medical schools. While Schepens and others in eastern medical schools were training sub-specialty fellows at the rate of up to six a year in the 1960s, however, the first ophthalmology subspecialty fellowships were being offered in San Antonio. Because of this timing, the order in which sub-specialization developed in South Texas was reversed. Sub-specialists were established in the community before sub-specialist faculty joined the Medical School. As a result, Medical

School sub-specialists were seen as competition in San Antonio and excluded from engaging in private practice from the very beginning.

Albert, Daniel M. and Diane D. Edwards, eds., 197;
Robert R. Hobson interview

A further disadvantage for Medical School sub-specialists arose from the fact that administrators made research an objective for the Ophthalmology Division later than elsewhere, just as they emphasized sub-specialty training relatively late in comparison with other parts of the country. Eastern medical schools with a strong commitment to research were benefiting from National Institutes of Health (NIH) support while the University of Texas Health Science Center and its Medical School continued to follow the original mandate of state legislators to focus exclusively on the basics of medical training. Ophthalmology Division faculty members were not encouraged to conduct research, despite the fact that a research infrastructure had been quickly established and salaries and space for research made available in other Medical School divisions. The Division had difficulty in attracting true academicians in subspecialty fields for some years since most academic sub-specialists of renown preferred working in established research centers where they might enjoy greater interaction with sub-specialist colleagues.

Dr. W.A.J. Van Heuven interview

Despite these challenges, however, the UTHSCSA Ophthalmology Division benefited from three unique advantages. First was the largest indigent population accessible to any medical school in the nation--almost double that of the next school on the list. Roughly 40% of all South Texas patients were totally un-funded; the next closest state had only about 20%. Translated in terms of medical education, this meant that ophthalmology residents in San Antonio had an opportunity to do more patient care and surgery than most others in the country. Eventually, their clinical experience ranked among the top 10% in the nation, and their experience of trauma cases at the very top of the profession. Second, because UTHSCSA residents regularly saw cases at local military facilities as part of grand rounds, they had more opportunities to learn about "*zebras*," or unique and unusual cases, than most of their counterparts nationwide. Third, the Medical School's affiliation with the Audie Murphy Veterans Administration Hospital provided additional opportunities for residents. Workers with the VA system had discovered that attaching veterans' hospitals to medical schools provided "*economies of sharing*" and

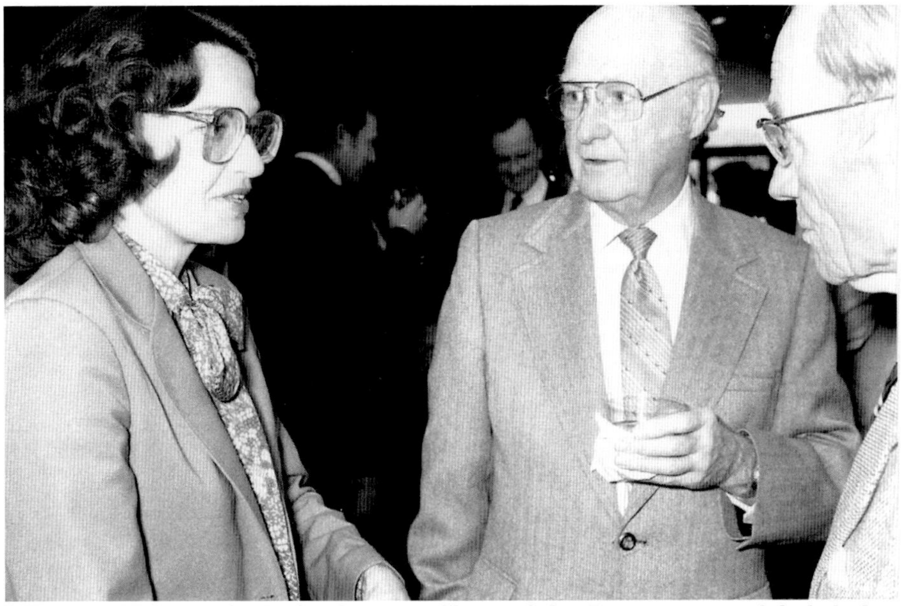

1981. Dr. Jean Holt (Left), Interim Chair of the Department of Ophthalmology 1979-1981, in discussion with Drs. Frank Weixel (Center) and "Jack" Matthews, both community ophthalmologists who shared a practice, at the welcoming reception for W A J van Heuven, the new chairman.

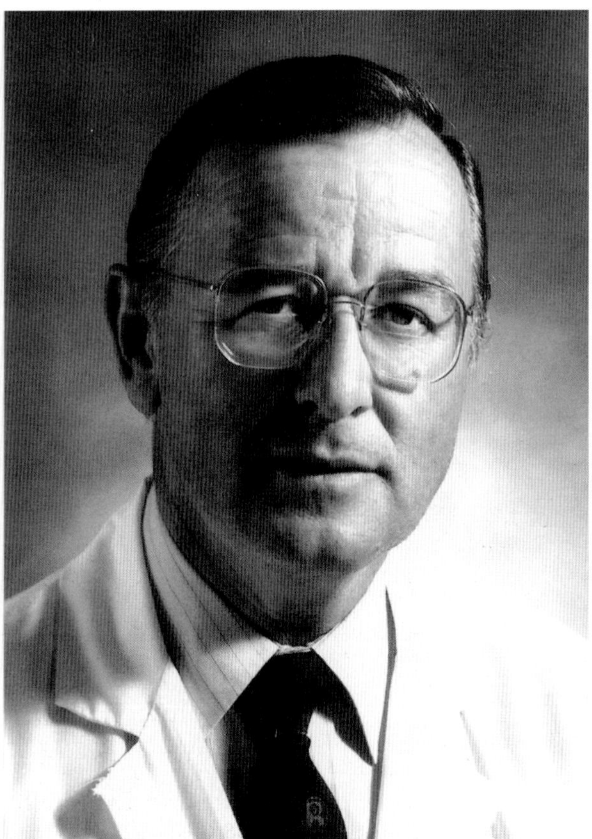

Wichard A. J. van Heuven, MD, first Chairman of the Department of Ophthalmology at UTHSCSA

improvements in veteran care. Over time, clinical teaching and medical education became a vital component of VA activity in a mutually advantageous system that enhanced the quality of medical school training. As medical schools provided house staff to the VA for supervision and seeing patients, the VA established a research branch that helped the Ophthalmology Division to attract sub-specialist faculty with research interests.

Mary Hicks, Drs. George Weinstein,
W. A. J. van Heuven interviews

In 1979, the Division of Ophthalmology was poised on the threshold of new developments when Medical School administrators at last reached the decision to create a separate Ophthalmology Department and to organize a search committee to find a new Chairman with the vision to build a more complete academic program, dedicated equally to teaching, research, and service. To meet interim staffing needs, the administration reverted to part-time staffing by community ophthalmologists, Drs. Robert Snip, James Speights, Judith Newman, Luis Taboada, and Mary Arno. Dr. Jean E. Holt, an outstanding teacher and cataract surgeon, clinical expert, and former Chief of Ophthalmology at the Audie Murphy Veterans Administration Hospital, was recruited to provide educational leadership until the new Chairman could be found.

UTHSC Department of Ophthalmology Archives;
Dr. George Weinstein, Mary Hicks interviews

## THE DEPARTMENT OF OPHTHALMOLOGY AND ITS FIRST CHAIRMAN

In 1981, after a nationwide search, the University of Texas Medical School at San Antonio announced the selection of its first Chairman to serve the new Department of Ophthalmology. Remarkably, this decision once more attracted to South Texas an individual who would serve as the instrument of important cultural transfer. The man chosen was not only a known academician, but also a physician whose roots linked Texas to the founders of ophthalmology in Europe. Wichard A.J. van Heuven, M.D., was born in Utrecht, the Netherlands, an important early center of ophthalmological advances, to a family with close ties to several of Europe's greatest practitioners.

UTHSC Department of Ophthalmology Archives;
UTHSC Department of Ophthalmology, Eye Report

The new Chairman was a graduate of Yale University and the New York Medical College. Trained at the Massachusetts Eye and Ear Infirmary, the Yale New Haven Medical Center, Albany Medical Center Hospital, and Harvard Medical School, he had served as a Professor of Ophthalmology at Albany Medical College and the University of Iowa and a faculty member of the American Academy of Ophthalmology

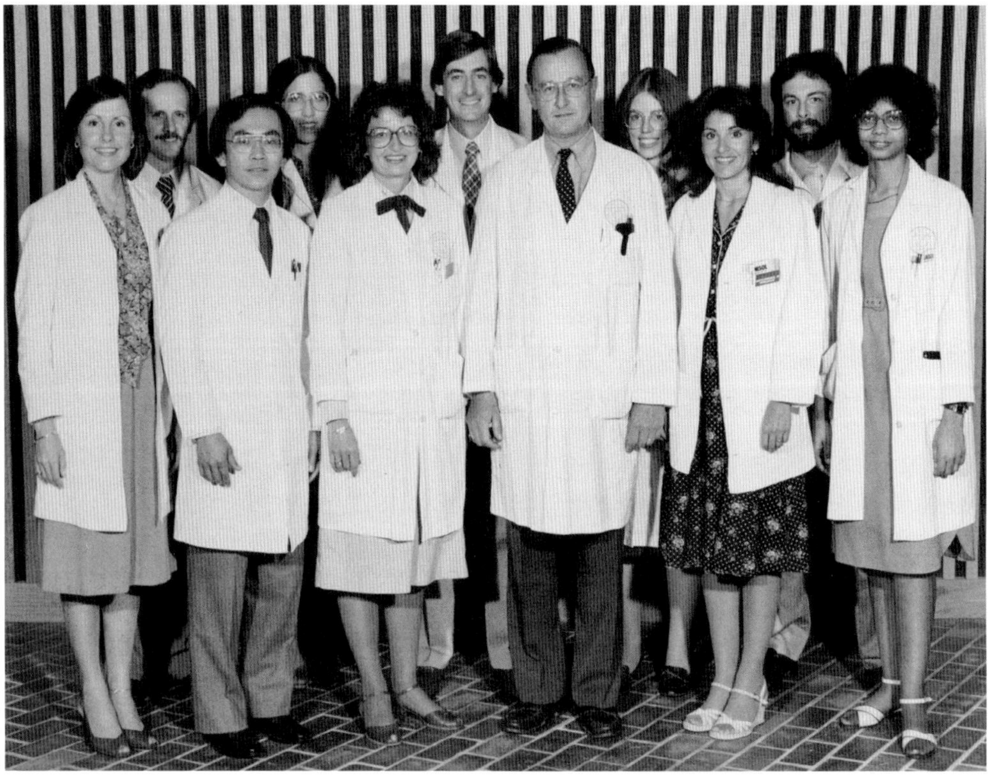

1982. Faculty and residents of the newly created independent Department of Ophthalmology. From L to R, front row: Jane L. Hughes, PGY2; Richard W. Yee, PGY3; Jean E. Holt, MD; W. A. J. van Heuven, MD: Loretta Miramontes, PGY3; Nancy Y. Bryant, PGY 4; back row: Arlo C. Terry, PGY3, Maureen M. Alexander, PGY4; Thomas J. Crawford, PGY2; MaryJo Locker, PGY4; Richard H. Blue, PGY2.

prior to coming to the Southwest. Of perhaps greater significance for the Medical School, he was an active sub-specialist with substantial research experience. In addition to his work as a principal investigator at Albany in the first NIH clinical trials to study diabetic retinopathy, Dr. van Heuven had been involved in experiments to test the value of lasers in postponing blindness from diabetes (D.R.S.) and in developing a large-scale model for subsequent evaluations. He had participated in studies of early treatment for diabetes (E.T.D.R.S.) and in efforts to determine the proper timing for vitrectomies (D.R.V.S.), and

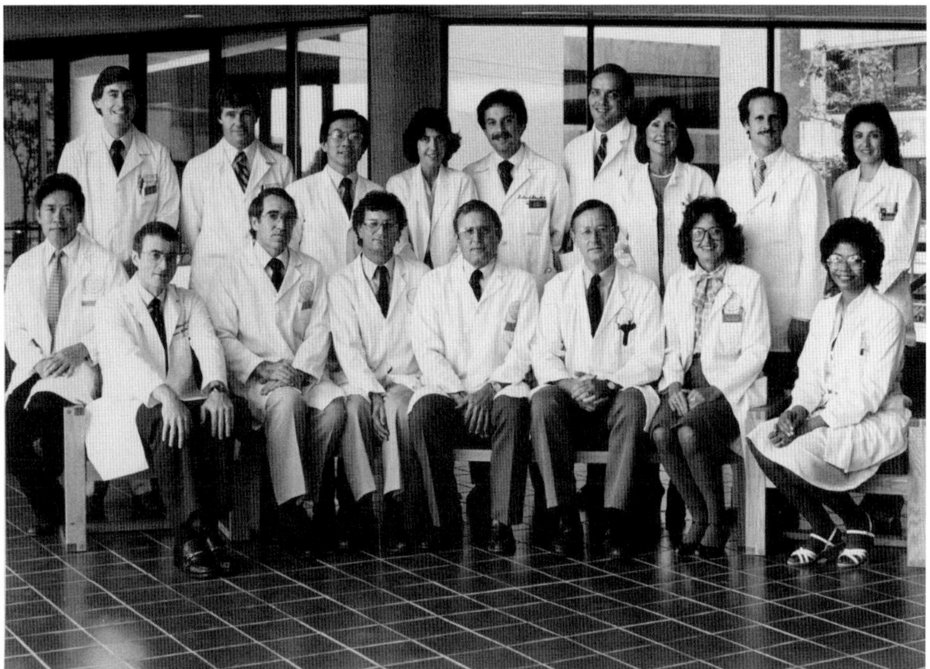

1983. The second year of the Department of Ophthalmology, when the faculty had increased and research had expanded.
From L to R, front row (faculty): Kwok-Wai Lam, PhD; Patrick S. O'Connor, MD; Charles H. Bonney, DVM, PhD; Joseph M. Harrison, PhD; David E. Shacklett, MD; W. A. J. van Heuven, MD; Jean E. Holt, MD; Nancy Y. Bryant, MD; back row (residents): Thomas I Crawford, PGY3; Michael M Alt, PGY2; Richard W. Yee, PGY4; Lori M. Ventura, PGY2; Richard H. Blue, PGY3; Clayton E. Whitney, PGY2; Jane L. Hughes, PGY3; Arlo C. Terry, PGY4, Loretta Miramontes, PGY4.

he was the first researcher to apply television technology to retinal angiography, a procedure that became the preferred method for angiographic imaging.

Dr. van Heuven curriculum vitae; Diabetic Retinopathy Study; Early Treatment Diabetic Retinopathy Study; Diabetic Retinopathy Vitrectomy Study.

Just as Dr. Ferdinand Herff and other European eye specialists had contributed their expertise to enrich South Texas medicine early in its history, Dr. van Heuven now expanded the Department's educational mission to usher in further progress by adding a new focus on research and the ophthalmic sub-specialty fields. He was attracted to South Texas by the opportunity to create an academic center with goals in research (both basic and clinical), in service, and in medical education, and promptly set out to increase the breadth and depth of the new Department's activities in each of these areas. He was espe-

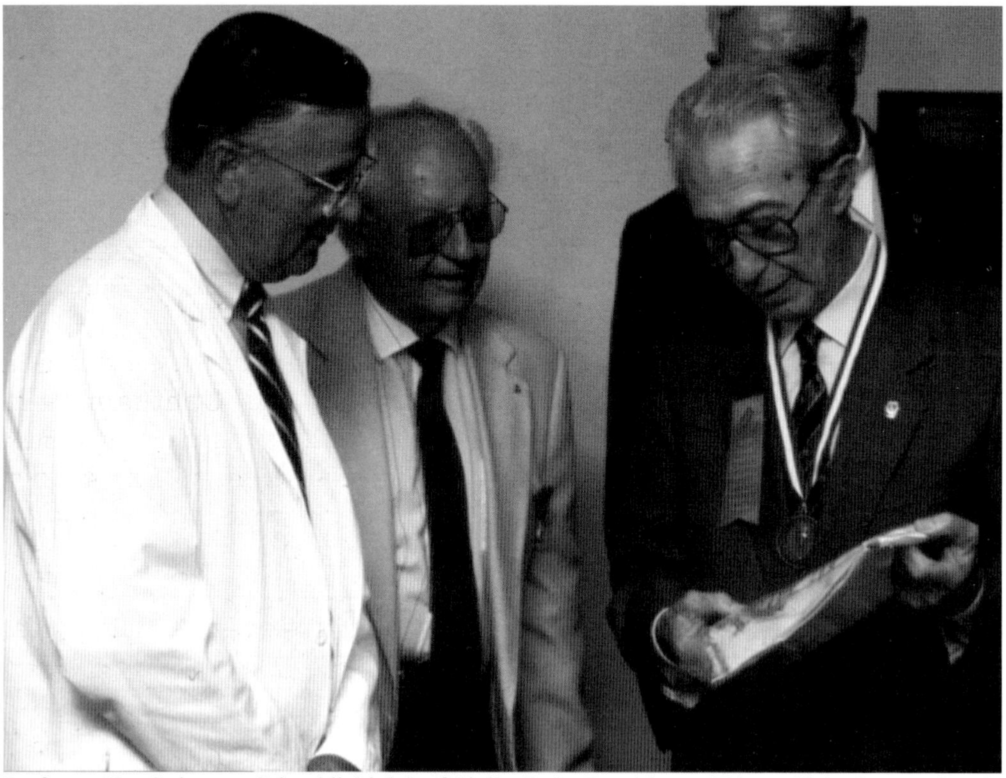

Professor Dr. Guiseppe Grimaldi (right) of Sicily, Italy, President of Lions Clubs International 1994-1995, presented a signed copy of the Grimaldi Family crest to Dr. W. A. J. van Heuven, Chair and Dr. Eugene Eberlin, leading member of the Board of the Lions Sight Research Foundation, which supported the development of eye research at UTHSCSA and funded much of the original equipment for the Ophthalmic Pathology Laboratory. Of historic importance may be the fact that an earlier Grimaldi (1618-1663) from Bologna also had an interest in ophthalmology (optics) by discovering the interference phenomenon. (The Grimaldi family rules Monaco today.)

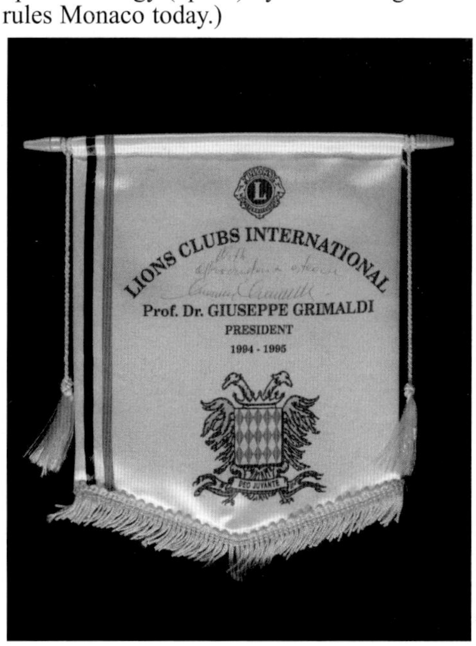


The Grimaldi Family crest

cially interested in the region's unique Hispanic population with its high prevalence of diabetes and related eye problems. Working with military and community ophthalmologists, he quickly designed and embarked upon an ambitious program that succeeded in placing the Ophthalmology Department in the top one-third of the nation's departments in under a decade.

Dr. van Heuven curriculum vitae;
UTHSC Department of Ophthalmology Eye Report

Under Dr. van Heuven's energetic leadership, changes and improvements were made in all aspects of the Ophthalmology Division. In teaching, he responded to the need to improve the curriculum by bringing together clinical sub-specialists in ophthalmology with other experts, particularly in areas underrepresented or not yet represented by the community practitioners who regularly shared their knowledge with the ophthalmology residents. To make the undergraduate Ophthalmology curriculum more comprehensive, he expanded the focus of its clinical experience to include a didactic course that covered the anatomy, physiology, and patho-physiology of the eyes. Residents gained expertise in the subspecialties by participating in the newly organized Alamo City Ophthalmology Residents Conference and in four-month long subspecialty rotations. The reward for these improvements came as program graduates filtered out across Texas and, increasingly, to other parts of the nation.

Among other early tasks, Dr. van Heuven set up new patient record systems and recruited essential personnel to support clinical research efforts in the Department of Ophthalmology. He also strengthened the program's research infrastructure by arranging for the faculty to participate in projects initiated by the Division of Clinical Epidemiology, a unit whose researchers already had established a national reputation as a center for diabetes research under the direction of Michael P. Stern, M.D. and his associate Steven F. Haffner, M.D. Bolstered by the existing track record of their colleagues, faculty of the Department of Ophthalmology subsequently found it easier to attract grants of their own.

Dr. van Heuven interview;
UTHSC Department of Ophthalmology, Eye Report

Soon after he arrived, Dr. van Heuven asked Drs. Patrick O'Connor and David Shacklett, two of the community ophthalmologists with special training in neuro-ophthalmology and retina respectively, to join the faculty. In choosing Dr. O'Connor, formerly of Brooks Air Force Base, the Chairman continued the tradition of close ties between military and civilian ophthalmology that had characterized San Antonio medicine throughout its history. He also hired eye pathologist Dr. Marilyn Kincaid, an expert in clinical research and a fine basic science teacher, and augmented the Department's strengths in basic research by hiring Dr. Kwok Wai Lam, a biochemist formerly of Albany Medical College. At the same time, to broaden their awareness of basic research issues, Dr. van Heuven encouraged second-year residents to attend annual meetings of ARVO, the Association for Research in Vision and Ophthalmology, a national organization for eye research.

Dr. van Heuven interview;
UTHSC Department of Ophthalmology Eye Report

To enhance the Department's community service, Dr. van Heuven established a diagnostic ultrasound service in the outpatient area at the Medical Center Hospital. He also made improvements in the ophthalmology clinic at the R.B. Green Hospital, and assigned Dr. David Shacklett, formerly of Wilford Hall, to serve as Deputy Chairman of the Department in charge there. After the 1979 passage of a statewide Vision Screening Law, the Department promoted vision screening, while the San Antonio Society of Ophthalmology added another important piece to the city's medical infrastructure with the creation of a Low Vision Clinic at the Santa Rosa Hospital Outpatient Clinic.

R. B. Green archives;
UTHSCSA Department of Ophthalmology Eye Report

By 1982, research projects underway in the Department of Ophthalmology had increased significantly. Joseph M. Harrison, Ph.D., a research scientist with Technology Incorporated in San Antonio, had been recruited to re-establish the visual function testing service in the Department and to initiate research projects in areas related to clinical visual physiology. Dr. Harrison had completed his training and conducted research in clinical visual function testing at the University of Florida Department of Ophthalmology, and had gone on to investigate the ocular effects of prolonged low-level laser exposure in rhesus monkeys using behavioral and electrophysiological techniques as part of a broad program of research under contract from the School of Aerospace Medicine. With the opening of reference laboratories for ocular angiography, eye pathology, and glaucoma evaluation facilitated further research activities, the Department henceforth was able to measure its success by its research output as well as its ability to attract a diverse and highly qualified group of residents each year.

Eye Report

By 1983, the Department of Ophthalmology had grown to a total of eight faculty members. Several of these individuals were involved in research as well as in private practice at the University Eye Consultants office housed at the Medical Center Hospital, a new facility on its way to becoming a community resource where South Texas physicians would increasingly refer patients for care involving newer treatments and techniques. To serve as Research Coordinator, Dr. van Heuven appointed Charles H. Bonney III, D.V.M., a new faculty member and former School of Aerospace Medicine researcher who had conducted studies on the ocular effects of electromagnetic radiations ranging from cosmic rays to lasers and also investigated the effects of short laser pulses for possible applications in surgery. Under the direction of Brian Berger, M.D. from Austin, the Department also set up a Uveitis Referral Service at University Eye Consultants in 1985 to offer complete care for problems relating to this condition.

UTHSCSA Department of Ophthalmology Archives

As internal advances were made, Dr. van Heuven and the Department of Ophthalmology also began to attract attention from the community. In support of eye research, the local Lions organization established a Sight and Tissue Foundation to raise funds for the cause and helped the Department to purchase, together with the San Antonio Area Foundation, most of the equipment for a new Eye Pathology Laboratory. Dr. van Heuven oversaw the creation of new biochemistry and electro-physiology laboratories, and enlisted thirty-six clinical faculty members from the surrounding community to support the Department's teaching and service agendas. To further fulfill the Department's research commitments, he was instrumental in the formation of the South Texas Association for Eye Research (STAER), an organization focused exclusively on research issues that created synergies by combining the expertise of Health Center faculty interested in eye research with that of vision researchers from Brooks Air Force Base, the University of Texas at San Antonio, and Wilford Hall.

Dr. van Heuven interview;
UTHSCSA Department of Ophthalmology Eye Report

Among those involved in STAER was Randolph D. Glickman, Ph.D., a physiologist by training and a researcher at Brooks Air Force Base who had obtained his doctorate in neuro-physiology and pharmacology from the University of Toronto and completed postdoctoral fellowships at the Schepens Eye Research Institute in Boston and the Biological Laboratories of Harvard University. In 1981, Dr. Glickman took a position as a Research Scientist with Krug International (formerly, Technology, Incorporated), where he conducted U.S. Air Force-sponsored research on laser bio-effects, especially the interaction of laser radiation with the eye and its effects on visual function, at the Laser Laboratory in the School of Aerospace Medicine at Brooks Air Force Base. (Later, when the Air Force reorganized its laboratories, the Laser Laboratory became part of the Air Force Research Laboratory). In 1983, Dr. Glickman joined the Department of Ophthalmology as an adjunct faculty member, lecturing the residents on laser safety and applications and mentoring those conducting research projects. To facilitate ophthalmic research, he developed an in vitro model of light-induced retinal degeneration for the U.S. Air Force that he used to evaluate pharmacological agents for potential use as prophylaxis for laser eye damage. This work attracted the attention of Alcon Laboratories, which awarded him a research contract to study the actions of experimental agents for use in the retina. His work was an excellent match for the research environment evolving at the time in the Department of Ophthalmology, and in 1989 Dr, Glickman accepted a part-time faculty position in the Department to carry out this research project. From 1989 to 1992, he maintained two laboratories--one at the UT Health Science Center and one at Brooks Air Force Base--and directed a separate research projects at each institution. Because the work of conducting projects at two different institutions simultaneously was physically demanding, Dr. Glickman took the opportunity in 1992 to become a full-time faculty member of the Department of Ophthalmology. Thereafter, he received consecutive grants from the Air Force Office of Scientific Research to study cellular mechanisms of response to laser and light exposure and the mechanisms of free radical generation in the retina and RPE that contribute to degenerative processes. He also obtained a grant from the Office of Naval Research to explore the use of a non-invasive spectroscopic technique to measure drug penetration in the eye. More recently, Dr. Glickman was "cross appointed" in the Departments of Physiology and Radiological Sciences, and held the rank of Professor.

Dr. Glickman interview

In the 1980s, however, Dr. van Heuven realized that despite significant progress in developing research and reaching other goals, the Department's academic growth would be hampered if it were not better known nationally as a clinical, educational, and research resource. To accomplish this growth, it needed to be able to attract future students and faculty from everywhere, not only Texas, and to produce graduates qualified to practice anywhere in the United States. With this in mind, the Chairman initiated several deliberate activities. The first was to publish a quarterly Eye Report for distribution to all ophthalmologists and optometrists in Texas and neighboring states, to all chairpersons, all program directors in the nation, all graduates of the residency program, and to national leaders in ophthalmology and eye research such as the staff of the National Eye Institute and the President and Staff of Research to Prevent Blindness. In addition, copies would be sent to members of subspecialty organizations to which the faculty belonged, such as The Retina Society and the Verhoeff Society.

Dr. van Heuven interview

As Dr. van Heuven conceived it, *The Eye Report* was designed not only to increase awareness of the Department's presence and academic direction, but also to communicate news of its faculty and resident research efforts. In addition to funding resident research and providing opportunities for collaboration with research faculty, the Department required each second-year resident to submit an abstract of their proposed research to ARVO, the Association for Research in Vision and Ophthalmology. To create higher visibility for its faculty on a national scale, the Department encouraged members to participate at national and international meetings, funded their travel to these events, and promoted research projects involving collaboration with faculty at other institutions. It also encouraged participation in clinical trials supported by the National Institutes of Health (NIH). (CRYO-ROP, Light-ROP, ETROP, COMS). Slowly, but surely, these activities in time succeeded, and the Department was able to attract both faculty and students more easily. By 1990, the faculty had become increasingly academic, and growing numbers of faculty and residents neither came from Texas, nor had received their previous training in Texas, and did not remain in Texas when they graduated or departed.

Dr. van Heuven interview

At the same time, South Texans could point to other significant advances in the region. Clinics at Wilford Hall in vitreoretinal disease, external eye disease, oculoplastics, and neuro-ophthalmology had expanded and been actively integrated into the UTHSCSA and Brooke Army Medical Center teaching programs. While sub-specialists nationally developed fellowships in their areas and formed new professional organizations, Dr. Charles (Chuck) Leone in San Antonio helped to create an organization for ophthalmic plastic surgery specialists (ASOPRS) that met before and after annual meetings of the American Academy. Subspecialty research in the Ophthalmology Department led to a new role as a clinical center for the study of Cryotherapy for Retinopathy of Prematurity in babies, a Corneal Research Laboratory was established at the VA Hospital, improvements continued to be made at the Brady Green, and a Medical School-sponsored San Antonio Glaucoma Symposium was held annually. The local Lions organization had now fully equipped the Department's Eye Pathology Laboratory, and it had become an important research resource.

Dr. van Heuven interview

As interests in eye research shifted once again to new clusters of problems, however, new challenges arose for the Department of Ophthalmology. Increasingly, the focus of research study moved below the scale of cellular biology to a more minute focus on molecular biology and biochemistry, facilitated by technological developments that paved the way for digitized imaging as a key to diagnosis, fiber optics as a new material for use in surgical tools, the use of laser light, and other improvements in research technology. Between the technology represented by the ophthalmoscope--the original imaging device used by ophthalmologists--and new computer-linked digitized imaging equipment lay a vast distance representing generations of doctors involved in learning and discovery. The use of fiber optic probes to illumine internal organs permitted new surgical techniques and treatment possibilities, while the use of columnated laser light created highly successful tools for surgery that allowed ophthalmologists to deliver energy in high density to small areas such as the retina. In order to remain on the cutting edge of the field, therefore, the Department needed to become increasingly effective and to acquire ongoing sources of support.

UTHSC Department of Ophthalmology Eye Report

Moving into the 1990s, South Texas ophthalmological resources provided a high level of eye care representing the work of a sophisticated medical community. The Ophthalmology Department moved to more spacious quarters in the McDermott Building on Floyd Curl Drive, which was constructed with support from Robert McDermott, an executive of the nation's largest military insurance provider, USAA, and Ross Perot, the famed Texas entrepreneur who became a candidate for the U. S. Presidency. Its yearly research budget, with a faculty grown to fifteen members, now totaled between one and two million dollars, including a significant level of NIH funding. Its goal was now stated as "*to generate, disseminate, and use knowledge to improve the quality of life of the public by enhancing eye health, detecting systemic diseases and increasing our understanding of the visual system. This mission would be actively pursued in the four interrelated areas of education, research, sub-specialty patient care and community service in a collegial atmosphere that optimized the potential of all participants.*" State, federal, and community support were in place to position the Department for a new century of advances as the Mayor of San Antonio, Henry Cisneros, and the President of University of Texas Health Science Center, Dr. John Howe, increased awareness of the economic importance of a strong medical school and support for a growing health care industry in the region.

UTHSC Department of Ophthalmology, Eye Report

As he looked back in 1990 over his years as Chairman, Dr. van Heuven observed that the Department of Ophthalmology was poised geographically and economically to take an academic leadership role in the hemisphere. On this occasion, he listed two key objectives for the coming years:

*- to increase the academic commitment to the region by obtaining increased endowments to sustain the academic effort and the conduct of research*

*- to increase the academic commitment relating to specific vision problems, not only in Bexar County and San Antonio but also in South Texas and the Americas, especially to improve indigent access to treatment for blindness and other diseases, including diabetic blindness*

Looking ahead to the future in 1990, with the realization that the Department of Ophthalmology would remain a key center from which further new advances would come, the following represents a summary of key accomplishments made during the first nine years of his history. They include:

*- the development of expertise in all the seven subspecialties within ophthalmology: the departments cornea, glaucoma, neuro-ophthalmology, orbits/plastics, pathology, pediatric ophthalmology, and retina.*

*- the development of a teaching curriculum for residents in each of these subspecialties, later leading to the development of post-residency fellowships*

*- the development of externally-funded basic research programs that became one third of the Departmental budget*

*- the initiation of efforts to create endowments for academic endeavors which by 1990 had reached over four million dollars*

*- advances as a regional resource for highly specialized clinical care, e.g., electro-physiology, ultra-sound, angiography, tumor diagnosis and treatment, etc.*

*- the creation of new opportunities for University of Texas at San Antonio undergraduate and UTHSCSA medical students to participate in vision research*

*- the creation of new venues of continuing education for South Texas ophthalmologists and optometrists*

*- the continuation of the tradition of cooperation between the military programs in San Antonio and the Medical School in research and teaching*

*- the development of increased interaction with other basic scientists in vision research at the Medical School and in the military community, e.g., in such areas as molecular biology, neuroscience, and laser technology.*

In his regular column in the monthly Eye Report, "*The View from the Chair*," Dr. van Heuven made the following comments in June of 1990. Summarizing his experience to date as Chairman of the Department of

Ophthalmology, he measured the distance covered in a significant period in its history and laid out a new agenda for the future. His remarks constitute a fitting close to, and the opening of future chapters in, the story of South Texas ophthalmology.

*"In 1981, after coming to San Antonio into the newly formed Department of Ophthalmology (Ophthalmology had been a division of General Surgery until then), it took me a few months to begin to understand the politics and economics of the University of Texas System, the Health Science Center, and the community itself. However, I was soon asked to prepare a "State of the Department" message, a yearly ritual given by chairmen to the Executive Committee of the U. T. Health Science Center. I took that opportunity to formulate a Seven Year Plan. This plan, which was completed during the subsequent seven years, was based on the simple premise that it was the goal of the Department to be a "balanced" department, equally involved with teaching, research, and patient care. This seemingly unarguable goal, however, made a conscientious decision that, without all three activities being strongly represented, the future of academic ophthalmology in South Texas would be uncertain. It was also a deliberate departure from the goals of many other clinical departments at UTHSC and also other departments of ophthalmology that frequently concentrate on only one or two of these endeavors. For example, some eye departments offer merely clinical preceptorships, with or without clinical research but with no basic research, while others are weighted heavily toward research."*

*"Trying to find out what makes departments of ophthalmology good is difficult. If one asks the medical students, the answer concerns the percent of the medical school class that was "turned on" to ophthalmology by enthusiastic teaching. If one asks the residents, the answer has to do with the volume of the eye surgery they perform. If one asks the fellows, subspecialty clinical expertise and one-to-one teaching in the operating room are important. If one asks the Dean, the answer may vary but often relates to being fiscally sound and fulfilling the basic teaching requirements for the medical school. If one asks the President of the Health Science Center, the answer relates to fiscal responsibility (a positive bottom line); to bringing insignificant outside monies to increase academic activities; or to being nationally prominent in research, patient care, and other academic pursuits. When one asks the San Antonio medical community, the answer has to do with taking care of the indigent patients of Bexar County. Looking at all these*

*answers, it is clear that they include all three activities of multilevel teaching, basic and clinical research, plus primary and tertiary eye care. All of this fits within the broad definitions of Academe (the garden near Athens where Plato taught), which has to do with teaching as well as advancement of knowledge."*

*"All these things are difficult to do well in a young department that is trying to become a major academic center. In teaching, we are fulfilling only slightly more than the minimum requirements for medical students. Clinical fellowships are only just now beginning. There is also a need for teaching ophthalmic assistants and technicians, of which there is an undersupply in South Texas. The number of continuing education programs for community physicians must also be increased to fulfill increasing demands. The teaching of students in Family Practice, Pediatrics, Internal Medicine, ENT - all need to be improved. Outreach programs to teach the South Texas population about the availability of medical care, particularly in diabetes, needs to be done on a grander scale. Finally, bilingual programs for health care professionals from Mexico and Central America need to be started."*

*"In research, while sustaining our efforts in basic biochemistry, cell culture, toxicology, electrophysiology, ultrasound, epidemiology, and psychophysics, programs need to be developed in molecular biology, genetics, microcirculation, and diabetes."*

*"In clinical practice, faculty positions need to be filled in ophthalmic pathology, ophthalmic plastic surgery, medical retina/immunology/AIDS, and vitreoretinal surgery."*

*"What are the present resources available to support this growth? Funding sources must come from the University of Texas, research grants, and patient income. As far as UT is concerned, it may surprise some to find out that only 8 of our 16 present faculty members are paid anything at all by UT, and those are paid a mere one-third of their salaries for the sole purpose of teaching. Thus, the Department must support two-thirds of those salaries, plus all benefits, plus the salaries of the remaining eight faculty members and most of the supporting staff from patient income and research grants. With research monies becoming increasingly difficult to acquire--we have been lucky so far--and with an overwhelming burden on the faculty to supervise the complex eye care of nonpaying indigent patients, it is clear that private patient*

*income also must continue to be an important revenue source. In our institution, which does not have the clinical track record of tertiary care expertise as do Johns Hopkins or Harvard, this is especially difficult to develop in an atmosphere of severe medical competition. In addition, it is not my personal goal to compete in clinical medicine with the San Antonio medical community, which is blessed with some exceptionally good ophthalmologists. Instead, I wish to concentrate on areas of clinical expertise not generally available in San Antonio, as the Department's recent involvement in the national Collaborative Ocular Melanoma Study illustrates. With the cooperation of local ophthalmologists, the Department could now truly offer patients comprehensive care in melanoma treatment and access to participation in a national clinical trial."*

*"It has been pointed out in the past that the presence of a strong learning center in a community is the single greatest stimulus to the economic development of that community. Hence, it should be the Department's goal to make the Health Science Center as strong as possible and let it fulfill all its academic goals maximally. In the Ophthalmology Department, with the fiscal constraints of insufficient UT funds and a shrinking national budget for research and increased clinical competition, it has now become necessary to acquire a substantial endowment to support research programs, education, and professorships in perpetuity. The establishment of the Whitehead Fellowship endowment, more than ten years ago, was the first endowment to our department and is now, after years of preparation, making it possible to start clinical fellowships. This year, the Herbert F. Mueller Professorship will be endowed, and an ophthalmic pathology professorship is being established by the District 2A-2 Lions Clubs of South Texas. This is just the beginning. It is my sincere hope that, during the next few years, we will be able to establish at least five $1,000,000 additional professorships so that we can attract the best academic minds to our campus to maintain what we have, develop new programs and make our department, and our medical school strong for the ultimate benefit of San Antonio and South Texas."*

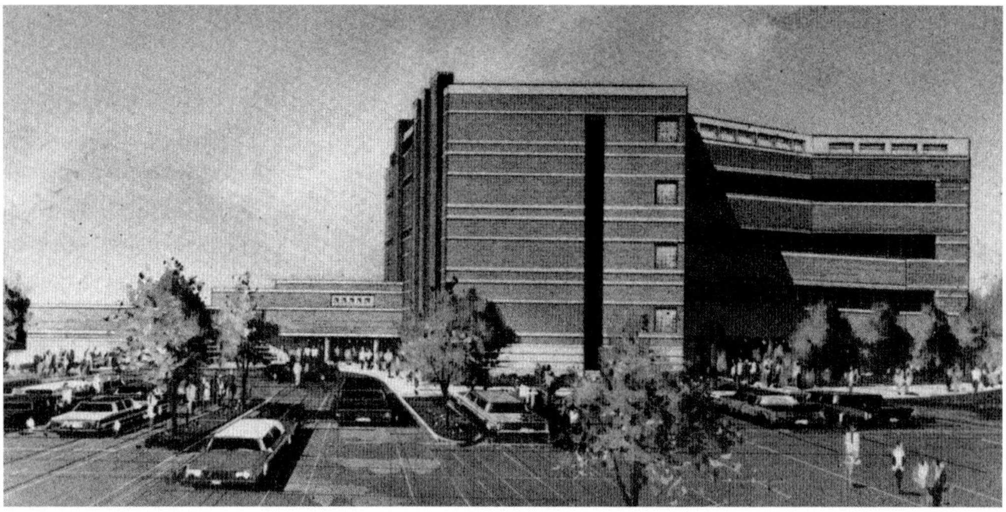

1990. Artist's rendition of the Robert F. McDermott Clinical Science Building, where the Ophthalmology Department would expand its research and teaching programs.

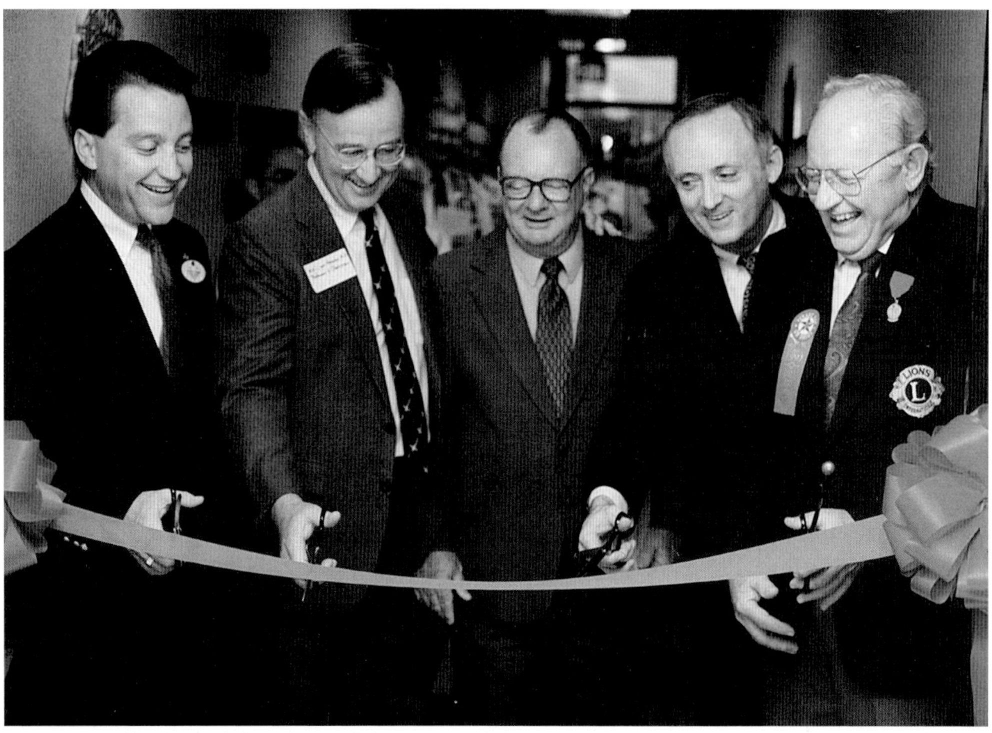

1991. Dedication of the Lions Sight Research Center in the newly completed Robert F. McDermott Clinical Science Building, the first expansion of the Medical School complex at the North Campus. The Ophthalmology Department was given the 4th floor for the expansion of its research and education missions.
From L to R: Kevin Dinnin, Lions Past District Governor; W. A. J. van Heuven, MD, Chairman; James J. Young, PhD, Dean; John P. Howe, III, MD, President of UTHSCSA; and Eugene Eberlin, MD, Board Member of the Lions Sight Research Foundation.

# Remembrance of Dr. Matthews

*Grand Rounds 4-14-1995*

From THE EYE REPORT, Vol. 13, No. 2
Published by the Department of Ophthalmology, UTHSCSA

As most of you know, John L. Matthews, M.D., our beloved Jack Matthews, died two days ago on April 12, 1995, at Methodist Hospital. That has given me, and could give all of us here, a moment to contemplate life and its opportunities.

To me Jack was a friend, an advisor, and an example. Although I selfishly guarded my special relationship with him, I had found over the years that he acted in that same capacity with others, including many of the leaders of our community. He was involved with everything and anything related to ophthalmology in South Texas and was either a founder or a past president of most regional organizations related to vision or to the prevention of blindness. He was also one of the founding fathers of this very medical school in San Antonio. Never, after helping start or presiding over any of these organizations, did he abandon them, but instead continued to watch over their welfare. His loyal attendance at almost every Friday morning Ophthalmology grand rounds was an example of his continuing interest in this department, and his presence helped assure that we would keep sight of our goals.

A few years ago, at one of the AUPO meetings, Ed Norton, then chairman at the Bascom Palmer Eye Institute, was asked what attributes made a good chairman. First on his list was integrity, or as Webster's Dictionary defines: having firm adherence to values, being incorruptible, the quality of being complete. Yesterday, when I asked Dr. Frank Weixel, Jack Matthews' partner for many years, how he would describe Jack, he said: "*He had integrity one hundred percent.*" I agreed and felt lucky to have had Jack's influence on me as I have chaired this department.

At the same time Jack also knew, and I quote Dag Hammarskjöld from his Markings, "*to be grateful as your deeds become less and less associated with your name, as your feet ever more lightly tread the earth.*" Jack demonstrated this sensitivity and humility by constantly diminishing himself while magnifying others and making sure that history remembered them correctly. He gave this department all the volumes of *The History of Ophthalmology*, by Hirschberg, so that we would remember our ophthalmic heritage. In addition, during the last few weeks, when he knew he might not live much longer, he called me to make certain that I would guarantee the continuing remembrance of people in our community who have been great supporters of our department. Specifically, he asked me to make sure that the Whitehead family was kept apprised of the work of their endowment, which was given many years ago for the support of fellowships. He also asked about the Hogan Professorship, which he had helped initiate, and was pleased to hear that we had raised nearly a quarter of a million dollars so far. In addition, he called Kittie and Rugeley Ferguson, the lead donors to the Hogan Professorship, to assure their continued support. Naturally, I promised Jack that I would continue to nurture these relationships.

And so now, at this moment of remembrance, I think that we may all wish to follow Jack's example of teaching and practicing integrity and humility and, as we do so on our walk through life, we may find Jack Matthews still walking with us, "*ever more lightly*."

# BIBLIOGRAPHY

## ARCHIVAL COLLECTIONS

AIRMED Museum Collections, Fort Sam Houston, San Antonio.
Baptist Medical Center Eye Bank Archives, "Historical Information," compiled February 1991.
Bexar County Medical Society Archives, including membership records on microfilm.
Briscoe Library Archives, University of Texas Health Science Center, San Antonio, including "Inventory of the Burns Memorial Library, May 1, 1962," and "Dedication of the Burns Collection."
Center for American History, The University of Texas at Austin.
Daughters of the Republic of Texas Library Archives, San Antonio, including biography and clipping files.
Department of Ophthalmology Archives, University of Texas Health Science Center, San Antonio.
Fort Sam Houston Museum Archives, Fort Sam Houston, San Antonio.
Hangar 9, Brooks Air Force Base, San Antonio, including Frederic H. Thorne journals and William C. Ocker materials.
Houston Metropolitan Research Center, Houston.
Institute of Texan Cultures Library, The University of Texas at San Antonio, including Strughold interview with Ingrid Kokinda, April 5, 1982, and vertical files.
Matthews, Dr. John L. papers in the Briscoe Library, University of Texas Health Science Center, San Antonio.
Robert B. Green Memorial Hospital Archives, San Antonio.
San Antonio Association for the Blind, including clippings and brochures.
San Antonio O&O Society Archives in Bexar County Medical Society Library.
San Antonio Public Library, Texana Collection, including Alamo Ironworks vertical file.
Strughold Library Archives, Brooks Air Force Base, San Antonio.
County Medical Society Records, Texas, including Cameron-Willacy Medical Society, Nueces County Medical Society Auxiliary, and Victoria-Goliad-Jackson Counties Medical Society.
Texas Medical Association, Austin, membership records.
Texas Ophthalmological Association records, Austin.
Wilford Hall Hospital Department of Ophthalmology Historical files, San Antonio

### INTERVIEWS

Ralph Allen, Ph.D., Technology, Inc., October 12, 1997
Andres Aquino, M.D., President, Kleberg-Kennedy-Kingsville Medical Society, February 6, 1996
Dor Brown, M.D., February 6, 1996
Fred B. Cooper, M.D., February 5, 1990
Pam Crane, Carl Crane's daughter, August 7,1996
Dorothy Crawford, Dr. Frederick Thorne's niece, December 16, 1996
James Fox Culver
Tom Folbre, M.D., interview submitted to Anne McCurdy, Chair of Committee of Research and Romance of Medicine in Bexar County, Bexar County Medical Society, 1984
Mauro Pat Gangai, M.D., Kerr-Kendall-Bandera Medical Society, January 26, 1996
Joseph DeGasperi, M.D., August 26, 1996
Richard Fixott, M.D., June 4, 1997
David Garrett, Former Executive Director, Baptist Memorial Hospital System, January 31, 1991
Mary Hicks, Senior Secretary, University of Texas Health Science Center Department of Ophthalmology, August 20, 1996
Robert R. Hobson, M.D., University of Texas Health Science Center Department of Ophthalmology, August 12, 1996
Pamela Lambden, Memorial Medical Center, Port Lavaca, January 18, 1996
Jack B. Lee, M.D., March 8, 1990
Col. William C. Lloyd, III, M.D., April 1, 1996
Ann McCurdy, January 10, 1997
Marion W. McCurdy, M.D., January 25, 1990
John Matthews, M.D., January 18, 1990
Mrs. John Matthews
Wilbur L. Matthews, author, History of the San Antonio Medical Foundation and South Texas Medical Center, August 12, 1998
James L. Mims, Jr., M.D., February 13, 1990, August 25, 1996
Doris Osborn, William Ocker's daughter, October 2, 1996.
Richard Poirer, M.D.
James Pridgen, M.D., April 23, 1997
Richard Ruiz, M.D., February 6, 1996
Dan A. Russell, Jr., M.D., April 25, 1997; January 30, 1990
William T. Sichi, M.D., February 6, 1990, May 17, 1996
Col. John R. Simmons, M.D., May 20, 1996
John Smith, M.D., April 5, 1996
Mrs. Bell Louise Stevenson (on Elizabeth Donaldson and Dr. John Burleson), May 14, 1991
Hubertus Strughold, M.D., interview with Ingrid Kokinda, April 5, 1982, typescript, Institute of Texan Cultures
Edwin M. Sykes, Jr., M.D., August 24, 1997
Thomas J. Tredici, M.D., August 8, 1990, November 18, 1991
W.A.J. Van Heuven, M.D.
Curtis Vaughan, Jr., December 12, 1996
Stephen G. Waller, M.D., Department of Ophthalmology, Wilford Hall, May 2, 1996
George Weinstein, M.D., September 4, 1996
Andy Weir, Texas State Commission for the Blind
Francis X. Weixel, M.D., February 21, 1990, May 22, 1996
Barney Williams, M.D., January 26, 1996

## NEWSPAPERS, PERIODICALS, AND DIRECTORIES

Appler's, Jules A., General Directory of the City of San Antonio, San Antonio, 1892-1902
Daniel's Texas Medical Journal, Austin, 1(July 1885)-8(1892-1893) Dictionary of American Medical Biographies, New York/London, D. Appleton and Co., 1928
Directory of Physicians in the United States, Chicago, American Medical Association, 1906-1989
Morrison and Fourmy's General Directory of the City of San Antonio (various publishers, 1877-1890)
Official ABMS Directory of Board Certified Medical Specialists, New Providence, N.J., Marquis Who's Who, 1994-
Ophthalmology Department, University of Texas Health Science Center at San Antonio, Eye Report, Quarterly Bulletin from the Department of Ophthalmology, June 1982-
Polk, R.L., and Co., Medical and Surgical Register of the United States, Detroit, Chicago, R.L. Polk and Co., Publisher, 1896
______. Polk's Medical Register and Directory, 1906, 1908, 1910
Red Book of Eye, Ear, Nose and Throat Specialists, 15th ed., Chicago, Professional Press, 1943
Red Book of Ophthalmology, 35th ed., Chicago, Professional Press, 1983
San Antonio Light
San Antonio Register
San Antonio Express News
South Texas Register of Specialists, 1943
State Medical Association of Texas, Proceedings and Transactions, 1869-1899; 1899 to date
Texas Medical Gazette 1(1901)-5(1905)
Texas Medical Record, Galveston 1(1881)-2(1882)
Texas Medical News, a Journal of Medicine, Surgery, and Hygiene, Austin, 5(1896)-25 (1915-16)
Texas State Journal of Medicine obituaries
Who's Who in American Medicine, New York, Who's Who Pubs., 1925.

### SECONDARY SOURCES

Acheson, Alex W. Texas Quackery. Denison, n.p., 1885.
Air Service Medical. War Department. Air Service Division of Military Aeronautics, Washington, D.C., Government Printing Office, 1919.
Air Training Command, Aerospace Medical Center, School of Aviation Medicine, United States Air Force, Brooks AFB, Texas, November, 1959.
"Airships to 'Burn' Air Are Predicted," November 7, 1951, San Antonio Express News.
Albert, Daniel M. and Diane D. Edwards, eds., History of Ophthalmology, Cambridge, Massachusetts, Blackwell Science, 1996.

_____. and Harold G. Scheie, History of Ophthalmology at the University of Pennsylvania, Springfield, Illinois, Charles C. Thomas, Publisher, 1965.

Alcott, Edward B., Aerospace Medical Division: 25 Years of Excellence 1961-1986, History Office, Aerospace Medical Division, Brooks Air Force Base, Texas, 1986.

_____. "Brief History of Brooks Air Force Base," typescript, Brooks AFB Hangar 9 Archives.

_____. "Col. William C. Ocker: Changing the Course of Early Aerospace Medicine," USAF Medical Service Digest, Summer 1991, 20-23.

Alliance for Eye and Vision Research, Vision of Hope for Older Americans: Progress and Opportunities in Eye and Vision Research: Official Report to the White House Conference on Aging, Washington, D.C., The Alliance, 1995.

"Antebellum fledglings," Sportsman Pilot

Armstrong, Harry G. Principles and Practice of Aviation Medicine, rev. ed., Baltimore, Williams and Wilkins Company, 1939, 1943.

"Army Plans for Fort Sam Big Question, San Antonio Light, October 21, 1945.

Arrington, George E., Jr. History of Ophthalmology, New York, M.D. Publications, 1959.

"ASF Medical Training to Occupy All of Fort Sam," San Antonio Light, November 2, 1945, 10-A.

Ashcroft, Bruce A. "Brief History of the School of Aviation Medicine, with an Emphasis on the Randolph AFB Years, 1931-1959," AETC History Office, April, 1996, typescript.

Atkinson, Donald T. External Diseases of the Eye, 1934; The Ocular Fundus in Diagnosis and Treatment, 1937; A Treatise on Cataract, 1921; Magic, Myth and Medicine, 1956.

_____. Texas Surgeon; an Autobiography, New York, Ives Washburn, Inc., 1958.

_____. Selected articles from the Eye, Ear, Nose and Throat Monthly, Chicago, Professional Press, Inc., Publishers):

"Management of Cataract in the Young," 5(October 1926)

"The Blow Upon the Eye," 9(1930), 227

"Cutaneous Cancer as Seen by the Ophthalmologist and Otolaryngologist," (1931), 408

"The Surgical Treatment of Strabismus," 23(1944), 97

"Pitfalls of Cataract Surgery," 23(1944), 487

"A Resume of Eight Hundred Cataract Extractions," 24(1945), 382

"Mechanics of the Etiology and Surgical Treatment of Glaucoma," 25(1946), 606.

"Controversial Steps in Cataract Operations," 26 (1947), 529.

"How Can We Improve the Management of Our Glaucoma Cases? 27(1948), 460

"Management of Incipient Cataracts," 33 (1954), 411

Aust, J.B., Letter to George Weinstein, November 17, 1969, UTHSC Department of Ophthalmology archives.

_____. Memorandum to George Weinstein, January 11, 1972, UTHSC Department of Ophthalmology archives.

"Aviation, Space Experts Arrive," November 6, 1951, San Antonio Express-News.

Barker, Eugene C. "Minutes of the Ayuntamiento of San Felipe de Austin 1828-1832," Southwestern Historical Quarterly, XXIII, 302-318.

Barksdale, Ethelbert Courtland. Genesis of the Aviation Industry in North Texas,

Austin, Bureau of Business Research, University of Texas, Texas Industry Series, 1958: No. 6.

Bartlett's Familiar Quotations. 16th ed. Boston, Little, Brown, 1992.

Bauer, Louis Hopewell. Aviation Medicine, Baltimore, Williams and Wilkins, 1926.

Baum, Alan C., President, Texas Ophthalmological Association, Letter to Dr. Jack B. Lee, May 14, 1981, TOA Archives.

Bell, J.H. "State Legislature and the Medical Profession," Transactions of the State Medical Association of Texas, 1900, 323-330.

Benford, Robert J. Doctors in the Sky: The Story of the Aero Medical Association, Springfield, Illinois, Charles C. Thomas Publisher, 1955.

_____. Heritage of Aviation Medicine: an Annotated Directory of Early Artifacts, Washington, D.C., Aerospace Medical Association, 1979.

Benjamin, G.G. Germans in Texas: A Study in Immigration, Austin, Jenkins, 1974 (1909).

Bexar County Medical Society Auxiliary Research Committee, "Anecdotes and Memoirs of Bexar County Doctors," typescript, 1984.

Biesele, Rudolph Leopold. History of the German Settlements in Texas, 1831-1861, Austin, Von Boeckmann-Jones, Co., 1930.

Bilstein, Roger E. Orders of Magnitude: A History of the NACA and NASA, 1915-1990, Washington, D.C., NASA Office of Management, Scientific and Technical Information Division, 1989.

Bisno, David C. Eyes in the Storm—President Hopkins's Dilemma: The Dartmouth Eye Institute. Norwich, Vermont, Norwich Publishing, 1994.

Bonnabeau, Raymond C., Jr., "Apprenticeship System and the Development of Early Medical Schools in America," Minnesota Medicine, 68(1985), 765-766.

Bonner, Thomas Neville. American Doctors and German Universities: A Chapter in International Intellectual Relations, 1870-1914, Lincoln, University of Nebraska Press, 1963.

_____. American Medical Association of Vienna, 1912.

_____. Becoming a Physician: Medical Education in Great Britain, France, Germany, and the United States, 1750-1945, Oxford University Press, 1995.

Boulay, Patrick. "Alamo is Also Cradle of Medical Care in San Antonio," San Antonio Light, March 1, 1981.

Bracht, Viktor. Texas in 1848, San Antonio, Naylor Printing Co., 1931.

"Brooke Army Medical Center History," BAMC Public Information Office, Fort Sam Houston, Texas, n.d., typescript

"Brooke Army Medical Center Training Activities, BAMC Public Information Office, n.d., typescript, Airmed Museum Archives.

Broussard, Ray F. San Antonio During the Texas Republic, El Paso, Western Press, 1967.

Brown, Clayton. "Medical Education in Texas: the Growth of Schools," Texas Medicine, 82(May 1986), 49-53.

Bryan, Sharon. Pioneering Specialists: History of the American Academy of Ophthalmology and Otolaryngology, San Francisco and Rochester, Minnesota, American Academy of Ophthalmology and American Academy of Otolaryngology: Head and Neck Surgery, 1982.

Burkhalter, Lois Wood. Marion Koogler McNay: a Biography, 1883-1950, San Antonio, Marion Koogler McNay Art Institute, 1968.

Burleson, John H., M.D. "First Aid to Injured Eyes," Read to Section on Railway Surgery at the State Medical Association of Texas Meeting, Houston, April 20, 1905.

_____. Letter from John Burleson, M.D. to August J. Streit, M.D., June 18, 1956, Texas Ophthalmological Society archives.

_____. "Standardization of Ophthalmology and the Ethical Attitude of Its Members," Texas Medical Association Journal, n.d., in Bexar County Medical Society records.

_____. "Texas O&O Society in the Beginning, as told by Dr. John H. Burleson, June 1956," typescript, Texas Ophthalmological Society archives.

Burrow, James G., M.D. "Economic and Political Policies of the Texas Medical Profession in the Progressive Era," Texas Medicine, 74(February 1978), 54-57.

_____. Organized Medicine in the Progressive Era, Baltimore, Johns Hopkins University Press, 1977.

Byrnes, Col. Victor A., Capt. D.V.L. Brown, H.W. Rose, M.D. and Paul A. Cibis, "Chorioretinal Burns Produced by Atomic Flash," AMA Archives of Ophthalmology, 53: March 1955: 351-364.

"Camp Travis: The National Army Cantonment at Fort Sam Houston, 1917-1992," 75th Anniversary, San Antonio, Fort Sam Houston Museum, 1992.

Carnegie Commission on Higher Education. Higher Education and the Nation's Health: Policies for Medical and Dental Education, New York, McGraw Hill, October 1970.

Cary, E.H., "EENT as a Specialty in Texas in the Past Century," Texas State Journal of Medicine, May 1953, 298-301.

"Centennial Record of the San Antonio Army Service Forces Depot, 1845-1945," San Antonio, Texas, The Depot, 1945.

Chabot, F.C. San Antonio and Its Beginnings. San Antonio, Artes Graficas, 1936.

_____. With the Makers of San Antonio. San Antonio, Artes Graficas, 1937

Chance, Burton. Ophthalmology (Clio Medica Series of Primers on the History of Medicine, edited by E.B. Krumbhaar, 20), New York, Hafner Publishing Co., 1962(1939).

Chestnutt, Lois, Bee County Families, Dallas, Curtis Media Corporation, 1992.

Chevreul, M.E. Principles of Harmony and Contrast of Colors and Their Applications to the Arts., Westchester, Pennsylvania, Schiffer Publishing, 1938.

"Chronology of the Texas Society to Prevent Blindness, typescript, n.p., The Society, September, 1992.

Clark, Archibald Fletcher, Sr. Autobiography, typescript, Prairie Lee, Caldwell County, December 1978, in Daughters of the Republic of Texas Library, San Antonio.

Cline, Isaac Monroe. Climate of Texas in its Relation to the Distribution of Diseases and the Effects of Climate and Weather Changes in Causing Diseases and Deaths, Galveston, Strickland Publishing Co., 1894.

Coates, John Boyd, Jr. Editor-in-Chief, Ophthalmology and Otolaryngology, Washington, D.C., Office of the Surgeon General, Department of the Army, 1957.

Coleman, James M., Aesculapius on the Colorado, Austin, Encino Press for the Friends of the Austin Public Library, 1971.

n.a., "Col. Ocker is Dead; Aviation Inventor," New York Times, September 18, 1942.

Conner, J.E. Centennial Record of the San Antonio Army Service Forces Depot, 1845-1945, San Antonio, The Depot, 1945.

Corner, William, comp. and ed. San Antonio de Bexar: a Guide and History, San Antonio, Bainbridge and Corner, 1890.

"Cosmic Rays Seen No Bar in Upper Air," November 8, 1951, San Antonio Express-News.

"Courses of Instruction at USA MFSS," typescript, Airmed Museum, Fort Sam Houston.

Crane, Carl, Letter to Mrs. T.E. McCray, August 20, 1967.
_____. "Spiral Dive," Airman, November 1964, 24-27.
Cranfill, J. B., M.D. Dr. J. B. Cranfill's Chronicle: a Story of Life in Texas. New York and Chicago, Fleming H. Revell Co., 1916.
Crew, F.A.E. Army Medical Services; Administration, vol. 2, London, Her Majesty's Stationer's Office, 1955, 514-523.
Culver, James F., "Contact Lenses for Flying Personnel, "Aeromedical Digest 12(7 July 1961).
n.a., "Brigadier General (Dr.) James F. Culver, USAF Biographical Sketch," 1980.
Curtis, Albert. Fabulous San Antonio, San Antonio, Naylor, 1955.
_____. Military San Antonio, San Antonio, Standard Printing Co., 1941.
Cushing, Harvey. Life of Sir William Osler. Oxford, Clarendon Press, 1940(1925).
Dammin, Gustave J. "Military Medicine and Its Influence on Medicine," Bulletin of the New York Academy of Medicine, New York, New York Academy of Medicine, 2nd series, 47(December 1971), 1455-1471.
DeWitt County Historical Commission. History of DeWitt County, Dallas, Curtis Media Corporation, 1991.
Dictionary of American Medical Biographies, New York and London, D. Appleton and Co., 1928.
Dixon, Charles D., MD. Menace: An Exposition of Quackery, Nostrum Exploitation and Reminiscences of a Country Doctor, San Antonio, Lodovic Printing Co., 1914.
Dunlop, Richard. Doctors of the American Frontier, Garden City, New York, Doubleday and Co., 1965(1962).
Engelke, Louis B. "The Doctors Study Over Time," San Antonio Express Magazine, February 17, 1952.
Everett, Donald E. San Antonio: The Flavor of Its Past, 1845-1898, San Antonio, 1975.
"Eye, Ear, Nose and Throat Hospitals in Texas," typescript, Historical Research Center, Houston Academy of Medicine-Texas Medical Center Library, Houston, February 1996.
"Eye of Horus," in Letters to the Editor, Australian Prescriber, 18: 4, (1995), 84.
Eye Institute Committee. "The Eye Institute," brochure, San Antonio, University of Texas Health Science Center, 1979.
"Fact Sheet," Bexar County Medical Society archives.
Farge, Emile J. "Eye Banking: 1944 to the Present," Survey of Ophthalmology, 33:4 (January-February 1989), 260-263.
Fehrenbach, T.R., Landmark Years, 1881-1981: 100 Years of San Antonio's History Reprinted from the Centennial Edition of the San Antonio Light, San Antonio, San Antonio Light, 1981.
Ferris, Sylvia Van Voast and Eleanor Sellers Hoppe. Scalpels and Sabers, Austin, Eakin Press, 1985.
Fisher, C.E., M.D. Queer Quaint Old San Antonio: Its Climate in Throat and Lung Diseases, San Antonio, n.p., 1895.
Flexner, Abraham. Medical Education in the United States and Canada, New York, 1910 (Ann Arbor, Xerox University Microfilms, 1970).
Fort Sam Houston Museum. "Camp Travis: The National Army Cantonment at Fort Sam Houston, 75th Anniversary 1917-1992". San Antonio, The Museum, 1992.
"Fort Sam Houston Troop List, vol. 2: World War I, 1916-1919," Fort Sam Houston Museum, San Antonio, 1994.
Frazier, J.M. "Evolution in the Study and Practice of Medicine in Texas in Sixty

Years," Texas State Journal of Medicine, 32 (1936), 300-305.
Fulton, John F., Phebe M. Hoff, and Henrietta T. Perkins. Bibliography of Visual Literature, 1939-1944. Prepared by the Committee on Aviation Medicine, Division of Medical Sciences, National Research Council, for the Medical Research. Office of Science Research and Development, Washington, D.C., 1945. Published by Yale University Press.
Garrett, David. "Growth of a Service," Eye Report, San Antonio, University of Texas Health Science Center Department of Ophthalmology, December 1984, 1-2.
Glasby, Clarence. Project Paperclip, New York, Atheneum, 1971.
n.a., "A Glimpse Into the Past," Texas Medicine 71(March 1975), n.p.
Goar, Everett L. "Ophthalmology," Texas Medicine 63(3), March 1967, 82-84.
Good, Pat, "Dr. John L. (Jack) Matthews," Community Relations Department, San Antonio Lighthouse, n.d.
Gorin, George. History of Ophthalmology, Wilmington, Delaware, Publish or Perish, Inc., 1982.
Goss, David A. "Eyes in the Storm—President Hopkins's Dilemma: The Dartmouth Eye Institute," Book Review in Optometry and Vision Science, 72:12(December 1995), 931.
Graham, Bill, "Med School to Add 'Eye Camera' Unit," San Antonio Express-News, 1971.
Greater Kelly Development Corporation. ""Brief History of Kelly Air Force Base," Office of History, San Antonio Air Logistics Center, Kelly AFB, Texas, 1995.
Gregory, H.B. "Centennial Record of the San Antonio Army Service Forces Depot, 1845-1945," typescript, Headquarters, Fifty U.S. Army, Fort Sam Houston, 108-115.
Greenwood, Allen. Military Ophthalmic Surgery, Philadelphia and New York, Lea and Febiger, 1918.
Gregory, R.L. Eye and Brain, the Psychology of Seeing, New York, McGraw-Hill Book Company, 1977.
Grimes, Roy, ed. Three Hundred Years in Victoria County, Victoria Advocate Publishing Co., 1968.
Grow, Malcolm Cummings and Harry G. Armstrong. Fit to Fly: a Medical Handbook for Fliers, New York, London, D. Appleton-Century Company, Inc., 1941.
Handy, Mary Olivia. History of Fort Sam Houston, San Antonio, Naylor Company, 1951.
Harris, Herbert H., M.D. "A Fifty Year History of the Texas Society of Ophthalmology and Otolaryngology," Speech before the Annual Banquet, November 5, 1976, in Corpus Christi, typescript, Houston, The Society, 1977.
Harris, Herbert, M.D., "Historical Notes of the Texas Society of O&O," n.d., typescript, in Bexar County Medical Society archives.
Herff, Ferdinand Peter, Laura L. Barber, eds. The Doctors Herff, A Three Generation Memoir, San Antonio, 1973.
Heusinger, Edward W., F.R.G.S. A Chronology of Events in San Antonio, San Antonio, Standard Printing Co., 1951.
_____. Heusinger Family in Texas, San Antonio, 1945.
Hill, Herbert, M.D. "Cooperation Between the Internist and Ophthalmo-Oto-Laryngologist," Southwest Texas Medicine, 14-21.
Hirsch, Sandy, Administrative Director, Texas Ophthalmological Association, Letter to Sue McDonald, January 15, 1990, TOA archives.
Hirschberg, Julius, translated by Frederick C. Blodi. History of Ophthalmology, Bonn, J.P. Wayenborgh, 1982.

"Historical Military Data on San Antonio and Fort Sam Houston," typescript, Fort Sam Houston archives.
"History of the Medical Training Center, Brooke Army Medical Center," typescript, Airmed Museum archives.
"History of the Robert B. Green—once neglected, now proud and strong," typescript, R.B. Green Memorial Hospital Archives.
Hoff, Ebbe Curtis and John Farquhar Fulton. Bibliography of Aviation Medicine, Springfield, Illinois, Charles C. Thomas, 1942.
Hubbell, Alvin A. Development of Ophthalmology in America, 1800 to 1870, Chicago, American Medical Association, 1908 (1907).
Hun, Henry. Guide to American Medical Students in Europe, New York, William Wood and Co., 1883.
Hunt, H.E. "Ophthalmology in Texas," Texas Medicine 63:6(June 1967), 67-70.
Hurtl, J., Letter, "Notes and Queries," Southwestern Historical Quarterly, XI (1956) no. 1, n.p.
International Postgraduate Medical Assembly of Southwest Texas, Minutes, 1955-1976.
"International Postgraduate Medical Assembly," copy from Special Newspaper Edition, January 25, 1949, in Briscoe Library, University of Texas Health Science Center, San Antonio.
Ireland, M.W., Surgeon General, U.S. Army, "Letter to Adjutant General, April 28, 1920," Airmed Museum archives.
"JFK's Visit to Brooks Recalled," San Antonio Express-News, November 1, 1987.
Janik, Allan and Stephen Toulmin. Wittgenstein's Vienna, New York, Simon and Schuster Touchstone Book, 1973.
Jones, Billy M. Health-Seekers in the Southwest, 1817-1900, Norman, University of Oklahoma Press, 1967.
Jones, Isaac H., "Flying Vistas," Aviation, 1958, 181-254.
Kaufman, Martin. American Medical Education: The Formative Years, 1765-1910, Westport, Connecticut, Greenwood Press, 1976.
n.a., "Kelly Field Medical Department," Kelly Air Force Base Office of History.
Kennedy, John F. "Address at Dedication Ceremony, Brooks Air Force Base, Texas," November 21, 1963, Brooks AFB Hangar 9 archives.
Kett, Joseph F. Formation of the American Medical Profession: The Role of Institutions, 1780-1860, New Haven, Yale University Press, 1968.
King, Edward. "Glimpses of Texas. 1: A Visit to San Antonio," Scribner's Monthly 7:3 (January 1874).
King, Lester S., "Medical Education: The AMA Surveys the Problems," Journal of the American Medical Association, 248:22(1982), 3017-3021.
Koenigsberger, Leo. Hermann von Helmholtz, Oxford, Clarendon Press, 1906.
Kroll, Harry David, ed. Kelly Field in the Great World War, San Antonio, Press of San Antonio Printing Co., 1919.
Lebensohn, James Elzar. Anthology of Ophthalmic Classics, Baltimore, Williams and Wilkins, 1969.
Lesky, Erna. Vienna Medical School of the 19th Century, Baltimore and London, Johns Hopkins University Press, 1976.
Link, M.M. and H.A. Coleman. Medical Support of the Army Air Forces in World War II, Washington, D.C., Surgeon General, 1955.
Lippmann, Otto, Letter to Dr. Jack Lee, June 10, 1981.
Littlejohn, M.D. "Southwest Texas as a Winter Resort," New York Medical Record,

XLII(November 19, 1982).
Lloyd, William C., III, M.D. "Brief History of the BAMC Ophthalmology Service, The Second Decade," typescript, University of Texas Health Science Center Department of Ophthalmology archives.
_____. "Founding of the BAMC Ophthalmology Residency Program," videotape, UTHSC Department of Ophthalmology archives.
_____. ". . . Seems Like Yesterday," presented at 10th Alamo City Ophthalmology Residents Conference, March 2, 1990, videotape.
n.a. "Louis H. Bauer Founders Award," Aviation, Space, and Environmental Medicine, 71(July 2000), 759.
MacMillan, Esther, ed. "People of San Antonio. Pt. II. The Cabildo and the People, 1731-1784" in San Antonio in the Eighteenth Century, San Antonio, 1976.
Macon, N. Don. Mr. John H. Freeman and Friends: A Story of the Texas Medical Center and How It Began. Houston, Texas Medical Center, 1973.
MacPherson, W.G., A.H. Bowlby, and Cuthbert Wallace, eds. History of the Great War. Medical Services. 2v. London, His Majesty's Stationery Office, 1922, with "Injuries and Affections of the Eye" in vol. 2: Surgery, 499-551.
Mann, Ida, Culture, Race, Climate and Eye Disease, Springfield, Ill., C.C. Thomas, 1966.
Matagorda County Historical Committee et al. Historic Matagorda County, vol. 1. Houston, D. Armstrong and Co., Inc., 1986.
Matthews, John A., M.D. "Absorptive and Reflective Filters for Spectacle Wear," paper given at III Pan-American Congress of Ophthalmology, Havana, Cuba, January 7, 1948.
_____. "Choroideremia," paper given at Texas Society of Ophthalmology and Otolaryngology, San Antonio, Texas, 1954.
_____. "Effect of Ophthalmic Filters on Color Vision," in Minutes of the 22nd Meeting of the Armed Forces-National Research Council Vision Committee, November 11-12, 1948, 21-28.
_____. "Eye Protective Devices," paper given at Memorias IV Pan-American Congress of Ophthalmology, 118-122, 1952.
_____. "Investigation of Certain Aspects of Color Vision," School of Aviation Medicine Research Report 168-1, July 1943.
_____. with William C. Brown, Robert E. Kollenberger, and Kenneth E. Hudson, "Leiomyoma of the Iris," American Journal of Ophthalmology, 43 (March, 1957), 457-459.
_____. "Observations on the Effects of Di-Isopropyl Fluorophosphate (DFP)," paper given at Texas Society of Ophthalmology and Otolaryngology, Dallas, Texas, December 1946.
_____. "Ophthalmic Injuries of War," War Medicine 4(September, 1943), 247-261.
_____. "Physical Standards for Selection of Radar Operators," School of Aviation Medicine Reserch Report 167-1, June, 1943.
_____. "Physiological Effects of Reflective, Colored, Polarizing Ophthalmic Filters," School of Aviation Medicine Research Report 21-02-040-1, March 1950.
_____. "Post Operative Care of Retinal Detachment," paper given at Symposium on Retinal Surgery, Sectional Meeting, American College of Surgeons, Dallas, Texas, January 10, 1958.
_____. "Some Considerations in the Selection of Flying Sun Glasses," Journal of Aviation Medicine, 20(February, 1949), 39-46.
_____. "Use of Absorptive Lenses: Facts for the Profession," Transactions of the

American Academy of Ophthalmology and Otolaryngology, (January-February, 1949), 274-277.

____. "War Injuries of the Eyes," given at Texas Society of Ophthalmology and Otolaryngology, Dallas, Texas, December, 1942.

Matthews, Wilbur L. History of the San Antonio Medical Foundation and South Texas Medical Center, n.p., 1988 (1983).

McBride, Captain Donald B., USAF, Kelly AFB, "Military Influences on the Economy and Municipal Government of San Antonio," San Antonio, Texas, Trinity University Research Paper printed by The San Antonio Light, 1950s, in San Antonio Public Library.

McGrew, Roderick E. "Ophthalmology," in Encyclopedia of Medical History, New York, McGraw-Hill, 1985.

n.a., "Medical Arts Hospital," San Antonio Express, June 21, 1927.

"Medical Field Service School" in Tousey, Lt. Col. Thomas G., Military History of Carlisle and Carlisle Barracks, Richmond, Dietz Press, 1939, 360-405.

"Medicine in Greater Houston, 1836-1956," typescript, Houston Academy of Medicine-Texas Medical Center Library, Houston.

Meyerhof, Dr. M. "Nightblindness as a War Disease," American Journal of Ophthalmology, 33 (1916-17), 139-43.

"Milestones," typescript, Wilford Hall Ophthalmology Department Archives.

Military Medical Manual, 4th ed. Harrisburg, Pennsylvania, Military Service Publishing Co., 1940.

"Minutes of Regular Meeting of March 28, 1918," Medical Annals of Southwest Texas, April 1918, 116ff.

Moursund, Walter H., Sr., M.D., LL.D. History of Baylor University College of Medicine, 1900-1953, Houston, Baylor, 1956?

____. "Medicine in Greater Houston, 1836-1956," edited by Mildred Moursun Essig, Baylor University College of Medicine, n.d., 442-448.

Naythons, Matthew, MD. Face of Mercy, New York, Random House, 1993, with narrative by Sherwin B. Nuland, M.D.

"New Clinic Honors Lady Brady," San Antonio Express, January 20, 1974.

Newcomb, W.W., Jr. Indians of Texas. Austin, University of Texas Press, 1961.

Nix Health Care System, "The Nix News," June 1993.

Nixon, Pat Ireland, M.D. Century of Medicine in San Antonio. San Antonio, privately printed by the author, 1936

____. History of the Texas Medical Association, 1853-1953. Austin, University of Texas Press, 1953.

____. Medical Story of Early Texas, 1528-1853. Lancaster, Pennsylvania, n.p., 1946.

Nueces County Historical Society. History of Nueces County. Austin, Jenkins Book Publishing Co., Inc., 1972.

Numbers, Ronald L. "History of American Medicine: A Field in Ferment." Reviews in American History (December 1982), 245-263.

____. "Medicine in New Spain," in Medicine in the New World, Knoxville, University of Tennessee Press, 1987, 12-63.

Ocker, William C. and Carl J. Crane. Blind Flight in Theory and Practice. San Antonio, Naylor Printing Co., 1932.

Olendorf, Donna, Christine Jeryan, and Karen Boyden, eds. "The Eye," Gale Encyclopedia of Medicine, Detroit, Gale Research, 1999.

Ophthalmic Research Foundation of San Antonio, Inc. "Articles of Incorporation" and "Bylaws." UTHSC Department of Ophthalmology Archives.

____. Minutes, Board of Directors Meeting June 19, 1980.
"Ophthalmology," in Oxford Companion to Medicine, New York, Oxford University Press, 1986.
"Ophthalmology in the American Expeditionary Forces"
see U.S. War Department. Surgeon General's Office. Medical Department of the U.S. Army in the World War.
"Organizational Meeting of the Texas Ophthalmological Association, April 23, 1956, 5:20 p.m., Terrace Dining Room, Hotel Galvez," typescript, n.d., in TOA Archives.
Osler, Sir William. Aequanimitas, with other Addresses to Medical Students, Nurses and Practitioners of Medicine, 3rd Ed., Philadelphia, P. Blakiston's Son and Co., Inc., 1932.
O'Toole, Marie T., ed. Encyclopedia and Dictionary of Medicine, Nursing, and Allied Health. 6th ed., Philadelphia, Saunders, 1997.
Panfield, Peter M. Wild Nights and Roaring Days in Old San Antonio. San Antonio, Kothman Publishing Co., 1968.
Pannill, F.Carter, "The University of Texas Medical School at San Antonio," in Lippard, Vernon W. and Elizabeth F. Purcell. Case Histories of Ten New Medical Schools. New York, Josiah Macy, Jr. Foundation, 1972.
Pastore, Nicholas. Selective Theories of Visual Perception, 1650-1950. New York, Oxford University Press, 1971.
Payne, Lt. Col. Brittain F. "Aviation Ophthalmology," Military Surgeon 100:6(June 1947), 488-497.
Pettey, Weston A., O.D. Optometry in Texas, 1900-1984. Austin, Nortex Press, 1985.
Peyton, Green, Fifty Years of Aerospace Medicine, 1918-1968. USAF School of Aerospace Medicine, Brooks AFB, Texas, 1968.
____. San Antonio: City in the Sun. New York, McGraw-Hill Book, Company, Inc., 1946.
n.a., "Physicians and Surgeons Hospital, San Antonio, Texas," brochure, 1978.
Pisano, Marina, "From Biplanes to 'Star Wars'," San Antonio Express-News, March 26, 1989, 8-T
n.a., "Pocket Guide to Historic Fort Sam Houston." Fort Sam Houston Museum, 1994.
Posey, William Campbell. Wills Hospital of Philadelphia, Philadelphia, Lippincott, 1931.
"Postgraduate Assembly Now 19 Years Old," San Antonio Express-News. January 25, 1949.
Pridgen, Joseph, M.D. "Henry Reuss, M.D., F.A.C.S., Founding Chairman, Texas Surgical Society, 1867-1919," unpublished manuscript.
n.a., "Program, Highland Hereford Breeders Association Conference, Marfa, Texas, August 24-25, 1951," in Briscoe Library Archives.
R.B. Green Memorial Hospital. "History" and "Fact Sheet," typescript.
Ramsdell, Charles. San Antonio: A Historical and Pictorial Guide. Austin, University of Texas Press, 1959.
"Randolph AFB celebrates 60th Anniversary This Year," San Antonio Express News, June 24, 1990, 25-R
Red, Mrs. George Plunkett (S.C.). Medicine Man in Texas. Houston, Standard Printing and Lithography Co., 1930.
"Research, Development Keep Brooks AFB Busy," Sunday San Antonio Express-News, June 25, 1989.
Richardson, Rupert N. et al. Texas: The Lonestar State. 6th ed., Prentice Hall, 1993.

Roemer, Dr. Ferdinand, Texas. San Antonio, Standard Printing Co., 1935.
n.a., "Romana Plaza in Evolution," North San Antonio Times, June 20, 1974.
Rosen, George. Specialization of Medicine, with Particular Reference to Ophthalmology. New York, Froben Press, 1944.
Rosenberg, Charles E. Cholera Years: The United States in 1832, 1849, and 1866. Chicago, University of Chicago Press, 1962.
Ross, A.A. "Stepping Stones in the Scientific and Social Progress of Medicine in Texas," Texas Medical Society Journal (June 1934), 70-75.
Rothstein, William G. American Medical Schools and the Practice of Medicine: A History. Cambridge, Oxford University Press, 1987.
_____. American Physicians in the Nineteenth Century. Baltimore and London, Johns Hopkins University Press, 1972.
San Antonio Association for the Blind, Assembler, vols. 1-2 (1980-81).
_____. Publicity Materials: History, Industrial Division, Rehabilitation Division, Employment Opportunities brochures.
Rucker, Charles Wilbur. History of the Ophthalmoscope. Rochester, Minnesota, Whiting Printers and Stationers, 1971.
"San Antonio Medical Arts Building," Texas State Journal of Medicine, December 1924, 462.
"Santa Rosa at Home in 'Cemetery,'" San Antonio Light, October 7, 1914.
Scheie, Harold, M.D., "Statistics and General Problems of Ophthalmology with Field Armies," Army Medical Service Graduate School, Walter Reed Army Medical Center, 1(1951).
Schier, Mary Jane. "24 Green Hospital Interns Live Fast Pace," San Antonio Express, March 9, 1964.
Schroeder, Clint, Jr. "Eye Program Strangled, Ex-Prof Says," San Antonio Express-News, n.d. in UTHSC Department of Ophthalmology archives.
Seifert, Josef. Back to "Things in Themselves:" A Phenomenological Foundation for Classical Realism. New York, Routledge and Kegan Paul, 1987.
Shastid, Thomas Hall. Outline History of Ophthalmology. Southbridge, Massachusetts, American Optical Company, 1927.
Silverthorne, Elizabeth. Ashbel Smith of Texas: Pioneer, Patriot, Statesman, 1805-1886. College Station, Texas A&M University Press, 1982.
Singleton, Albert O. Account of the Early History of Surgery in Texas. Galveston, Texas Surgical Society, 1932.
Soresby, Arnold, N.D., F.R.C.S. Short History of Ophthalmology. London, Staples Press, Ltd., 1933.
"Space Ship Given Many Descriptions," November 9, 1951, San Antonio Express-News.
Speer, William S. Encyclopedia of the New West. Easley, S.C. Southern Historical Press, 1978 (1881).
Spraycar, Marjory, ed., Stedman's Medical Dictionary, Baltimore, Wiliams and Wilkins, 1995.
Starr, Paul. Social Transformation of American Medicine. New York, Basic Books, Inc., 1982.
"Statistical Report on the Sickness and Mortality in the Army of the United States," compiled from the records of the Surgeon General's Office, 1855-1860, Washington, D.C., George W. Bowman, Printer, 1860.
Sykes, Edwin Meredith, Jr., M.D. Faith in Education: A History of the Sykes Family, 1805-1975. San Antonio, published by the author, 1993.

"TOA Honors Past Officers," Perspectives of the Texas Ophthalmological Association, The Association, September 1981.
Texas Ophthalmological Association. Brochure. n.d.
_ ____. "By-Laws" and "Minutes," published by the Association, 1956.
"Texas Ophthalmologists," extracted from the Gazetteer of Texas Physicians database developed by the Historical Research Center of the Houston Academy of Medicine-Texas Medical Center Library, Houston, Texas, February 1996.
Texas Society of Ophthalmology and Otolaryngology. Annual Meeting Programs with lists of members, 1950.
____. Correspondence, in Texas Medical Association Archives.
____. Historical Notes. typescript, Texas Medical Association archives.
____. Membership Rolls, 1926-1975.
____. Minutes of the First Annual Meeting, 1926, and 1926-1975, in 3 volumes, The Society, n.d.
Texas Society to Prevent Blindness, "Chronology of the Texas Society to Prevent Blindness," n.d., in TSPB archival materials.
Texas State Commission for the Blind. "The First Fifty Years in Review," photocopy, n.d., n.p.
Texas State Eye, Ear, Nose and Throat Society. "Minutes of the Meeting of the Pre-Organization for the Formation of a Texas State Eye, Ear, Nose and Throat Society, Medical Arts Building, San Antonio" September 26, 1926, in Texas O&O Society Archives.
Thorne, Frederick H. "Ophthalmology in Aviation," Archives of Ophthalmology, 1938, Series 2, 19: 253-277.
Tidy, Sir Henry Letheby. Inter-Allied Conferences in War Medicine. New York, Staples Press, 1947.
Tomlinson Lone Star Book of Texas Records. Fort Worth, Lone Star Book of Texas Records, Inc., 1977 ed.
"Towering Nix Building Is Medical Landmark," San Antonio Express, January 25, 1949;
Tredici, Thomas J., M.D. Aerospace Ophthalmology: Contributions of the Ophthalmology Branch, USAF School of Aerospace Medicine to Visual Science and National Defense, USAF SAM, n.d, 1-6.
Turner, Leo. Story of Fort Sam Houston. San Antonio, L. Turner, 1936.
"Twenty-Four Green Hospital Interns Live Fast Pace," in San Antonio Express, March 9, 1964.
Tyler, Ron, editor-in-chief. New Handbook of Texas. Austin, Texas State Historical Association, 1996.
U.S. School of Aviation Medicine. Manual of Medical Research Laboratory. War Department. Air Service. Division of Military Aeronautics. Washington, D.C., Government Printing Office, 1918.
U.S. War Department. Surgeon General's Office. Historical Notes Concerning the Medical Department of the U.S. Army from 1775 to 1873. U.S., Government Printing Office.
U.S. War Department. Surgeon General's Office. Manual of Ophthalmology, prepared by the subsection of ophthalmology, section of surgery of the head, division of surgery. Washington, D.C., Government Printing Office, 1917.
U.S. War Department. Surgeon General's Office. Medical Department of the U.S. Army in the World War. VIII: Training; XI: Surgery, including "Ophthalmology in the American Expeditionary Forces," 659-728. Washington, D.C., GPO, 1923-29.

U.S. War Department. Surgeon General's Office. Report, Washington, D.C., GPO, 1919.
UCLA Tissue Typing Laboratory. "History of Transplantation: 35 Recollections," Los Angeles, Regents of the University of California, 1991.
University of Texas Medical Branch, Galveston. Faculty and Staff. University of Texas Medical Branch at Galveston: A Seventy-Five Year History by the Faculty and Staff. Austin, University of Texas Press, 1967.
Vail, Derrick T. "Rise and Fall of EENT," Transactions of the American Academy of Ophthalmology and Otolaryngology, 74 (January-Februrary 1970), 11-17.
Vanzant, T.J. "Texas Ophthalmological Association," Texas Medicine 63:3 (March 1967), 85.
Von Braun, Werner and Frederick I. Ordway, III. Rockets Red Glare. Garden City, Anchor/Doubleday, 1976.
Wagener, Elaine Hoffman, compiler and editor. George C. Vaughan: Early Entrepreneur, San Antonio, Watercress Press, 1984.
n.a. "War and the Future of Our Societies," Annals of Southwest Texas (December 1917), 21.
Weinstein, George W., M.D., Curriculum Vitae.
Weinstein, George, M.D., Letter to J. B. Aust, M.D., November 21, 1969, UTHSC Department of Ophthalmology files.
Weisman, Joseph S., Major, USAF, MC, Chief, Neuro-Ophthalmology Service, Residency Program Director. Report, 1992.
Wharton, Clarence R. Republic of Texas. Houston, C. C. Young, 1922.
White, Elizabeth Borst. "Eye, Ear, Nose and Throat Hospitals in Texas," Historical Research Center, Houston Academy of Medicine-TMS Library typescript.
_____. "Patterns of Development in Texas Hospitals, 1836-1935: Preliminary Survey," Texas Medicine 82(December 1986), 55-60.
Wiener, Meyer, M.D. Ophthalmology in the War Years. 2 v., Chicago, Year Book Publishers, 1946.
Woolford, Sam and Bess. San Antonio Story. San Antonio, Joske's of Texas, 1950.
Wygant, Larry J. Medicine and Public Health in Galveston, Texas: the First Century, Ph.D. Dissertation, University of Texas Medical Branch at Galveston, 1992.
Young, James Harvey. Medical Messiahs: A Social History of Health Quackery in 20th Century America, Princeton University Press, 1967.

# Photograph Acknowledgements

*The authors wish to thank the many individuals who generously shared their stories, photographs and other memorabilia. Photos were provided by several libraries through their archival collections, by websites, by South Texas ophthalmologists and/or by their descendants. The following list documents (to the best of the writer's ability) the sources of the photographs and illustration used in this book.*

John Larkin Matthews i
(Photo Courtesy — Sally L. Buchanan)

1887 Map of Texas and detail of South Texas ii
(Photo Courtesy - UT Arlington Virginia Garrett Cartographic History Library)

Chester R. Burns, M.D. 2
(Photo Courtesy - UT Medical Branch Archives- Galveston)

P. I. Nixon, M.D. 12
(Photo Courtesy - Briscoe Library Archives, UT Health Science Center at San Antonio)

Cabeza de Vaca 18
(Photo Courtesy - Thayer Watkins, San José State University, http://www.sjsu.edu/faculty/watkins/cabeza3.htm)

Detail Map of South Texas Counties 18
(Photo Courtesy - UT Arlington Virginia Garrett Cartographic History Library)

Stephen F. Austin 29
(Photo Courtesy - The Lone Star Junction– http://www.lsjunction.com/people/austin.htm)

George Joseph Beer, M.D. 34
(Photo Courtesy - The History of Ophthalmology, Vol 4, Julius Hirschberg, p 206;)

Carl Ferdinand von Graefe, M.D. 34
(Photo Courtesy - The History of Ophthalmology, Vol 7, Julius Hirschberg, p 239)

George Frick, M.D. 36
(Photo Courtesy - Briscoe Library Archives, UT Health Science Center at San Antonio & Wayenborgh Collection)

Hermann von Helmholz, M.D. (as a young man) 61
(Photo Wayenborgh Collection)

# INDEX

Impresión/Printer
A.G. Zamphirópolos S.A.
www.agz.com.py